German Sports, Doping, and Politics

Doping und Anti-Doping in der Bundesrepublik Deutschland 1950 bis 2007

Genese – Strukturen – Politik

M. Krüger, C. Becker, S. Nielsen, M. Reinold

German Sports, Doping, and Politics

A History of Performance Enhancement

Michael Krüger
Christian Becker
Stefan Nielsen

ROWMAN & LITTLEFIELD
Lanham • Boulder • New York • London

Published by Rowman & Littlefield
A wholly owned subsidiary of The Rowman & Littlefield Publishing Group, Inc.
4501 Forbes Boulevard, Suite 200, Lanham, Maryland 20706
www.rowman.com

Unit A, Whitacre Mews, 26-34 Stannary Street, London SE11 4AB

British Library Cataloguing in Publication Information Available

Library of Congress Cataloging-in-Publication Data

Kr?ger, Michael, 1955-
German sports, doping, and politics : a history of performance enhancement / Michael Kr?ger, Christian Becker, and Stefan Nielsen.
pages cm.
Includes bibliographical references and index.
ISBN 978-1-4422-4920-2 (cloth : alk. paper) — ISBN 978-1-4422-4921-9 (ebook)
1. Doping in sports—History—Germany. 2. Athletes—Drug use—History. 3. Sports—Moral and ethical aspects. 4. Sports—Political aspects—Germany. I. Title.
RC1230.K783 2015
362.29088'7960943—dc23
2014046967

∞™ The paper used in this publication meets the minimum requirements of American National Standard for Information Sciences Permanence of Paper for Printed Library Materials, ANSI/NISO Z39.48-1992.

Printed in the United States of America

Dedicated to Ommo Grupe (1930-2015)
and his vision of a fair and better sport

Contents

Acknowledgments ix

Introduction: Basics and Problem Definition xi

Abbreviations xxxiii

Chronology xxxvii

1 From Common Practice to Prohibition: The Beginnings of Doping and Anti-Doping in German Sport of the 1950s and 1960s 1

2 Cold War and the Climax of Doping in Germany: From the Munich Olympics of 1972 via Montreal 1976 to the Introduction of Out-of-Competition Controls in the 1980s 53

3 Doping and Anti-Doping in the Process of German Reunification 135

Conclusion 189

Bibliography 203

Index 215

About the Authors 223

Acknowledgments

The book is the result of teamwork. We want to say thank you to those who supported its genesis.

The Federal Institute of Sports Science in Germany financed the project. Namely, Dr. Carl Müller-Platz and Ruth Luetkehermölle assisted the work.

At Muenster University various colleagues and assistants contributed to the work, foremost Marcel Reinold, and Nils Niemeyer, Lukas Rehmann, and Justus Kalthoff.

Dr. Brian Bloch worked hard editing the English version of the text, which was translated and adapted by Michael Krüger.

Introduction

Basics and Problem Definition

This book presents the results of a research project dealing with the history of doping and anti-doping in (West) Germany from 1950 to the beginning of the twenty-first century (2007). The original German text has been translated, with parts of it newly written and formulated especially for American readers.[1] Certain additional explanations and diversions have been necessary to clarify some Germany-specific aspects. The project was initiated by the umbrella organization of German sports federations, the German Olympic Sports Federation (Deutscher Olympischer Sportbund, DOSB). The report providing the main results of the work was completed at the beginning of 2013. Three official and public meetings were held in Leipzig and Berlin to present the interim results. During the research process, some specific aspects and results were published in national and international specialist journals.[2]

The Bundesinstitut für Sportwissenschaft (BISp, Federal Institute of Sports Science), a governmental institution for the promotion of sports science in Germany, supported the research project. An academic advisory board consisting of independent experts from science and sports supervised the research work.

The general intention behind this research project can be attributed to the fact that the German public has paid close attention to the history of the German Democratic Republic (GDR, East Germany) since reunification in 1989/90. In this context, many studies have been conducted on the characteristics of sports within the GDR. Doping plays an important and even essential role in this history. The evaluation and analysis of various sources of information and documents on the history of sports in the GDR has revealed an alarming degree of doping. Doping was systematically propagated in sports policies, and there was even an official program from the state and sports authorities for researching and applying doping (Staatsplanthema 14.25). However, all this was concealed from the public, as well as from the arenas of international sports and politics. Additionally, these revelations about doping and top-level sports in the GDR, which became progressively more conspicuous and obvious after the breakdown of the GDR and the subsequent German reunification, provoked debate and controversy on doping procedures in the Federal Republic of Germany (FRG; Bundesrepublik Deutschland, BRD).

In fact, doping was a common practice on both sides of the Iron Curtain. But why and how, and how many athletes were involved in the misuse of medication to enhance achievements, performance, and sporting success? Who knew about these practices? Who was responsible? What were the differences between East and West?

These were just some of the fundamental questions motivating a research project on doping and anti-doping and their backgrounds within the culture, society, and politics of West Germany. The project is unique in that, to the best of our knowledge, it was the first time a state had sponsored scientific research to investigate its own doping history.

Initially, the research project was limited to German doping issues. However, it soon became clear that doping and anti-doping in sports cannot be limited to a national context. Doping and anti-doping raise fundamental questions about sports worldwide. German sports, in both East and West, have always been part of global sporting or the "Olympic family" (the official denomination in the Olympic charter), organized in the form of Olympic organizations and the international sports federations. Within this large family, many members have not only been tempted to cheat by using forbidden substances, they have duly succumbed to the temptation. Sports are not a world in isolation, however, but are connected globally to broader political and economic interests and—very importantly—communicated consistently by the international (as well as national) media.

Sports organizations in East and West Germany were antagonistic toward each other in all essential dimensions. Sport in the West was genuinely free, self-responsible, independent of state politics, and autonomous. By contrast, sport in the East was organized and controlled by the all-powerful and unchallengeable state party, Sozialistische Einheitspartei Deutschlands (SED). The only really common issue between East and West German athletes was the sporting activity itself. Furthermore, the common sporting rules of the games and competitions were universally valid. "There are no capitalist handstands or Marxist chin-ups," as the first president of the FRG, Theodor Heuss, once said in a speech held on the occasion of the founding of the German Gymnastics Federation in 1950 (Deutscher Turner-Bund, DTB).[3]

However, all other aspects of sports differed between East and West, extending to the cultural, social, and political orientation and functions, organizations or governing bodies, concepts, and structures. Despite these antagonistic sporting structures in East and West, several elements of the different systems were nonetheless closely related to each other, especially with respect to sports and training practices, international sports policies, sports science, and the support of international top-level sports, sports medicine, and sports promotion. The contest between East and West Germany led to an adaptation of ideas and structures on each side. Socialist Germany in the East became the most professional and, somewhat ironically, capitalist sporting nation. For athletes, coaches, and officials, only the outcome was important—winning. The openly capitalist West German sports organizations that tried, at least until the early 1980s, to keep their sports as an autonomous *Eigenwelt*—a world of its own—adopted many methods and structures of the GDR step by step, aiming to gain as many Olympic medals as the smaller but much more successful GDR. In fact, the superiority of GDR sport was limited to a few essential Olympic disciplines. In any event, West German sports organizers and politicians were keen to imitate the methods and structures of the GDR sports system. According to the criteria of "modern sports," as Allen Guttmann defined them in his internationally well-known book *From Ritual to Record*, the GDR sports system was by far the most modern in the world in the 1970s and 1980s.[4]

These issues and insights explain why, roughly twenty years after German reunification and subsequent digging into the history of the GDR, the focus has turned to the West. The present research project analyzed the West German sports system and its involvement with doping and anti-doping from the early 1950s until 2007. The year 2007 marks the preliminary end of the process of implementing, reforming, and integrating the National Anti-Doping Agency (NADA) into German and international sports. The historical analysis of West German sports was clearly reflected in the East German model and captured by original sources and documents.

The results of the project were discussed extensively in public and by the media in Germany and even worldwide.[5] Apart from the above-mentioned three public conferences devoted to presenting and discussing the interim results, the parliamentary Sports Commission (Sportausschuss des Deutschen Bundestags) frequently requested up-to-date information about the project. This broad public and political interest can be attributed to several factors. First, this project was financed by tax money, and it should be noted that top-level sports in general are also mainly tax-financed. However, the critical interest of the parliamentary commission in spending a lot of public money in this context seems far less than that of the doping research project. In any event, it is the duty of the elected representatives to control the budget and monitor the outcome. Therefore, the request of the representatives to account for the way public funds were spent was legitimate. The main reason for the interest in this project was actually political. The second and more important fact is that the project concerns institutions and sports personalities who still serve on administrative bodies, or have other functions within sports administrations and formulate sports policies, or have had a lasting effect on German sport in general. Due to the potentially sensitive results of the project, it was necessary to ensure that the research project remained independent and free (unobstructed), despite the governmental subsidy. The elected representatives of the opposition and governing parties of the Bundestag wanted to ensure this independence.

Furthermore, the project had important effects on German home affairs. Even twenty years after the breakdown of German communism, it could be shown that doping was not only a "black spot" in the "empire of evil," as Ronald Reagan denounced the USSR (rightly or wrongly) and its satellite states inside the Eastern bloc behind the Iron Curtain, but this "black spot" was even evident on the allegedly clean slates of the free West and Federal Republic of Germany, considered by East Germans as the land of milk and honey. Therefore, the project contributes to a more realistic view of the West. It can also be regarded as a moderate symbol of social and national hygiene and historical justice to demonstrate to former inhabitants of the GDR that not only their former homeland GDR had such black spots, but so too did the West. The people in the GDR were therefore no more morally degenerate than their West German "brothers and sisters," who were fortunate enough to live on the "right and bright" side of the Iron Curtain.

The book is divided into three parts. Part 1 deals with the history of doping in the postwar period of the 1950s and 1960s. Part 2 focuses on the climax of doping with anabolic steroids, as well as on the beginnings of a coordinated anti-doping movement. The last part considers the development of doping and anti-doping from the reunification of 1989/90 to the foundation of the World Anti-Doping Agency (WADA) and the National-Anti-Doping Agency (NADA) in Germany, including the problems of anti-doping policy up to recent years.

The fundamental issue that this book confronts is whether and to what extent the problem of doping had an impact on the relationship between sports and German policy, or whether this relationship itself contributed inversely to supporting or combating doping. Doping and anti-doping are thus two sides of the same coin, both of which need to be considered in equal measure.

This chronology correlates to the social "figuration," which changed as doping and anti-doping processes developed. The expression "figuration" is one of Norbert Elias's theoretical concepts of "figuration and processes."[6] The doping figuration—or the specific interdependency of sports, policy, science, doping, and its actors—contributed to the specific dynamics of doping and anti-doping. These figurations also differ according to the type of sport. For example, in cycling, swimming, athletics, etc., social figurations vary according to the superordinate context. Therefore, there are different social figurations in weight lifting than in gymnastics. The processes leading to or supporting doping are as varied and complex as those of anti-doping. Figurations are formed by individuals. Sports figurations consist of the interdependencies between sportsmen and athletes, including parents, friends, and relatives (these individuals often remain in the background of the events but play a relevant role in training and recreation processes) as well as coaches, doctors, and scientists. All can be involved in these specific social figurations in sport, which also produce doping and anti-doping, and the associated acts yield more than the sum of their individual behavioral parts.

Such figurations are rooted in social processes that extend back into the past much further than we do so here. In addition to this basic figuration, which generally characterizes sports developments in the early Federal Republic of Germany, there are other essential bodies, such as the media and its journalists, as well as state officials and politicians, who shaped the social construct of sports, doping, and the associated communication.

As a consequence of the 1972 Olympic Games in Munich, as well as of the participation of German athletes in the Olympic Games and World Cups in general, a modification of the doping figuration became considerably more apparent. International bodies in different kinds of sports, in the Olympic movement, and in European and international institutions took center stage in this figuration. National limitations were a thing of the past. Due to the essential fact that the Cold War affected Germany directly, with the division of the country and the reunification in 1989/90, Germany underwent a completely different process of international politics and society from other countries. Therefore, the approach to doping and anti-doping changed in response to international dimensions in a manner that would have been unthinkable and impossible under the old terms.

THE ROLE OF DOPING IN THE RELATIONSHIP BETWEEN POLITICS, SPORTING POLICIES, AND SPORTS

Since their foundation, the relationship between politics and sports were defined differently by the Federal Republic of Germany and the German Democratic Republic. After German reunification in 1990, the different sports systems and sports organizations developed to form a new and unique one. The issue of doping played an important and complex role in the formation of this relationship. One major research objective was therefore to highlight, analyze, and interpret this role. In order to fully comprehend doping and anti-doping, it is necessary to establish the context of the relationship between politics and sports in general, on the basis of proven facts. The original consideration was that a certain passivity on the part of the sports clubs, resulting from the extraordinary challenge of doping, ultimately compelled the government to deal with the question of anti-doping policies. Institutional innovations, such as the National Anti-Doping Agency and the rudiments of anti-doping law, seem to reflect this development.

The relationship between politics and organized sports, or sports associations, is based on a mixture of autonomy and partnership. This partnership, which is intended to guarantee the autonomy of sport, is the result of a historical process and consideration of the experiences of the Third Reich, when sport itself was exploited politically. This partnership not only meant that the sports clubs and associations were (and still are) responsible for sports in Germany, but also that state politics explicitly had to support the organizations in the proper discharge of their duties, which were considered to contribute to the welfare of the whole population. The term "subsidiary partnership" is used to describe this special relationship. One central political function of top-level sports is the representation of Germany at international sporting events like the Olympic Games, as well as the European or World Championships in various different sports and disciplines. The amateur sports organizations themselves were and still are unable to finance competitive teams without the financial support of the federal state.

Direct political intervention by the state and its governing bodies has not played a role in terms of organized sports. This political restraint can be attributed to the aspect of sports autonomy, which means the independence and self-responsibility of sports clubs and associations, considered a sports policy guideline in West Germany. In Germany, sports are not part of the federal constitution (*Grundgesetz*), which implies that sports are regarded as a personal affair, based principally on self-organization and self-responsibility. The state is not obliged to organize and finance private sports. However, the state can and must intervene in cases of violation of the law. With respect to doping, this occurs only when illegal drugs are used or distributed, but there is no state law in Germany that forbids and sanctions the actual doping process. Sports federations, not the state, are responsible for sanctioning doping. In that respect, at least in theory, the state has no reason or need to interfere in sports activities.

In practice, the state finances sports activities for many practical reasons, especially top-level sports at an international level, as mentioned above. This creates the opportunity for the state to influence sports positively by supporting top-level athletes, and negatively by sanctioning them or their clubs and associations when they violate sporting rules and the moral standards of sport and society.

In fact, doping is a problem that is not only related to sports and their fundamental principles of health and fairness, but also to society as a whole, especially when the state is financing sports with tax money. Therefore, the autonomy of sports and the prevention of intervention by the state (and other institutions like the media and the economy) is ensured, but that autonomy is based on the premise that it is possible to exclude any kind of abuse by any power through self-regulatory processes. In other words, this means that if the autonomous and self-responsible sports organizations are neither able nor willing to prevent athletes from doping, their autonomy will be limited and controlled.

In fact, for a long time, all bodies of sports and politics respected the principles of autonomy and subsidiary partnership. Political issues concerning sports remained limited to a financing role. It was left to the governing bodies of the sports organizations and the sports clubs and associations to specify the sports policy guidelines and the criteria for spending tax money on athletes, coaches, sports facilities, and so on. Sports associations assume specific public functions within this partnership and therefore receive state assistance, mainly in the form of money. In the following respects, this arrangement is practicable for both sport and state. The state acknowledges the monopoly of sports associations in matters of organization, representation, and self-control, and the state, as well as the public as a whole, benefits from the ability of sports clubs to activate voluntary commitment. Furthermore, the leading representatives of sports associations, as well as of sports policy, identify with the fundamental values of the European sports model. This model includes the social-integration and health-related functions of sports, as well as the relationship between amateur or mass sport, on the one hand, and high-level sports, on the other.[7] In Germany and various other European countries, more intensive interventions in sporting organizations have always been considered dysfunctional, because a political functionalization of sport could endanger the politically required voluntary commitment.

With regard to doping and anti-doping, the partnership between state and sport raises some awkward questions. On the one hand, sporting associations feel exposed to contradictory performance expectations from the public and the state. Given its high identification potential and role-model effect, politicians and the public expect maximum sporting performance. On the other hand, this maximum performance has to be achieved without any performance enhancers, so that the health of the athletes can be preserved and negative role-model effects prevented. This is again a condition for governmental support of sport. If maximum performance can be reached solely by using performance enhancers, sports associations find themselves in a dilemma, which can affect their willingness to ban doping. Either way, they risk losing governmental support.

Additionally, public reactions to detected doping cases are ambivalent. Such cases are regarded not as evidence of effective anti-doping policies, but as reflecting widespread misbehavior in sports in general. In addition, sports associations have always been unable to combat doping successfully. An effective anti-doping policy would require adequate powers for sports associations to compel coaches and athletes to implement anti-doping procedures. However, this was not ensured within the complex structures of West German sports for a long time. Even today the situation remains unsatisfactory.

The German sociologists Karl-Heinrich Bette and Uwe Schimank assume that sports organizations are typical examples of those faced with contradictory public expectations and, at the same time, unable to achieve them because of a lack of resources.[8] Organizational sociologists deal with the difficulty of converting theoretical concepts into organizational practice, with rhetoric and action often being poles apart. The politically interesting question is whether this gap between talk and behavior is part of a political strategy or simply the result of ignorance about what really happens in the world of sports. In fact, this seems to be precisely the problem within German (and international) sports organizations. The history of the anti-doping policies of German sports organizations, as well as of international sports federations, is also a history of impressive statements against doping, followed by considerably less effective measures. The British sports scientist and sociologist Barrie Houlihan maintains that the history of doping is one of inadequacy, indifference, and subversion, rather than of consistent anti-doping activities.[9]

The history of failed anti-doping policies from sports organizations implies that the "state," that is, any governmental or other parliamentary authority, is supposed to intervene in sports because state authorities cannot and should not, in the long run, accept such an important part of public life and attention being beyond public and political control. According to the sociology of figurations and processes, modern, "civilized" societies (in the sense of Norbert Elias) are characterized by processes of centralization and monopolization. Individual behavior is reciprocally related to collective power.

Elias referred to the link between "psychogenesis" and "sociogenesis." Related to sports and doping, this distinction means that individual sports practices, in accordance with doping, have been progressively socialized, publicly discussed, and ultimately become a matter of state politics. This process of transformation of private affairs into public and political matters of society and state power seems to be symptomatic of the history of sports and doping. In the meantime, sports and doping have become centralized and monopolized to such an extent that supranational institutions like the WADA are ultimately responsible for anti-doping worldwide.

The development of monopolies in sport could include both doping and anti-doping. As the example of the GDR demonstrates, the state established a monopoly over sport. Sports and doping were organized systematically by state organs, and doping was truly "Staatsdoping." However, the formation of different institutions and measures for anti-doping, from national as well as international perspectives during the last thirty years, shows that monopolization in sport is not necessarily a product of the state alone. The rise of international sporting federations, with the International Olympic Committee (IOC) at the top, confirms that such processes are initially social. The history of the WADA reveals that doping and anti-doping policy is indeed a process, and the result of private and public actors of sports organizations as well as national, transnational, and international organizations and, last but not least, governments and parliaments.

According to process and figurational sociology, the foundation of monopolies is also related to changes in individual emotional sentiments, thinking, and acting. In the words of Norbert Elias, there is a changing threshold of shame and pain (*Scham- und Peinlichkeitsschwelle*). With respect to sports and doping, it is evident not only that doping has spread throughout sports worldwide, but also that the awareness on the part of all actors has increased that they are doing something morally wrong or bad. Whereas in earlier times anything was allowed to improve performance, in current sport there are many rules and regulations about what is allowed and what is not. The process of civilization is characterized by the phenomenon that things which were once allowed are now expressly forbidden. Whereas athletes used to dope without shame or a bad conscience, modern athletes still do it, but with varying degrees of shame and a conscience. They know that what they are doing is against the rules and the spirit of sport, but the desire to win is often irresistible and overpowering.

Additionally, the responsibility of the state concerning anti-doping seems quite clear. The fundamental values and social functions of sports in general are jeopardized by doping, especially the role of top-level athletes as idols for young athletes. Society in general also has a right to morally acceptable behavior. State politics has to protect sport from the danger of doping, because sports organizations are obviously unable to do so on their own. Furthermore, as the largest sponsor of top-level sports, the state is also guilty of some form of misbehavior if it fails to prevent doping or at least to combat it seriously and consistently. Therefore, doping has the potential to delegitimize not only sport, but also the state and its responsibility for ensuring the health and security and ethics of the people.

The example of GDR doping victims reveals that, in the end, not only the doped athletes had to pay a high price, sacrificing their health. The state, too, was partly responsible and had to pay compensation for the inhuman practices in the former GDR. The reunited German Bundesrepublik took over the responsibilities of the GDR for its unethical doping practices, although, according to West German politicians, the sports authorities were in fact responsible for that disaster and not the state.

In summary, the central questions concerning the relationship between state and sport, or between state and sports authorities in terms of doping and anti-doping, can be formulated as four subquestions:

1. How and to what extent was German politics actively concerned with the doping problem (i.e., public bodies, governmental institutions, and parliamentary commissions)? What were the consequences and what was in fact done by the various state authorities?
2. How and to what extent did sports organizations and sports officials influence the sports policies of state authorities—for example, in order to finance top-level sports and anti-doping policies?
3. How and to what extent did existing doping practices influence the anti-doping activities of sports organizations and state authorities? What structures and decisions in the sports process, especially concerning doping and anti-doping, were ultimately changed?
4. How and to what extent were political initiatives concerning doping and anti-doping successful? Did political discussions in public and parliament really change the balance between state and governmental institutions, on the one hand, and the autonomous sports organizations, on the other? Has the doping problem proven to be a suitable arena for influencing sports policies as a whole? Does the doping problem create an opportunity for politics and politicians to benefit from the cultural, media-related, and popular image of top-level sports?

Indeed, the basic assumption could be confirmed that the doping problem is the main reason for questioning the traditional relationship between state and sport in matters of autonomy and subsidiary partnership. Meanwhile, the autonomy of sports, at least in the context of top-level sports and doping, is no longer a reality. New institutions such as anti-doping agencies, which can be defined as organizations in public-private-partnership, signal a new balance of power between the state and top-level sports. The debate on an anti-doping law in Germany makes it obvious that on the one hand, the pressure exerted by the public and state politics on sports organizations is increasing, and on the other hand, the influence of sports and sporting networks is still strong enough to prevent doping in Germany from being forbidden outright by state law and not only by sports rules.[10]

In the Federal Republic of Germany, *Staatsdoping*—doping organized by the state, as in the GDR—did not exist.[11] In contrast, West German sports policy and politics were (and still are) ambivalent. On the one hand, doping is rhetorically and morally rejected. On the other hand, top-level sports were pushed and supported by tax money, as well as by political and public expectations of top-level performance and success. Especially during the Cold

War, West German top-level sports were heavily politicized. Politicians, sports officials, journalists, media, and the public expected top performances and success from "their" athletes. The athletes were expected at least to be competitive in international sports, especially at the Olympic Games, and not to always lose against the doped East Germans. Everybody knew what was going on, but nobody (or at least far too few) really protested and accused the dopers of betrayal. However, cheating with doping was very difficult to prove at that time, and the GDR officials were good at keeping their system secret. In West Germany, there were many dopers, but nobody knew exactly how many, and, as indicated, there was no broader "system." When doping became public, however, sports officials often remained morally ambivalent and tried to make doping cases look harmless in public. Yet this behavior of the officials, and the increasingly objective social and sporting constraints of West German athletes, can be regarded as factors that indirectly supported the misuse.

Another important aspect should be mentioned. The present research project clearly demonstrated that the development of sports and doping, as well as anti-doping, is integrated into an international context. Doping and anti-doping history cannot be explained sufficiently without considering the process of internationalization or globalization of sport. The battle against doping is undoubtedly part of this general development. German sports organizations and German sports politics are embedded in international organizations, with the IOC and the international sports federations at the top of the hierarchy. However, political institutions like the European Council, the International Conference of Ministers and Senior Officials Responsible for Physical Education and Sport (MINEPS), and UNESCO are also part of international efforts against doping, generally together with the sports organizations, and sometimes also against them. The international dimensions of doping and anti-doping modify the German perspective of doping and anti-doping to some degree. Germany was a pioneer of neither doping nor anti-doping. But especially during the Cold War, both Germanies played—more or less—a major role in doping, and after German reunification, in anti-doping policies.

METHODOLOGICAL BASICS: SOURCES AND DOCUMENTS

To answer the complex questions raised above, numerous written sources in various archives and depots of sports federations and associations in Germany, as well as international archives like the IOC archive, were researched and analyzed. So too were national and international scientific or academic publications and documents from and about politicians and sports officials, including protocols, minutes, reports, and memoranda of official commissions of sports and government. This basic research on these sensitive issues was conducted more systematically and intensively than ever before in Germany. Although the research project was originally intended to be limited to a national perspective, it rapidly became clear that this would be too narrow an approach to describe and explain the complex networks of modern top-level sports including doping and anti-doping. As a result, the sports policy development led to the foundation of the WADA in 1999/2000. Therefore, it was necessary to intensively study the international "state of the art" of doping and anti-doping in the context of international sports. At international meetings and congresses, our research group contacted various international working groups researching doping and anti-doping.[12]

The focus on authentic written documents as the methodological basis of our analysis is justified in several respects. First, the analysis and hermeneutical interpretation of written historical documents is an established methodological instrument in the historical sciences. The wide variety of written documents, such as minutes or protocols, memoranda, legacies of deceased sport officials and politicians, letters and correspondence, statements, and so on, ensure a high degree of objectivity in a field characterized by personal, subjective emotions, notions of political and moral correctness, social and cultural values, socially expected behavior and communication, bad consciences, dogmatism, and assorted other motives, which make it difficult to distinguish facts from personal opinions and ideologies. However, our scientific interest is to find out what "really happened." This is an appropriate and sufficient requirement of serious historical research, in contrast to other objectives of investigation, such as journalistic ones. In short, what was written down constitutes a stable and reliable foundation. In contrast to the GDR, where nearly everything important about sports and doping was protocolled officially, or unofficially by the Ministry of State Security (Stasi), West Germany was very different. The "secrets" of GDR sport can be found in archives of the Stasi and others and, since the reunification, in the Bundesarchiv (central archive of the FRG), collected and arranged in proper (Prussian) order according to the rules and regulations for public archives. However, that did not apply to West Germany and still does not in the FRG. Due to the West German process of development and its traditions, sport was a matter of private life, not public life. Nobody was obliged to collect and meticulously file important documents in public archives, rather than in private depots of the sports organizations. Because doping was forbidden, and everybody knew that, all responsible persons tried to avoid any traces or "paper trails." In contrast to anti-doping, it is difficult to find written evidence of doping and doping practices in the FRG. Yet documents about anti-doping can be interpreted as indicators of doping. After all, only where there is doping is there anti-doping. However, we could not find any concrete, written proof that any sports officials or sports politicians compelled West German athletes to take forbidden medication to enhance sports performance. In fact, this definitely did not occur. As mentioned above, there was an indirect message that doping is not really wrong, that doping controls and sanctions do not really work, and that athletes were expected to be successful rather than to avoid doping by all means and at any cost.

There can be no serious doubt that the secret services on both sides of the Berlin Wall were interested in each other's knowledge and practices of sports, sports structures, personalities, and doping. This fact became evident during our studies in the archives of the East German Stasi and the West German spying service, the Bundesnachrichtendienst (BND). The East German secret service, the Stasi, did everything to keep the doping system of the GDR secret, to prevent the defection of athletes, coaches, and other crucial persons of the GDR top-level sports system, and, finally, to collect information on the West German sports policies. The West German BND was mainly informed about East German sports, practices, concepts, athletes, and whatever else political refugees from the East pointed them toward. However, it is probable that the BND also had agents or spies of its own working in this field of sport. There are numerous documents that confirm the hypothesis that both sides acquired enough information about what the other side did or knew. Additionally, it seems unrealistic to believe that this knowledge did not find its way to politicians and sports officials.

In fact, the situation described in written documents provided good reasons to talk to selected contemporary witnesses, using the methods of oral history, about their knowledge and memories and the effect of the various issues on doping and anti-doping history. However, after some initial checks, we abandoned this additional method of finding out the historical truth about doping and anti-doping.

The following reasons were relevant for our methodological decision. First, personal memories did not yield quantitatively more and more accurate knowledge beyond what we already knew from the written documents. Second, all important witnesses were somehow and in some way themselves involved in doping and anti-doping activities in the past. It is undoubtedly very difficult (or even impossible) for a witness to be objective and to avoid personal views, socially desirable responses, or politically correct statements and opinions. Furthermore, this is in a field that is not only loaded with various social and cultural values, but constitutes a highly sensitive target of media opinion. Such witness statements seemed rather to confuse and devalue the knowledge obtained from written documents than to clarify and supplement it. After intensive discussions and (self-)critical evaluation, we were convinced that our central objectives of collecting value-free facts and information about doping and anti-doping and enriching scientific knowledge without ideological and moral influences could be achieved more effectively without contemporary witnesses than with them.

STATE OF THE ART

Doping and the growing public and political debate on this topic are indeed phenomena of the second half of the twentieth century. However, this is not to say that the use of drugs or other means of enhancing performance in sports or other fields of bodily demands was not a reality before. It is well known that professional and commercialized sports and athletes in the 1920s and 1930s were familiar with various means of enhancing or improving achievement and performance, for example in cycling, boxing, and athletics, as well as in football and other team games like ice hockey.[13] The use of drugs and medication was not limited to professional sports, either. Notorious incidents include the Olympic marathon races in Saint Louis in 1904 and in London in 1908, when the winners Thomas Hicks (USA) and Pietri Dorando (Italy) presumably used amphetamines, strychnine, and other dubious substances.[14] Marathon races and cycling tours like the famous Tour de France are examples of extremely demanding and indeed exciting events, in which athletes feel unable to succeed through their own "natural resources" alone.

The use of stimulants like caffeine, cocaine, alcohol, and strychnine, and also the application of oxygen or certain types of radiation, has been practiced in modern sports from the beginning. Yet their use did not seem to be regarded as a problem, given that there was no critical debate at that time, neither inside the world of sport nor among the public as a whole, neither about the risks for athletes' health nor about violations of the sporting ethos of fair play. These drugs and other means of improving athletic achievement and performance were not forbidden by rules, laws, or even public opinion. Pietri Dorando, for example, was disqualified after his marathon race in London in 1908 not because he used drugs, but because he was physically supported by coaches and friends during the last steps before the finish line. However, he was indeed confused and disorientated, probably because of both exertion and drugs. The historical irony is indeed that according to the rules of the first marathon race at the Olympic Games in London, taking drugs was explicitly forbidden in rule 4: "No competitor either at the start or during the progress of the race may take or receive any drug. The breach of this rule will operate as an absolute disqualification." However, there were no controls after the race, but a medical commission had to establish the fitness of the competitors before the race.[15] The case of Dorando can therefore be regarded as one of the first undetected-doping cases in sport history. There was an anti-doping rule in London 1908, which Pietri Dorando duly breached, but without being controlled or caught. He was disqualified only because of other rules.

Pierre de Coubertin, the *spiritus rector* of the Olympic Games and the Olympic spirit of fair play, praised the achievements of Dorando and regretted his disqualification.[16] For him, Dorando was a hero and idol because he had fought like the legendary soldier who brought the message of the victory of the Greeks over the Persians from Marathon to Athens in 490 BCE. According to the legend, he cried, "We won," collapsed, and died. Nobody knows whether he took drugs or not.[17] If we can believe modern medical science, it is unlikely that a well-trained soldier would die merely from overexertion. The Greek hero probably came under the influence of unhealthy, dangerous drugs or had an undetected cardiac disease.

In short, there was no doping in early sports because there were no anti-doping rules and no sanctions against doping by any authority, or indeed by anyone at all. It is evident that the story of drug-free early sport is just not true, as John Hoberman and other historians emphasize.[18] What is currently considered to constitute forbidden doping was usually practiced at that time without punishment or any pangs of conscience.

The anti-doping rule at the marathon race in London in 1908 shows that officials and organizers of international sporting festivals like the Olympic Games, and especially the members of the IOC, were indeed aware of the practice of taking performance-enhancing substances. The IOC even reacted to these practices. "The IOC did have a rule that expressively forbade doping as a criterion for competition which had been accepted as early as 1938," John Gleaves and Matthew Llewellyn found as a result of their analysis of IOC documents.[19] This first anti-doping rule, handwritten by Avery Brundage in 1937, became part of the eligibility code of the IOC, which governed the admission of amateur athletes to Olympic competitions. Gleaves found that IOC anti-doping policies focused on drug-free amateur athletes, whereas professional athletes took drugs. Apparently, normal practice in sports was to take drugs. The anti-doping policies of the IOC are therefore related to the ethos of amateur sports, which had been a strong differentiator from professional sports. Amateur sports were for those athletes who "loved" (from the Latin origin of the word *amateur*) sports and games for the games' sake, whereas professional sports were for athletes who had to work in the field of sports. The one should be drug free, and the other not necessarily.

In Germany, the famous Olympic sportsman and Mister Olympics 1936, Carl Diem, a close friend of Avery Brundage, stated that professional sports are not sports at all: "Professional sport is not sport [. . .] but the opposite: Business, especially part of show business. Professional sport and business have in common the discipline and constraints of work and profession. The distinction between sport and professional sport is not a value judgment but a fact."[20]

According to this spirit of amateur sports, the anti-doping rule was included in the charter of the IOC in 1946, in the chapter on "Resolutions regarding the Amateur Status." Rule 6 defines clearly "Doping of athletes." Amateur athletes participating at "amateur meetings or Olympic Games" are not allowed to "use drugs [. . .] or artificial stimulants of any kind." Using such drugs or stimulants "must be condemned most strongly."[21]

A new era of sports and doping, as well as of anti-doping history, started after World War II, with the new beginning of international sports relations, including the Olympic Games and world championships. International doping historians generally agree that the experiences of athletes with drugs since the 1930s, and mainly of soldiers during World War II, were a major contributing factor in the spread of drug use and doping in the 1950s. These years are regarded as the formative period for the misuse of new types of drugs in sports, mainly stimulants such as amphetamines, which were also used systematically in World War II, especially by the German Air Force.[22] In Germany, the early fifties were also crucial for initial anti-doping activities, such as the attempt to define doping in the rules of the sports federations so as to ban the misuse of drugs and pharmaceuticals as a means of enhancing sporting performance (see chapter 1). Sports officials were becoming increasingly concerned about the health problems that were plaguing athletes.

In the early days of the phenomenon, doping in sports was limited exclusively to stimulants. This changed in the 1960s, when hormone doping was practiced systematically, at first in (heavy) athletic disciplines like discus, javelin, and shot put (and the bodybuilding community), and then in other sports. This development has been characterized by the continuous development and use of new types of drugs and doping methods in different sports and disciplines until today. Parallel and related to the spread of doping—metaphorically referred to as the doping-helix—the development of anti-doping began. A public debate emerged on doping in sports and on the need to prevent it. Doping was regarded as a problem associated with sports and their development that had to be solved and that could no longer be considered as acceptable, especially in top-level sports. This rise in public awareness of doping as a problem in sports was evident internationally.[23]

The 1960s mark a historical change in anti-doping policies. The approach changed from a mainly theoretical one of recognizing and defining doping to the practical challenge of solving the problem. Therefore, doping was no longer the exclusive terrain of doctors and scientists, but of sports policies in general. New actors emerged in the international and national sporting networks (or communities) of sports federations and governmental sporting politics. The latter gained progressively more influence in sporting affairs, parallel to the increasing importance of sports in society as a whole, including their role as an international means of political representation and propaganda.[24]

In essence, taking forbidden drugs to improve performance and achievement in high-level sports is not "natural," but rather a social construction of sporting practice. Considering doping in a narrow sense of the word implies banning such practices by the rather informal common-sense treatment of doping as a morally wrong and unhealthy practice, and by written sporting (and other) rules (or laws).

SCIENTIFIC DEBATE ON DOPING AND PUBLIC MORALIZATION

Doping has been part of the genesis of modern sports since the late nineteenth century.[25] Therefore, doping seems to be a side effect of sports development, quite apart from other characteristics such as striving for better achievement and breaking records or—at another level—professionalization, commercialization, and international competitiveness.

Research on the historical development of doping and anti-doping after World War II requires a clarification of the essential theoretical basics. The philologist Schnyder emphasizes just such a basic problem of historical research on doping:

> In earlier times, methods were known and practiced which we retrospectively refer to as doping. From a historical point of view, this is not correct, because these methods were embedded in a completely different context compared to today. This context differs not only in cultural, political and social respects, but also in relation to different discursive and institutional settings. These methods could be evaluated as bad for the athletes' health and/or as eroding fair competition, but the modern discourse on doping began when the medical discourse was supplemented by legal and ethical public debate. From then onwards, older methods of taking drugs in some sports and cases changed to doping.[26]

Sociological research on doping tends to neglect or level out historical differences. However, a historical perspective demonstrates that doping cannot be separated from anti-doping, which are two elements of the same issue. Doping can be explained and understood only against its background as illegitimate, forbidden methods of performing and winning. "Where there are no rules one cannot cheat."[27] Doping is defined essentially by its moral and public condemnation, by the discussion of doping "scandals," by condemning and criminalizing doping through written rules and laws in the statutes of the sports federations (or even in state laws), and, finally, by controlling and sanctioning doping in competitions and—subsequently—even "out of competition" during training or at home. It is obvious that doping and anti-doping are also part of a social process of bureaucratization in sports, as shown by the wide range of doping and anti-doping clauses in the rules of the sports federations.

Therefore, with respect to historical research on doping and anti-doping, Dimeo describes the following problem:

> The consumers of drugs have always been the rebels, the underground deviants, while those in charge of anti-doping have had the moral authority and social power. They have recorded meetings, conferences, scientific analyses and been supported by media reportage. [. . .] So, popular perception tends to reflect the ways in which anti-doping ideology and publicity has worked.[28]

In sum, historical research on doping is in danger of viewing doping teleologically, influenced by current knowledge on anti-doping. It is difficult to perceive this history and evaluate it "as it really was," because we know about its development largely through anti-doping. In consequence, the continuity between past and present prevails, rather than the differences. Teleological historical research in this field is also in danger of regarding the past as dichotomized between morally "good" and "bad" actors: those who doped, and those who did not or who actually prevented doping, stopped or tried to stop doping, and pushed anti-doping.

With these theoretical reflections and the knowledge that anti-doping was not established in sports and in the public awareness before the late 1960s in mind, a retrospective moralization of doping in the 1950s, early 1960s, and before seems distinctly inadequate and inappropriate from the perspective of scientific historical research. As Dimeo and Møller lament, this teleological and sociological ideology of history arguably originated in false, dubious, and one-sided research and interpretation of doping and anti-doping history.[29] This is also one of the experiences and findings of the present German research study about doping and anti-doping.

Doping is the result not only of an increasing number of highly sophisticated technological and pharmaceutical products and methods, but perhaps more importantly of the will to use them. Motivation and individual thinking and action do not take place in a social vacuum, but are embedded within a broader social context. Individual motivation to use forbidden methods in order to perform better varies within the context of the social and historical contingency that drives this behavior. A major objective of this project was therefore to identify these socially produced systems of motivation for doping (and anti-doping). Therefore, sports and sports medicine are not autonomous systems. They develop within a social context and are social constructions.

PROBLEMS OF EMPIRICAL EVALUATION AND PROVING DOPING

In contrast to the fact that the percentage of positively tested athletes in doping controls is constantly at the same low level (only about 2 percent test positively), doping researchers generally suspect that the misuse of forbidden drugs in sports has increased considerably.[30] In that respect, doping is not a new phenomenon, but an increasingly social and sporting one. However, empirically clear and sound evidence of this assertion is lacking. There is only indirect evidence to indicate the spread and increase of doping in sports. Very often, incidents that are interpreted as doping cases are basically anecdotal:

> Until the mid-1970s, all that was known regarding the incidence of performance-enhancing drug use in sport was based on anecdotes, testimonials, and rumors from journalists and others.[31]

Knowledge about doping in sports is essentially based on four main sources, all of which are characterized by methodological problems:[32]

1. Statements from athletes and coaches who are for the most part no longer active. The problem is that such testimonies often are generalized. Therefore, they are in danger of overestimating the use or misuse of doping substances. A good example is the statement of Jacques Anquetil, five-time champion of the Tour de France, who declared in 1967: “I dope. Everyone dopes. Those who claim they don’t are liars. For 50 years, bike racers have been taking stimulants.”[33] However, it is just not possible to prove this statement empirically. Other examples refer to quotes like the following in the famous book *Doping Dokumente*, by Brigitte Berendonk.[34] This book was and still is fundamental for anti-doping campaigns in Germany. “I remember the days when I became aware of the fact that women’s athletics was completely poisoned by pharmaceuticals or male hormones. During the European championships of 1971 in Helsinki, I met female javelin throwers and shot-putters. Their bodies, voices and behavior had changed so dramatically that everybody who had eyes was immediately aware of the fact that the end of (real) women’s sports had come.”[35]
2. Contemporary articles in magazines, written by investigative journalists. Statements and allegations in these articles are very often not sufficiently proven. The journalists and their outlets are, all too often, only interested in scandals, or at least many of their readers are.
3. Records and minutes of investigative commissions established by sports organizations or state authorities. These documents are based mainly on individual statements by athletes, coaches, officials, and others who have been involved in doping. Therefore, they will probably deny or play down any active involvement.
4. Drug tests. Since the 1960s, drug tests and controls have been introduced step by step, but the methods of testing and controlling drugs have never been sufficiently sound. Furthermore, those who really want to cheat invariably have found ways to remain undetected.

> Therefore, the results of these tests are not representative of the true extent of doping. Denying and obfuscating doping is part of the doping genesis and the social structure of doping, and its fundamental reality.

Common to all these sources is the fact that they do not provide a complete and clear overview of doping, either past or present. However, Manfred Donike, the famous doping and anti-doping expert, for many years head of the Doping-Control Laboratory in Cologne, stated that there are no rumors about doping in sports without some degree of truth.[36] In other words, there is no smoke without a fire. However, this popular saying is not always true, especially not with respect to doping, in which context smoke can also be produced or invented by communication alone (without the presence of a fire). Furthermore, results and interpretations are perceived as more true, the more individual evidence is gathered from different sources.[37] Despite this, generalization in the field of doping tends to be wrong, or at least incomplete and insufficient, without sound empirical proof. Therefore, it seems impossible, even today, to present comprehensive and scientifically valid research about the development, increase, and spread of doping in sports. Researchers in this field cannot do more than approach reality.

NOTES

German bibliographic information: Krüger, Michael; Becker, Christian; Nielsen, Stefan; Reinold, Marcel (2014): Doping und Anti-Doping in der Bundesrepublik Deutschland 1950 bis 2007. Genese - Strukturen - Politik. 1. Auflage 2014. Hildesheim: Arete Verlag.

1. We are grateful to the Bundesinstitut für Sportwissenschaft and its director, Jürgen Fischer, for their interest and support in publishing the results of the project in cooperation with Rowman & Littlefield. The official report can be downloaded on the website of the BISp (www.bisp.de/). We also thank Dr. Brian Bloch for his help in translating and editing the text into good academic English.

2. A list of publications in national and international journals produced by the research group of Münster is attached in the bibliography.

3. Theodor Heuss, in his speech on Whitsun 1950 in St. Paul's Church in Frankfurt am Main, quoted in Michael Krüger, "Die Neugründung des deutschen Turner-Bundes 1950," in *200 Jahre Turnbewegung—200 Jahre soziale Verantwortung* (Frankfurt: DTB, 2011), 118–22, quote on 118.

4. Allen Guttmann, *From Ritual to Record: The Nature of Modern Sports*, updated, with a new afterword (1978; New York: Columbia University Press, 2004).

5. See "Research Finds Wide Doping; Study Withheld," *New York Times*, 23 August 2013.

6. Especially see Norbert Elias, *What Is Sociology? European Perspectives* (New York: Columbia University Press, 1978), in German as Norbert Elias, *Was ist Soziologie? Grundfragen der Soziologie*, 10th ed. (Weinheim: Juventa-Verl, 2004), 139–45.

7. See sporting reports of the federal government, such as those from 2002 and 2006. Bundesministerium des Inneren (BMI), *Sportberichte der Bundesregierung* (Bonn, Berlin, 1973–2010).

8. Karl-Heinrich Bette and Uwe Schimank, *Doping im Hochleistungssport: Anpassung durch Abweichung,* Edition Suhrkamp 1957 (Frankfurt am Main: Suhrkamp, 2006).

9. Barrie Houlihan, *Dying to Win: Doping in Sport and the Development of Anti-Doping Policy*, 2nd ed. (Strasbourg: Council of Europe Publications, 2002); Barrie Houlihan, "The World Anti-doping Agency and the Campaign against Doping in Sport in Europe," *European Yearbook.* In *Council of Europe Handbook* (Council of Europe Publishing, 1998), pp. 8–21.

10. See among others Martin Nolte, *Staatliche Verantwortung im Bereich Sport: Ein Beitrag zur normativen Abgrenzung von Staat und Gesellschaft,* Schriftenreihe des Lorenz-von-Stein-Instituts für Verwaltungswissenschaften Kiel 23 (Kiel: Lorenz-von-Stein-Institut für Verwaltungswissenschaften, 2004); and Udo Steiner, "Schutz des Sports: Verbands- oder Staatsaufgabe?" in *Wettkampfmanipulation und Schutzmechanismen* (Stuttgart: Boorberg, 2012), 45–52, with respect to a possible German anti-doping law. For an international political perspective, and regarding the WADA, see Barrie Houlihan, "The World Anti-Doping Agency: Prospects for Success," in *Drugs and Doping in Sport: Socio-Legal Perspectives*, ed. John O'Leary (London: Cavendish, 2001), pp. 125–145.

11. The name *Staatsdoping* is generally used for the system and practice of doping in the GDR. Klaus Latzel, *Staatsdoping: Der VEB Jenapharm im Sportsystem der DDR* (Cologne: Böhlau, 2009), used the title *Staatsdoping* for his book about the pharmaceutical factory Jenapharm, which produced medication like anabolics (Turinabol) specifically and only for sports use and by order of the governmental authorities.

12. We are grateful to our colleagues John Hoberman, Thomas Hunt, Verner Møller, Paul Dimeo, and others for their inspiring contributions and discussions.

13. Concerning football, see Ivan Waddington and Andy Smith, *An Introduction to Drugs in Sport: Addicted to Winning?* (London: Routledge, 2009), 136; for French sports, especially boxing and cycling, see C. Brissonneau and F. Depiesse, "Doping and Doping Control in French Sport," in *Doping and Doping Control in Europe: Performance Enhancing Drugs, Elite Sports and Leisure Time Sport in Denmark, Great Britain, East and West Germany, Poland, France, Italy*, ed. Giselher Spitzer, Edition Sport & Freizeit 15 (Aachen: Meyer & Meyer, 2006), 145–67, esp. 145; and on heavy athletics with anabolic steroids, see Terry Todd, "Anabolic Steroids: The Gremlins of Sport," *Journal of Sport History*, no. 14 (1987): 87–107.

14. David E. Martin and Roger W. H. Gynn, *The Olympic Marathon* (Champaign, Ill.: Human Kinetics, 2000), 46ff., 72–75. Paul Dimeo, *A History of Drug Use in Sport, 1876–1976: Beyond Good and Evil* (New York and London: Routledge, 2007), 27ff., also supposes that Dorando took drugs.

15. *Official Report of the Olympic Games 1908*, 72. Available at *IOC-Archives*, http://olympic-museum.de/o-reports/report1908.htm.

16. Coubertin, in his report on the London Games in *Revue Olympique*, August 1908, 115–18, in Pierre de Coubertin and Norbert Müller, *Olympism: Selected Writings* (Lausanne: International Olympic Committee, 2000), 417ff.

17. Wolfgang Decker, *Sport in der griechischen Antike: Vom minoischen Wettkampf bis zu den Olympischen Spielen,* Beck's archäologische Bibliothek (Munich: Beck, 1995), 73.

18. John M. Hoberman, *Sterbliche Maschinen: Doping und die Unmenschlichkeit des Hochleistungssports* (Aachen: Meyer & Meyer, 1994); John M. Hoberman, *Testosterone Dreams: Rejuvenation, Aphrodisia, Doping* (Berkeley: University of California Press, 2005), 179.

19. John Gleaves and Matthew Llewellyn, "Sport, Drugs and Amateurism: Tracing the Real Cultural Origins of Anti-Doping Rules in International Sport," *International Journal of the History of Sport* 31, no. 8 (2014): 850, doi:10.1080/09523367.2013.831838.

20. Carl Diem, *Wesen und Lehre des Sports und der Leibeserziehung*, 4th ed. (Berlin: Weidmann, 1964), 25. The first edition of this book was published in 1949.

21. *Olympic Rules* (1946), Olympic Charter through Time, http://www.olympic.org/Documents/Olympic%20Charter/Olympic_Charter_through_time/1946-Olympic_Charter.pdf, 28. Accessed 3 July 2014.

22. Dimeo, *A History of Drug Use in Sport, 1876–1976*, 46–49; C. E. Yesalis, A. N. Kopstein, and M. S. Bahrke, "Difficulties in Estimating the Prevalence of Drug Use among Athletes," in *Doping in Elite Sport: The Politics of Drugs in the Olympic Movement*, ed. Wayne Wilson and Edward Derse (Champaign, Ill.: Human Kinetics, 2001), pp. 43–62; Marcel Reinold and John Hoberman, "The Myth of the Nazi Steroid," *International Journal of the History of Sport* 31 (2014): 1–13, doi:10.1080/09523367.2014.884563.

23. See Waddington and Smith, *An Introduction to Drugs in Sport*, 64; Dimeo, *A History of Drug Use in Sport, 1876–1976*, 103.

24. With respect to the chronological structure in an international perspective, see John M. Hoberman, *Mortal Engines: The Science of Performance and the Dehumanization of Sport* (New York: Macmillan, 1992); Hoberman, *Testosterone Dreams*; Rob Beamish and Ian Ritchie, *Fastest, Highest, Strongest: A Critique of High-Performance Sport,* Routledge Critical Studies in Sport (New York: Routledge, 2006); Patrick Laure, "Zur Entwicklung von Dopingregeln und Antidoping-Gesetzen," in *Dopingprävention in Europa: Grundlagen und Modelle; Erstes internationales Expertengespräch 2005 in Heidelberg*, ed. Wolfgang Knörzer, G. Spitzer, and G. Treutlein (Aachen and Graz: Meyer & Meyer, 2006), 121–32; Dimeo, *A History of Drug Use in Sport, 1876-1976*; and Waddington and Smith, *An Introduction to Drugs in Sport.* With respect to cycling history, see Rüdiger Rabenstein, "Some Facts about the History of Doping in Cycling History Competition," *Proceedings 8th International Cycle History Conference, 1997*, 119–30. For France, see C. Brissonneau and F. Depiesse, "Doping and Doping Control in French Sport," 145–67; for the UK, Ivan Waddington, "Changing Patterns of Drug Use in British Sport from the 1960s," *Sport in History* 25, no. 3 (2005): 472–96; and for the IOC, A. Wrynn, "The Human Factor: Science, Medicine and the International Olympic Committee, 1900–1970," *Sport in Society* 7, no. 2 (2004): 211–31; Thomas M. Hunt, *Drug Games: The International Olympic Committee and the Politics of Doping, 1960–2008*, Terry and Jan Todd Series on Physical Culture and Sports (Austin: University of Texas Press, 2011); and Kathryn Henne, "The Emergence of Moral Technoentrepreneurialism in Sport: Techniques in Anti-Doping Regulation, 1966–1976," *International Journal of the History of Sport* 30 (2013): 1–18, doi:10.1080/09523367.2013.817990.

25. Dimeo, *A History of Drug Use in Sport, 1876–1976*, 9.

26. P. Schnyder, "Erfundene Ursprünge und sprechende Bilder: Historische, etymologische und metaphorologische Bemerkungen zum Dopingkurs," in *Doping: Spitzensport als gesellschaftliches Problem*, ed. Michael Gamper, Jan Mühlethaler, and Felix Reidhaar (Zurich: NZZ Verlag, 2000), 69–88, esp. 73.

27. Waddington and Smith, *An Introduction to Drugs in Sport*, 38.

28. Dimeo, *A History of Drug Use in Sport, 1876–1976*, 7.

29. Dimeo, *A History of Drug Use in Sport*, 6–9; and Verner Møller, *The Ethics of Doping and Anti-Doping: Redeeming the Soul of Sport?* Ethics and Sport (London: Routledge, 2010), 32–48.

30. Waddington and Smith, *An Introduction to Drugs in Sport*, 48, 64, 205.

31. Yesalis, Kopstein, and Bahrke, "Difficulties in Estimating the Prevalence of Drug Use among Athletes," 44.

32. See Yesalis, Kopstein, and Bahrke, "Difficulties in Estimating the Prevalence of Drug Use among Athletes," 45–56; Waddington, "Changing Patterns of Drug Use in British Sport from the 1960s," 472–96.

33. Cited by Dimeo, *A History of Drug Use in Sport, 1876–1976*, 60.

34. Brigitte Berendonk, *Doping Dokumente: Von der Forschung zum Betrug*, 2nd expanded edition, Rororo Sport 8677 (Reinbek: Rowohlt, 1992).

35. Ibid., 11.

36. Andreas Singler and Gerhard Treutlein, *Doping im Spitzensport,* Sportentwicklungen in Deutschland 12 (Aachen: Meyer & Meyer, 2000), 43.

37. Waddington, Ivan. "The Development of Doping and Doping Control in Britain". In Doping and Doping Control in Europe. Performance enhancing drugs, elite sports and leisure time sport in Denmark, Great Britain, East and West Germany, Poland, France, Italy, Oxford, edited by Giselher Spitzer, 115-144. Aachen: Meyer & Meyer, 2006.

Abbreviations

Abbreviation	Name/Organization	English
ADK	Anti-Doping-Kommission	Anti-Doping Commission
AMG	Arzneimittelgesetz der Bundesrepublik Deutschland	Drug Law of the Federal Republic of Germany
ATSB	Arbeiter- Turn und Sportbund	Workers' Gymnastics and Sports Federation
BA-L	Bundesausschuss Leistungssport	Federal Committee for Achievement Sport
BAköV	Bundesakademie für öffentliche Verwaltung	Federal Academy of Public Administration
BAMF	Bundesamt für Migration und Flüchtlinge	Federal Office for Migration and Refugees
BASM	British Association of Sport and Medicine	British Association of Sport and Medicine
BDR	Bund Deutscher Radfahrer	German Cycling Federation
BISp	Bundesinstitut für Sportwissenschaft	Federal Institute of Sports Science
BLZ	Bundesleistungszentrum	Federal Training Center
BMI	Bundesministerium des Inneren	Federal Ministry of the Interior/ Home Office of FRG
BND	Bundesnachrichtendienst	Secret service of the FRG
BRD/FRG	Bundesrepublik Deutschland	Federal Republic of Germany
BVA	Bundesverwaltungsamt	Federal Office of Administration
BVDG	Bundesverband Deutscher Gewichtheber	Federal Association of German Weightlifters

CDU	Christlich Demokratische Union Deutschlands	Christian Democratic Union of Germany (political party)
CSU	Christlich-Soziale Union in Bayern	Christian Social Union of Bavaria (political party in Bavaria)
DABV	Deutscher Amateur-Boxverband	German Amateur Boxing Federation
DBVG	Gesetz zur Verbesserung der Bekämpfung des Dopings im Sport	Act to Improve the Fight against Doping in Sport
DDR/GDR	Deutsche Demokratische Republik	German Democratic Republic (East Germany)
DKS	Doping-Kontroll-System	Doping Control System
DLV	Deutscher Leichtathletik-Verband	German Athletics Federation
DM	Deutsche Mark	German Mark
DOSB	Deutscher Olympischer Sportbund	German Olympic Sports Federation
DRV	Deutscher Ruderverband	German Rowing Federation
DSÄB/ DGSP	Deutscher Sportärztebund/ Deutsche Gesellschaft für Sportmedizin und Prävention	German Sports Doctors Association/ German Association for Sports Medicine and Prevention
DSB	Deutscher Sportbund	German Sports Federation
DSV	Deutscher Schwimm-Verband	German Swimming Federation
DSHS	Deutsche Sporthochschule, Köln	German Sports University, Cologne
DTB	Deutscher Turner-Bund	German Gymnastics Federation
DTSB	Deutscher Turn- und Sportbund der DDR	German Gymnastics and Sports Association of the GDR
EC	Europarat	European Council
EPO	Erythropoetin	Erythropoietin
EU	Europäische Union	European Union
FDGB	Freier Deutscher Gewerkschaftsbund der DDR	Free German Labor Union of the GDR
FDJ	Freie Deutsche Jugend der DDR	Free German Youth of the GDR
FIE	Fédération Internationale d'Escrime/ Internationaler Fechtverband	International Fencing Federation
FIMS	Fédération Internationale de Médicine du Sport	International Federation of Sports Medicine

	(Internationaler Verband für Sportmedizin)	
FINA	Fédération Internationale de Natation (Internationaler Schwimmverband)	International Swimming Federation
FMSI	Federazione Medico Sportiva Italiana (Italienischer Verband für Sportmedizin)	Italian Federation of Sports Medicine
FN	Fédération Équestre Nationale, Deutsche Reiterliche Vereinigung	National Equestrian Federation of Germany (FRG)
IAAF	International Association of Athletics Federations (Internationaler Leichtathletikverband)	International Association of Athletics Federations
IOC	Internationales Olympisches Komitee	International Olympic Committee
LSB	Landessportbund	Regional Sports Association
MINEPS	UNESCO-Weltkonferenz der Sportminister	International Conference of Ministers and Senior Officials Responsible for Physical Education and Sport of the UNESCO
NADA	Nationale Anti-Doping Agentur	National Anti-Doping Agency
NADC	Nationaler Anti-Doping Code	National Anti-Doping Code
NGO	Nicht-Regierungsorganisation	Nongovernmental organization
NOK/NOC	Nationales Olympisches Komitee für Deutschland	National Olympic Committee for Germany (FRG)
NS	Nationalsozialismus	National Socialism
OS	Olympische Spiele	Olympic Games
OSP	Olympiastützpunkt	National Olympic Training Center
ReSpoDo	Rechtskommission des Sports gegen Doping	Juridical Commission of Sport against Doping
SBZ	Sowjetisch besetzte Zone	Soviet-Occupied Zone (East Germany)
SED	Sozialistische Einheitspartei Deutschlands	Socialist Unity Party of Germany (GDR)
SPD	Sozialdemokratische Partei Deutschlands	Social Democratic Party of Germany (FRG)
Stasi	Ministerium für Staatssicherheit der DDR	Ministry of State Security of the GDR
UCI	Union Cycliste Internationale (Internationaler Radsportverband)	International Cycling Association

UdSSR/ USSR	Union der Sozialistischen Sowjet Republiken	Union of Soviet Socialist Republics
UIPM	Union Internationale de Pentathlon Moderne Internationaler Fünfkampfverband	International Pentathlon Union
UNESCO	United Nations Educational, Scientific, and Cultural Organizations	United Nations Educational, Scientific, and Cultural Organizations
USOC	US-amerikanisches Olympisches Komitee	United States Olympic Committee
UVI	Unione Velocipedistra Italiana Italienischer Radsportverband	Italian Cyclist Union
WADA	Welt Anti-Doping Agentur	World Anti-Doping Agency
WADC	Welt Anti-Doping Code	World Anti-Doping Code
WHO	Weltgesundheitsorganisation	World Health Organization

Chronology

The 1950s

- Amphetamines and doping definitions are at the center of the doping discussions
- Sporadic und unorganized anti-doping policies (hardly any regulations, control, prosecution, and sanctioning)

1950

- Founding of the German Sports Federation (Deutscher Sportbund, DSB), the umbrella organization of West German sports associations and federations
- Start of the (West) German Sports Doctors Association (Deutscher Sportärztebund, DSÄB)

1951

- International Amateur Boxing Federation adopts doping regulations

1952

- USSR participates in the Olympic Games for the first time
- "Brustmann case" becomes the first publicly discussed doping case in the Federal Republic of Germany (FRG) before the Olympic Games in Helsinki
- DSÄB develops definition of doping

1953

- DSB adopts DSÄB's doping definition

1955

- Establishment of the Council for Sports Medicine Research in Cologne

The 1960s

- Cold War on the track
- Process of "totalization" of top-level sports becomes more dynamic
- List of banned substances developed
- Increasing international integration of anti-doping actors
- Increasing use of testosterone and anabolic steroids
- Increasing introduction of doping tests

1960

- Death of Danish cyclist Knud Enemark Jensen at the Olympic Games in Rome is attributed to doping

1962

- Opening of the world's first independent doping laboratory in Florence by the Italian Federation of Sports Medicine (FMSI)

1963

- European meeting on the problem of doping in Uriage-les-Bains
- Decree of the Austrian Federal Ministry of Education imposed to punish doping in sports

1964

- Establishment of national training centers in West Germany

1965

- International expert conference of the Council of Europe Committee for Out-of-School Education in Strasbourg, among other conferences to combat doping in sports
- First anti-doping activity of the West German Ministry of the Interior (Bundesministerium des Inneren, BMI)
- Doping Symposium of DSÄB in Berlin

- Establishment of full-time national coaching bodies

1966

- Cyclists strike in the Tour de France because of doping controls
- Munich awarded the 1972 Olympic Games

1967

- Death of British cyclist Tom Simpson during the Tour de France due to the amphetamine Tonedron
- Establishment of the West German Sports Aid Foundation (Stiftung Deutsche Sporthilfe)

1968

- West German Swimming Federation conducts first urine tests
- Death of professional boxer Jupp Elze triggers debate on doping in West German professional sports
- First official doping tests at the Olympic Games in Grenoble and Mexico

1969

- Responding to a BMI initiative, DSB requests forty-two associations to add anti-doping policies to their constitutions (only four had included the policies)
- Establishment of the Federal Committee for Achievement Sport (Bundesausschuss Leistungssport, BA-L) as crucial organization in the DSB to organize top-level sports and distribute government financial support to the sports associations and federations
- Foundation of the first Special Committee for Sports and the Olympic Games, later the Sports Commission of the German Bundestag (Sportausschuss des Deutschen Bundestages)

The 1970s

- Nomination criterion *Endkampfchance* (chance of participating in the finals) begins to govern selection for the Olympics in the early 1970s
- Anabolic steroids are at the center of the doping problem
- Construction of a doping laboratory in connection with the Olympic Games in Munich, whose structures and instruments are later transferred to Cologne

- Significant increase in number of doping controls in the FRG in the second half of the decade

1970

- Doping Symposium in Freiburg
- DSB adopts Framework Guidelines to Combat Doping
- Establishment of the Federal Institute of Sports Science (Bundesinstitut für Sportwissenschaft, BISp) as an office of the Ministry of the Interior in order to support sports science for top-level sports

1972

- Doping controls at the Olympic Games in Munich under the direction of Manfred Donike

1974

- Flight of GDR sports doctor Alois Mader to West Germany
- IOC puts anabolic steroids on the doping list after a validation process is developed

1976

- Luftklistier (air clyster) and Kolbe-Spritze (Kolbe injection) affairs, and obvious anabolic-steroid use at the Olympic Games in Montreal

1977

- Anabolic steroids are integrated as banned substances in the Framework Guidelines to Combat Doping
- Declaration of Principles for Top Sport (Grundsatzerklärung für den Spitzensport) of the Tripartite Commission, headed by Ommo Grupe
- Sports Commission of the German Bundestag consults experts on the topic "affecting performance and performance-enhancing measures in high-performance sports"

1978

- Federal government support for sports federations is made formally dependent on their observance of the anti-doping rule

The 1980s

- End of amateur sports
- Medicalization of sports and society becomes more dynamic
- New doping substances based on hormones

1981

- Amateur paragraph deleted from the statutes of the IOC

1983

- Resolution on the Declaration of Principles for Top Sport of the DSB, with stronger sports medicine promotion

1984

- “Strittmatter case” before the Olympic Games in Los Angeles

1985

- BISp assigns the so-called regeneration study

1987

- Death of the West German heptathlete Birgit Dressel because of “multiple organ failure”
- Sports Commission of the German Bundestag holds public hearing on “humanity in top-level sports”

1988

- Doping case of Canadian sprinter Ben Johnson at the Olympic Games in Seoul

1989

- Start of the pilot project “Training Testing” in West Germany
- Council of Europe adopts Convention against Doping

The 1990s

- End of Cold War in politics and on the track
- Process of German reunification begins

- Commercialization, professionalization, and medicalization of top-level sports
- EPO becomes new challenge for anti-doping policies
- Out-of-competition testing

1990

- Doping in the media; simultaneous reports of past doping in the old West Germany

1991

- Ten percent budget freeze on key measures in the field of elite sports until the presentation of an anti-doping proposal
- Work and report of the Tab Commission
- Work and report of the Richthofen Commission

1992

- Establishment of the Anti-Doping Commission in Germany (Anti-Doping-Kommission, ADK)
- "Krabbe case" involving the training group of Thomas Springstein

1994

- Ratification at national level of the Council of Europe's Convention against Doping

1998

- Intensification of the pharmaceutical law
- Processes against doping loaded GDR sports officials, coaches and medic charged with doping of athletes
- Festina scandal at the Tour de France

1999

- Doping World Conference in Lausanne
- Establishment of the World Anti-Doping Agency (WADA)
- Establishment of the doping-victim assistance association

The 2000s

- New international and national anti-doping structures
- Diversity of doping and anti-doping
- Hormone and gene doping

2002

- Establishment of the National Anti-Doping Agency (Nationale Anti-Doping Agentur, NADA)
- Doping Victims Aid Act comes into force

2003

- NADA officially begins its work

2004

- WADA Code goes into effect
- Publication of the NADA Code

2005

- Session of the General Conference of UNESCO in Paris: "International Convention against Doping in Sport" (goes into effect in 2007)

2006

- Unification of DSB and the National Olympic Committee for Germany under the new German umbrella organization for sports, called the German Olympic Sports Federation (DOSB)
- DOSB adopts "anti-doping action plan"
- German government submits "measures against doping in sport"

2007

- Doping scandal involving the Telekom professional cycling team
- Minister of the interior establishes Project Group to Investigate Doping
- NADA crisis because of the lack of financial support from sports associations and the government

Chapter One

From Common Practice to Prohibition

The Beginnings of Doping and Anti-Doping in German Sport of the 1950s and 1960s

After the defeat of Nazi Germany in World War II and the "bedingungslose Kapitulation" (unconditional surrender) of the Third Reich on May 8, 1945, Germany no longer existed as a sovereign nation-state.[1] The German people were governed by the Allied forces, namely the United States, Great Britain, the Soviet Union, and France. The territory was divided into four occupation zones in which the various governors of the Allied armies represented and executed state power. Specifically, there was the USSR in the east, the United States in the west and south of Germany, Great Britain in the west and north, and France in the southwest. Despite the increasing ideological differences between the Allies, between the "capitalist" Western powers on the one hand and the socialist Soviet Union (including its dependent states) on the other, the Allies were united in their common will to fundamentally destroy Nazism and militarism in Germany. Prussia was regarded as the heart of German militarism. Therefore, Germany was divided into new regions (*Länder*) without Prussia, which had been by far the greatest and most powerful regional state in Germany in the recent past since the German *Kaiserreich*. German organizations and institutions that were part of or closely affiliated with the Nazi Party and Nazi ideology were to be reorganized. German people should be reeducated in order to prevent a revival of German Nazism and militarism and to reintegrate the German people and a future German nation-state into the community of free and peace-loving countries. Of course, opinions were divided between the Western and the Eastern Allied forces as to how this should be done. The Soviet Union and its dictator, Joseph Stalin, attempted to secure complete political and economic power over their occupied territories, and demanded that East Germany become part of the socialist empire. According to the teleological Marxist ideology of history, socialism and communism are predetermined to defeat capitalism. Therefore, Stalin was eager to prepare his empire for this final battle of world history.

The Western Allies attempted to retain their ideals of a free and democratic world. A free economy, a peaceful civilian society, independent institutions, and a republican state, all based on a democratic charter, were essential objectives of Western Allied politics from the end of the war until the official foundation of the Bundesrepublik Deutschland (BRD; Federal Republic of Germany, FRG).

Step by step, these fundamental differences between the Western and Eastern blocs concerning future German society and the nation-state became all too obvious. They were in fact all also relevant for establishing different sports systems in East and West Germany. In East Germany since 1949, sport in the German Democratic Republic (GDR; Deutsche Demokratische Republik, DDR) was organized according to the communist principles of the Soviet Union. In the free West Germany, officially the FRG after 1949, sport was to be an equally free part of the new and democratic civil society. This was the initial basis of the Cold War, which lasted until the breakdown of the communist Soviet Union and the fall of the Berlin Wall in 1989/90.

Both sporting models can be regarded as results of the war and of Nazi politics. Socialist or communist principles of sport and its organization, "body culture" and "body education"—the official *termini technici* in the GDR—seemed to be the best guarantee for a better future, at least from the perspective of socialism and communism. After the victory of the Soviet Union over Nazi Germany, it seemed quite clear to convinced socialists that the world of the future would and should be a socialist one, that or nothing. With this thinking, sport was closely connected to the socialist state, its ideology, and its institutional structures.

By contrast, in the Western world, the main message of the victory over Nazi Germany was that the principles of liberalism, democracy, and a strong civil society, based on classic bourgeois morality, had triumphed over the terrorist regime of Hitlerism and Nazism, with its militarism, racism, anti-Semitism, and assorted other "-isms" that belonged to the now-conquered "empire of the devil." The alternative could only be a liberal and democratic state with the independent institutions of a free, liberal, and democratic society. Therefore, sport was initially regarded as a private, personal, and free activity. The state must not interfere in this private sphere of citizens, who are free to organize their sporting interests and needs by themselves, and not by the state or its administrations. This was the underlying principle according to which sport was understood and organized in the United States and Great Britain, and how the Olympic organization of amateur sports worked and had worked since its beginnings at the end of the nineteenth century. Consequently, the manner in which the Western Allies attempted to rebuild sports and sporting organizations in their area of influence in West Germany and the FRG was driven from the bottom up by the citizens themselves, and not from the top down by the state and its various organizations, as in East Germany and the Soviet Union.

A common consequence in both East and West Germany during the early 1950s was sympathy with sports-for-all concepts. They corresponded with the German traditions of *Turnen* and gymnastics, as well as with the traditions of the workers' sports movement and the international ideas and ideals of amateur sport.[2] However, this initial and fundamental concept changed radically in the process of the Cold War, when top-level sports at the Olympic Games, as well as at European and world championships, became symbols of the overall achievement and performance of the Western or Eastern world, of socialism or capitalism, and of the power of nation-states in general. For Germany, this development peaked during the process of preparing for and implementing the Olympic Games in Munich in 1972.

In this context, doping also became relevant for sports policies and, in the long run, for state politics as well. Although doping had already been a familiar phenomenon in international and national sports since the beginning of the Olympics, it was not really regarded as a problem, at least not for amateur sports. Sports officials, functionaries, and representatives of sports-for-all, *Turnen*, gymnastics, physical education, and physical health criticized more the excesses of professional sports, like six-day cycling races or professional boxing matches, where athletes seemed to be treated like slaves and forced to perform to the limits of human endurance or beyond. Some German "Turners" also criticized Olympic amateur sports in a similar manner, but in general, doping was not discussed in the amateur-sports organizations and their publications.

After World War II, however, new experiences with drugs and medications of various kinds were starting to influence the world of sports. Soldiers on all sides, mostly young men, had taken drugs like amphetamines to cope with exertion, pain, hunger, and other hardships, as well as to enhance their strength and aggression in combat.[3] On the one hand, these experiences seemed to be relevant for the further development of doping in the context of sports. On the other hand, there was the tendency to impose higher standards of morality on the postwar development of sports. Both are reasons why doping practices became a real and socially constructed problem in sports in Germany and worldwide, at least since the 1960s. Doping was known but not regarded as relevant to amateur sports in the 1950s, neither publicly worldwide, nor specifically in Germany, nor in the relationship between state and sport.

In terms of Norbert Elias's figurational and process sociology, as mentioned in the introduction, doping and the process of "sportization" took steps toward higher standards of performance and achievement, more political and functional instrumentalization, more rationality and bureaucracy, and also more social control and higher levels of moral behavior—that is, stricter mechanisms of self-control.[4] Things that had been allowed before and without restriction or a bad conscience were now forbidden and moral taboos.

SPORTS IN THE FEDERAL REPUBLIC OF GERMANY AFTER THE SECOND WORLD WAR

The Allies were somewhat amazed how quickly the Germans had distanced themselves from their Nazi past. Obviously, they were enormously relieved to be free from the nightmare of war and Nazi dictatorship, and most Germans tried to make a new beginning under control of the Allies. This certainly applied to all parts of society, politics, economy, culture, and indeed sports and the associated policies. In East Germany, in accordance with the politics and ideology of Joseph Stalin, who was the dictator not only of the Soviet Union, but also in effect of East Germany and the Eastern bloc, sports were kept under strict control of the state and its state party, the Sozialistische Einheitspartei Deutschlands (SED). The former gymnastics and sports clubs were not allowed to be refounded, even those that were closely connected to the former Social Democratic Party, the political party of the majority of the working class. The SED in East Germany was founded in 1946 as a result of massive political pressure placed on the former Social Democratic Party by the Soviets. The unity of the left was the result of compulsion, not of volition. This history is in fact responsible for the deep distrust that the Social Democratic Party in Germany holds toward left-wing communist parties even today, such as the party Die Linke (The Left), which was created after German reunification out of the dissolved SED.

In West Germany, officially established in 1949 as the Bundesrepublik Deutschland, sport was intended to be strictly separated from state politics. This was a precondition of the Western Allies, as well as a desire of both old and new German sports representatives, motivated by their experiences during Nazi dictatorship, when gymnastics and sports clubs were marginalized step by step by the state. At the latest after the (self-)liquidation of the Deutscher Reichsausschuss für Leibesübungen (DRA) in 1934/35 and the Olympic Games of 1936, the so-called Massenorganisationen der Partei (Mass Organizations of the Nazi Party) attempted to replace the classic German *Vereine* (clubs). However, they were basically unable to fulfill the public duties and social functions of these clubs in democratic societies, like spending free time together, organizing their sporting, health, cultural, and societal interests, and—last but not least—acting independently of state control and constraint, at least with respect to sports activities, and according to the democratic traditions and structures of German *Vereine*.

The strong position and revival of the club system for the development of sports seems to be one distinctive criterion, among others, of West German sports development after the war, as a result of the role of sports under the Nazi dictatorship and in contrast to the new German dictatorship in East Germany. This characteristic also seems to constitute a major difference from structures of sports in the Anglo-Saxon world, specifically the United States and Great Britain, where school sports, college and university sports, and private and commercial sports dominate the system.

The self-perception or self-image of sports, represented by sportsmen and sports officials in the early years of the Federal Republic of Germany, entailed the notion that sports ought to be free, based on the decisions of individuals, and not molded by exterior constraints and least of all by the state. Free individuals should be free to organize themselves into independent and free clubs, as had been the case in Germany before the dictatorship of Hitler and his Nazi Party. In consequence, the rebuilding of a sporting club system for everybody was a major objective and motivation during the early years of the Federal Republic. As Willi Daume, the first elected president of the Deutscher Sportbund (DSB) always used to mention, as part of the new German society, club sports had to work hard to regain its reputation after the deep crisis of war and Nazi dictatorship.

However, German sportsmen in both East and West also wanted to participate again in top-level sports and rejoin the international and Olympic sports family. At the end of the war in 1945, the spectacular Berlin Olympics of 1936 were not even a decade past. Memories of the outstanding performances and successes of the German athletes were still vivid. However, they were now associated more with the competent training and diligent efforts of the stable German club system and its sports experts than the centralism of Nazi sports politics. There was clearly substantial interest in and motivation to tap into these successes and be reacknowledged in the world of international sports. Nonetheless, this objective could not be achieved earlier than 1952, when a German Olympic team was finally able and allowed to take part again in the Olympic Games of Helsinki, and in 1954, when the German national soccer team won the World Cup in Bern, Switzerland. This victory seemed so amazing that it was glorified by the press as the "Wunder von Bern"—the miracle of Bern.[5] However, this victory was in fact no miracle at all, but a late or postwar product of the high level of German sports and especially soccer skills since the late 1920s. Some historians have asserted that the postwar German nation-state was born after this event, but the foundation of the Bundesrepublik Deutschland in 1949 was not really affected so much by the national German soul as by historical and political facts, including rational power and legal considerations.

Below is a detailed description of the (re)building of West German sporting structures. This analysis is necessary in order to portray the further development of doping and anti-doping within German sports and in the context of the changing relationship between sports and sports organizations, on the one hand, and state authorities on the other.

STRUCTURES AND SELF-PERCEPTIONS OF THE GERMAN FEDERAL SPORTS ORGANIZATIONS

The Allied occupying forces in Germany, officially named Allierter Kontrollrat, and their High Commission took only eight months after the unconditional surrender of Nazi Germany to release an edict concerning sports and sports organizations. The Allies issued an order, referred to as Kontrollratsdirektive No. 45, on December 17, 1945, that all clubs and sports organizations had to be suspended. All had been members of the Nationalsozialistischer Reichsbund für Leibesübungen (NSRL) and were therefore forbidden. This procedure was part of the Allied policy of denazification, and the sports clubs, federations, and associations were in fact regarded as part of the Nazi Party and the centralized state system of the Third Reich. New clubs were allowed only by permission of the responsible officers of the Allied forces. Federations and associations extending beyond local or regional boundaries were not allowed, and neither were associations between clubs in different occupation zones. Despite this strict order, many gymnastics and sports clubs were reestablished in the Western zones during the summer and autumn of 1945. However, they had to be reapproved and prove that no previous Nazi officials or politicians continued to influence or play a role in these clubs. Yet this was extremely difficult in reality, because sports had, on the one hand, been heavily infiltrated by Nazi ideology, and on the other hand, many German sportsmen, officials, and functionaries asserted during their denazification that they had merely been *Mitläufer* of the regime, that is, more or less blind and passive followers who were only interested in sports and not in Nazi politics. This argument conformed precisely to that of apolitical sports that had been functionalized or instrumentalized by Nazi politics.

The question was, Who would be able, as well as morally and politically equipped, to lead the German sports clubs into a better future? Better, that is, for all those who wished to do sports in clubs, and better for athletes wishing to participate in international and Olympic performance sports. The former officials of the workers' gymnastics and sports clubs and associations were intended to play a major role in this process. Their working-class sports clubs had been suspended and destroyed by the Nazis, and many leading officials had to emigrate, had been imprisoned, or had died in concentration camps or in combat. Some representatives of the previous working-class clubs like Oscar Drees, Heinrich Sorg, or Fritz Wildung, the well-known manager of the German Arbeiter-Turn- und Sportbund (ATSB), previously the greatest and most important workers' sports organization in the world, favored the model of local clubs, including several sports or sports sections, and, therefore, regional *Landessportbünde,* which are associations of these clubs. Such *Landessportbünde* were established as soon as the American and British occupation forces authorized their foundation in 1946/47.

Some remaining officials of *bürgerliche Sportbewegung*, the middle-class sports clubs and federations, were very eager to prepare for the reentry of German top athletes into international events or tournaments, especially the Olympic Games. The most famous and important representative of these groups was Carl Diem, manager of the previous Deutscher Reichsausschuss für Leibesübungen (DRA) and manager of the 1936 Olympics in Berlin. Accordingly, he was called Mister Olympics, and was, by the way, the first dean (*Rektor*) of the West German Sports University in Cologne, which was established in 1947 by the British army officer John Dixon. Diem was also the only German guest at the London Games of 1948, the first after the war and after the two cancelled Olympic Games scheduled for 1940 and 1944. A German Olympic team was not and could not be invited to these "Austerity Games," because a German Olympic Committee did not yet exist. The High Commission did not allow its foundation as long as there was no sovereign German nation-state. The Bundesrepublik Deutschland was formally founded on May 23, 1949, and as a consequence of this political precondition, the German National Olympic Committee, or NOK für Deutschland, was founded on September 23, 1949, in Bonn.

One year later, on December 10, 1950, the Deutscher Sportbund (DSB; German Sports Federation) was founded in Hannover. This umbrella organization of the West German gymnastics and sports clubs included fifteen *Landessportbünde*—one for each newly founded West German *Bundesland*—and, at that time, twenty-five *Spitzen- oder Fachverbände*, which are organizations for specific sports like soccer, gymnastics, athletics, and so on. This was the concept of sports organization favored by the middle-class sports representatives, whereas the model of *Landessportbünde* had been favored by previous working-class representatives. Accordingly, the structure of newly organized West German sport was a compromise between two historical models of German sports federations and associations. However, both groups agreed that this compromise was based on the notion of freedom for all. The unity of German sport should be voluntary and not the result of compulsion. The emphasis on the unity of German sport being based on the "free will" of its participants, as expressed in the charter of the DSB in 1950, signaled the very deliberate contrast to the totalitarian sports organizations of the Third Reich, as well as to the totalitarian sports system of East Germany.

Every club and every association was and is free, sovereign, and independent to join or leave the umbrella organizations DSB and NOK für Deutschland, which, since 2006, have been united into the new Deutscher Olympischer Sportbund (DOSB). However, it goes without saying that athletes can participate in events, competitions, tournaments, championships, or Olympic Games only if they are members of sports clubs that are members of a federation or association of the DSB or NOK. After all, the Olympic charter prescribes that only the NOK, acknowledged by the IOC, is able to appoint athletes for participation in the Olympic Games.

There is another aspect that ought to be mentioned concerning the structure of West German sport. The historical compromise leading to the foundation of the DSB also included the principle that only one federation can represent one sport. This means, for example, that only one federation can award the title of "German champion" in a given sport, and not, as in the Roaring Twenties, that champion athletes were named by the German Turners, as well as by the German Athletics Federation and the workers' sports association. To give another example, at that time, soccer championships were organized by various sports organizations.

In sum, the West German umbrella organization of sports, the Deutscher Sportbund, was in fact politically weak, basically comprising various independent members. The DSB has no real authority over its members, its policies being based on discussion, agreement, and compromise. Its "institutional members" are free and autonomous in financial, organizational, and sporting respects, as the charter has prescribed since 1950. However, the historical compromise of 1950 included a good prevention mechanism against the fragmentation of sport, which had been regarded as one of the reasons for the *Gleichschaltung* of sports organizations during the Third Reich. This *Gleichschaltung* (literally: making equal) refers to the complex process by which the Nazi Party and state succeeded in getting sports under their totalitarian control, without any noteworthy opposition.

The West German DSB was constructed in deliberate opposition not only to the past, but also to the East German model. At the same time as West Germans were attempting to rebuild new sports organizations according to democratic and liberal principles, in East Germany, the state and its so-called mass organizations, including the state party, the SED, assumed complete power and responsibility for sport. The most important were the Freie Deutsche Jugend (FDJ; Free German Youth), the youth organization of the SED, and the Freier Deutscher Gewerkschaftsbund (FDGB), which was the leisure-time organization of the trade union in the GDR, controlled by the SED. These organizations signaled that in the early days of the GDR, organized sports for the whole population, specifically for the mass of working people, were fundamental to self-perceptions of body culture and sports in the GDR, the first German state for peasants and workers, as the communist ideologists of the SED propagated. This conception then changed when the Eastern bloc and leaders of the GDR decided to take part in the Olympic Games—in other words, to compete against the capitalist West on the track.

Whereas body culture and sports were mentioned in the charter of the GDR, this did not apply to the *Grundgesetz*, the charter of the Bundesrepublik. Incidentally, the latter was called the *Grundgesetz* because it was intended to constitute a provisional charter, in expectation of having one for a subsequent unified German nation-state. Physical education at schools was organized within the sphere of influence and responsibility of the *Bundesländer*, the regional states in the federal union. The Federal Republic of Germany was and is a federal state composed of strong regional states like Bavaria and North Rhine-Westphalia.

The decision for the autonomy of the West German sports clubs and federations and their independence from the state made common sense to the West German public. The charter of the DSB proclaimed not only that the DSB and its members had to be "neutral" on "political, religious, and racial" issues, but that all members had the "absolute right to self-determination and self-organization." The DSB should merely work publicly and with respect to the state authorities to support their members. In the early years of the Bundesrepublik, the new president, Willi Daume, a businessman from the Ruhr area with little experience in sports administration, constantly explained to the public these basics of autonomy and self-determination in sport. On the occasion of the third assembly of the DSB in 1956:

> The Turn- [gymnastics] and sport movement has to be pure, with no objective beyond promoting sport itself [. . .].The Turn- [gymnastics] and sport movement needs *1.* the absolute right of self-determination and self-organization [. . .] *3.* free decision-making on ideals and ethical principles in their clubs.[6]

This concept of autonomy was justified by the *Eigenweltcharakter* of sport. Sport ought to be a world of its own.

> The deeper sense of the sport concept is the elimination of all its non-sport functions. Gymnastics [Turnen] and sport are not practiced because of any external logic or function. The process itself is their only meaning and aim.[7]

This traditional ideology of sport was not only in accordance with that of amateur sports, represented by the International Olympic Committee. At the same time, Daume deliberately contrasted the West German model of free and independent sport with the functionalized concept of state sport in East Germany. Ultimately, by arguing in this manner, he managed to fend off the state authorities.

SPORTS POLICY

Sports in the Federal Republic of Germany include two essential components. First, the *Sport-Selbstverwaltung* (self-organization and management) of clubs and associations, and, second, the limited public management of sports by state authorities, to varying degrees by the Federal Republic *(Bund)*, the regions *(Bundesländer)*, and the communities *(Städte und Gemeinden)*.

In principle, the *Bundesländer* are powerful and responsible for all educational issues, including physical education at schools. They also have to pay salaries to teachers. The communities, on the other hand, provide and look after buildings and equipment. The *Bund* itself and its federal administration have no ministry responsible for sporting issues. Various ministries assume responsibility for sports and physical education—for example, the Ministry of Defense, which was established in 1955, provides physical education and sports for soldiers. Step by step, when top-level sports and top-level athletes became more relevant for representing the new West German state in international events or contests, the Ministry of the Interior assumed a leading role, for national reasons, in the administration and financing of these high-performance sports.

At the beginning of the Federal Republic of Germany, Carl Diem, the dean of the sports university at Cologne, was asked to advise the new federal government under the leadership of Chancellor Konrad Adenauer on general issues concerning sports. Diem had a part-time job as a *Sportreferent* (sports consultant) from 1949–1953, and as he mentioned himself, he could handle it during the short ride from Cologne to Bonn, the new and provisional capital of West Germany.[8]

Diem's successor for this function was the former decathlete Hans-Heinrich Sievert. He was given a full-time job as *Sportreferent* inside the Ministry of the Interior, which was to be responsible for federal issues concerning sports. In 1954, Sievert repeated the familiar perception of sports and sports administration in the early years of the Federal Republic. Sport is an "activity," he stated, "which belongs to the private sphere of the citizen." Therefore, he continued, "it is logical that sport, with millions of members in clubs, in principle manages itself. In a democratic state like the Federal Republic of Germany, this seems a matter of course."[9]

This statement once again underlined the autonomy and self-responsibility of sport. Sievert also emphasized the voluntary work of sports clubs and federations for the public and community. The first president of the Federal Republic, Theodor Heuss, did likewise when he defined the relationship between state and sport. The state ought to be a "good friend but not the manager of sports, and not damage its freedom and voluntary nature," he added.[10]

However, this doctrine had to be modified when West German athletes returned to the international stage and later to top-level sports, which really began with the Olympic Games in Helsinki in 1952. The state and public of the FRG were very keen to send an outstanding team to the Olympics and to other international sports events. The sports organizations, which are financed only through membership fees, were not able to finance these expensive excursions, not to mention the increasing investment in coaching, training camps, equipment, medical care, and so on. German athletes were less affluent than ever and there were few if any wealthy athletes like the gentlemen athletes in the early days of British amateur and gentleman sport. Therefore, the German public logically had to support top-level sports, not only rhetorically, but also monetarily. This support seemed to be a duty of the federal state. The principle was called "subsidiarity," a *terminus technicus* borrowed from the Catholic doctrine of social sponsorship, which means "helping people to help themselves." Applied to sports, subsidiarity in the context of the solidarity and partnership between state and sport includes financial support for public achievements and the efforts of sporting organizations. Top-level sports is one of them.

The sports consultant Hans-Heinrich Sievert defined subsidiarity rather reluctantly as follows:

> Sport, at least free sport for adults, must always be self-financed. [. . .] The state—especially the federal government—agrees to support sport for really important enterprises or activities, but only on condition that the sport organizations contribute adequately.[11]

This was the beginning of financial support for sports, especially at the top level, by the federal government of the FRG. From then on, intensive discussions were held every year between the Ministry of the Interior and sporting organizations about the exact level of financial support. The first budget of the FRG in 1950 included the modest sum of DM 300,000 "for essential processes and procedures of sport and physical activity [*Leibesübungen*]." In fact, some training camps and the events of sports associations, such as championships, received a grant from the federal state. The DSB in fact received a jump start of around DM 20,000.

Sievert specified the nature of support for sports by the federal government as follows:

> Only associations at a national level can be financially supported if a concrete and direct motivation for the federal government is evident. Those events and measures can be supported which are in the national interest, like international or European championships or Deutsche Turnfeste [German gymnastics festivals] or equivalent events. International exchange can also be supported, as well as scientific and medical research with respect to sport and sports medi-

> cine. [. . .] The federal government offers its support to all worthy projects when other sponsors are not available and when such projects could not otherwise be realized.

The sports budget increased every year, from DM 425,000 in 1951 to DM 600,000 in 1952 and rising to DM 900,000 by 1955. In 1960, the sum amounted to DM 2 million. The longtime manager of the DSB, Karlheinz Gieseler, asserted that starting in the 1960s, it was appropriate to talk of "systematic support for sport."[12] In 1969, the budget was DM 11.3 million. However, this sum was not really all that high, given the economic growth in West Germany and the rate of inflation during that period.[13]

How to finance sports arenas, stadiums, sports halls, training camps, sports centers, and so on, which all gradually became more relevant for the improvement of training conditions, emerged as a central issue in the sports policy dialogue between sports organizations and state authorities at the levels of *Bund* (federal government), *Ländern* (regions), and *Gemeinden* (cities and communities).

Sports consultant Sievert had already stated in 1954 that it should be clear that the state and public have a duty to provide good sports facilities and conditions for training and contests. Yet it took until 1957 for the federal budget to include an amount of DM 5 million to finance buildings and training centers for top-level sports. Even so, the amount was in fact ridiculously low. At that time, Willi Daume, president of the DSB, calculated that cities and communities had been spending more than DM 335 million on sports arenas, swimming pools, and sports halls from 1948 to 1953.

In 1959, the Goldener Plan für den Sportstättenbau (Golden Plan for the Construction of Sports Sites) was concluded after intensive discussions between sports organizations and sports authorities at all levels. The budget was set at DM 10 million in 1960 and increased to DM 30 million by 1962/63.

Despite the increasing systematic support of sports by the state, both state authorities and sporting organizations persisted with the principles of autonomy and subsidiarity, which were also to apply to Olympic Games. The costs of preparing and sending delegations to the Olympic Games were not to be paid as a matter of course. Therefore, the foundation of the Deutsche Olympische Gesellschaft (DOG, German Olympic Society) as a private organization aimed to support the Olympic athletes by fund-raising.

Sports officials agreed unanimously to oppose excessive financial support by the state. As Willi Daume stated in 1958, "only the most essential requirements should be financed by the state. Liberty and independence are more important and valuable than victories and medals. No price is too high to ensure the autonomy of sport."[14]

PHYSICAL HEALTH AS A COMMON OBJECTIVE—A LEGITIMATION FOR STATE SPONSORING

Sports and physical-education ideologists argued very much in accordance with politicians on at least one basic issue, namely the contribution of physical education, fitness, recreation, and sports to individual and public health. The DSB always emphasized the role of sports and physical education for the promotion of public health. The representatives of the sports organizations traditionally argued that the level of bodily or physical fitness of the population, and especially of children and the youth, is generally poor. This seems to have remained the case up to the present, if one believes the various health surveys in Germany and worldwide. In any event, this line of reasoning is generally a successful strategy for seeking the support of public and political authorities for sports and public-health programs, including physical fitness and preventive and recreational programs associated with sports and movement. This form of legitimation goes back to the 1920s and earlier, when gymnastics and *Turnen* were recommended as a means of countering *Zivilisationsschäden* (diseases or other damage imposed by civilization) and for improving the *Volksgesundheit* (public health). In the 1950s and 1960s, these arguments were still common.[15]

In 1954, the DSB delivered a "Denkschrift über die Gegenwartsprobleme und Aufgaben des deutschen Sports" (Memorandum on Current Problems and Responsibilities of the German Sports Movement) to the federal government and members of parliament (Deutscher Bundestag). In addition to the above-mentioned health-and-fitness issue, the DSB paper lamented the poor conditions for physical education at schools and the lack of suitable sports and swimming halls, arenas, stadiums, and so on. For the first time, this paper included a comparison with the (allegedly) generous support of sports and sports science in East Germany.

The lobbying efforts of the sports officials were ultimately successful. The additional governmental support (always justified according to the principle of subsidiarity) for the sports-club movement increased year by year. A milestone of the health-policy offensive of the DSB was the foundation of the Kuratorium für die sportmedizinische Forschung (Curatorship for Medical Research on Sport) in Cologne. This institution was led by the DSB but financed by the federal government. At least 80 percent of its budget was tax-financed, about DM 700,000 annually from 1955 to 1961.[16]

Two associated issues seem particularly noteworthy. First, the mere fact that medical research on sports was sponsored by the federal state speaks volumes. Second, there was the beginning of specific support for research on sports or, more generally, sports sciences, especially sports medicine, by the state and the taxpayer. However, it was not clear what kind of medical research on sports and sports sciences was intended, either by the DSB or by the government. The suspicion may well be justified that on the "front page," the traditional argument about the poor level of fitness and health of the population was rampant, but on the "back page," the sports officials, as well as sports politicians in government and parliament, were well aware of the need for better medical research and support for the performance of top-level athletes, in order to prevail at international contests, especially against the athletic "brothers and sisters" of East Germany. The Cold War was just beginning, also "on the track."

In general, the lobbying activities of the DSB were intensified steadily. As early as 1951, the newly elected president of the Federal Republic of Germany, Theodor Heuss, agreed to take over the patronage of the German sports movement. In 1953, after the retirement of Diem, the part-time job of the sport consultant to the government in the Home Office (Ministry of the Interior) was increased to a full-time position. It is also worth noting that the Home Office had always been the ministry mainly responsible for sports issues, as early as the era of the Weimar Republic as well as during the Third Reich.

The DSB also expanded its lobbying to members of parliament. At the same time, in the early 1950s, a so-called Kreis der Freunde des Sports im Deutschen Bundestag (Circle of Friends of Sport in Parliament) met informally but regularly. This group of sports-friendly members of parliament was an ideal contact for the lobbying of the DSB. It was also the basis for the formal establishment of the Sportausschuss des Deutschen Bundestages (parliamentary Sports Commission) in 1969, in the context of preparing for the Munich Olympics of 1972.

Willi Daume asserted in 1958, in his statement to the DSB, that this circle was very helpful for more effective "subsidiarian" support of the German sports movement:

> If we are talking about productive cooperation between sport and state, I especially emphasize the Circle of Friends of Sport in Parliament with deep gratitude. The efforts of the DSB, as well as the increasing motivation of many members of parliament, have resulted in this group gradually becoming an avid supporter of sport in Germany. This group in particular is responsible for the rapidly growing allocation to sport in the federal government budget from DM 1 million to DM 1.8 million, as well as for the "special budget" of over DM 5 million for sport facilities.[17]

Guido von Mengden,[18] full-time manager of the DSB, argued in the same way some years later in 1962:

> The budget of 1957/58 was in some way a breakthrough. The Circle of Friends of Sport in Parliament and the chair of the DSB succeeded in gaining a regular item in the government budget. After careful preparation and hard work, mem-

> bers of the budget commission agreed to define item 0602, title 973 of the budget of the Home Office to spending DM 5 million on sport facilities (by the federal government).[19]

Nonetheless, sports officials of the DSB and other sports associations, as well as their management, were constantly criticizing the ignorance of state policies towards sporting needs and interests. An example was the fact that just one political party represented in the Deutscher Bundestag employed a specific sports consultant—namely, the Social Democratic Party (SPD). Another criticism was that during the 1950s, sporting issues had never been discussed during a party assembly or in parliamentary debates in Bonn or in regional parliaments.

Guido von Mengden argued as follows:

> The government will not be able to ease its bad conscience by arguing that it is not legally responsible for sport. [. . .] We have no state sport, and we do not want it either. In fact, we detest such a sport system. [. . .] We want sport to be free and private.[20]

He continued his speech with various compelling statements about the relationship between sport, state, and politics in the future for Germany:

> However, modern sport is unable to develop without the state. Sport needs public support from the *Bund, Länder* und *Gemeinden*. [. . .] The question is not whether there are links between sport and politics, but rather what constitute the limits to liberty, self-government and self-responsibility on the one hand, and on the other hand, what guarantees both the idealistic and material support of sport by the state and by tax payers.[21]

In essence, during the 1950s, the newly formed sports organizations were seeking rapid help from the state and the public. Uta Andrea Balbier argues that the sports organizations tried to push their own agenda. However, both sports officials and politicians agreed on the principles of autonomy, liberty, and self-responsibility for organized sports in Germany.[22] These principles were supplemented by that of subsidiarity, in order to fulfill all the needs and responsibilities associated with sports and health for the German population. In fact, after the war there was an enormous need to rebuild sports and sports facilities. Therefore, the lobbying of the DSB was motivated not only by its own interests or egoism, but also by objective national needs. Step by step, a further and fundamental issue became evident to the public, namely parallel developments in East Germany. Rather ironically, the GDR became a positive ideal to be imitated, because of its generous support of sports. However, at the same time, it constituted a negative ideal, because of the totalitarian system that extended to the world of sports.

COMPETITIVE SPORTS AND NATIONAL REPRESENTATION: THE DELAYED START—GERMANY IN THE CONTEXT OF INTERNATIONAL SPORTS DEVELOPMENT

Sports politics in West Germany at the time of rebuilding the nation during the 1950s and 1960s aimed mainly at improving the general conditions for sports and physical education (in Germany, also called physical training, gymnastics, or *Turnen*) in general. Sports facilities had to be rebuilt and renewed, physical educators and coaches had to be educated, and the system of physical education at schools and in private clubs reestablished. As mentioned above, this restitution of West German sports had been based essentially on concepts, people, and experiences from the 1920s and early 1930s, while the period of the Nazi regime was ignored or implicitly considered as little more than an accident of history. However, many of those who were active in and responsible for gymnastics and sports in the 1920s also played a major role in Nazi Germany.

German athletes in the East, as well as in the West, were eager to return to the international arena and to the Olympics. Former and experienced Olympians like Carl Diem, "Mister Olympics 1936," as well as German members of the IOC Karl Ritter von Halt and Herzog Adolf von Mecklenburg succeeded in founding a National Olympic Committee "for Germany" as early as 1949, even before the official foundation of West Germany and East Germany. The historical fact was that two German states had been established on the territory of Germany and populated by what was clearly one German nation. In fact, this terminology of two states and one nation was the political dogma of the 1950s and 1960s in the Bundesrepublik Deutschland. However, a bias gradually became apparent. The Germans wanted to return to the international sporting stage as soon as possible, on the one hand, and to be appreciated and successful. But on the other hand, the Bundesrepublik Deutschland did not want to spend much tax money on the international activities of West German athletes. Sport should be independent and autonomous—at least in the West, and in contrast to East Germany. The GDR government had decided, in accordance with the sports politics of the USSR, to support its athletes extensively in order to compete successfully in international top-level sports and prove the superiority of its system.

The prevailing sentiment of the Cold War period concerning sports was that success in international sports events, especially at the Olympics, was related to the broader performance of the states (and governments) where the successful athletes originated. This argument was not used at the beginning in the 1950s in West Germany. If the state were to sponsor sports with public funds, this should be limited to the rebuilding or renewal of sports sites or sports facilities "for all" and intended less, if at all, for top-level athletes. In West Germany, the responsible politicians, as well as the representatives of the sports organizations, were critical toward any state influence in sports, especially given the still omnipresent Nazi past. The president of the DSB, Willi Daume, warned several times of "regarding the number of gold medals at Olympic Games [. . .] as a criterion of the sporting performance or even of the status of health and well-being of a country." In a speech in 1958, Daume referred explicitly to the GDR when he argued: "We know that top-level performance in sport is neither an argument in favor of, nor against any specific political system or regime. The athlete's achievement prevails as a phenomenon of the single person, of the personality of the athletes. Any forms of state-amateurism (as in the GDR and in the USSR) or pretense at amateurism (as in capitalist countries) cannot challenge this principle."[23]

At the general meeting of the National Olympic Committee (NOK für Deutschland) in 1959, he again clearly expressed the notion or ideology of early West German sport: "Sport is not a means of foreign policy. Sport is a world of its own. Therefore, sport cannot and should not follow the laws and constraints of politics. When sport is told what to do by the state and politicians as it used to be in the Zone,[24] this is to the detriment of sport and—ultimately—to politics as well."[25]

The opinion of Daume and other sports officials corresponded with the statements and behavior of leading politicians. The fact that no minister of the federal government was present at the "Wunder von Bern," the miracle of Bern in 1954, when the West German soccer team had rather surprisingly (at least on the surface) won the World Cup, was neither coincidental nor just a freak event, but the result of governmental sporting policies. Only with great delay was the team officially received and honored by the president of the Federal Republic, Theodor Heuss, who, incidentally, was very much in favor of sports but was one of the most fervent proponents of this form of nonpolitical sports policy, as he had stated many times. He and the liberal-conservative governments under the leadership of Konrad Adenauer and his followers rejected any ambitions to use sports as propaganda for the political system, the state, or the government.

In sum, performance and success in top-level sports were not regarded as an expression of achievement and success for the people, state, or nation in West Germany, at least not at the beginning. Therefore, the progress of top-level or high-performance sports was slow compared to other states that really pushed their athletes. If athletes were successful, their achievements were attributed to support from their clubs and sports comrades. Gymnastics and sports in clubs were seen as the base of a so-called performance pyramid (*Leistungspyramide*). The best athletes could thrive only on this stable foundation of clubs in a civil society, produced by the voluntary work of their members. The top-level athletes were intended to serve as idols for the mass of sporting people at lower levels, but the top athletes should also be aware of the fact that this "sporting family" was the social as well as the sporting fundament of their achievement and success.[26] This German club ideology of the "third sector" between the capitalist economy and state socialism accorded fully with the ideology of Olympic amateurism, especially as preached by Avery Brundage. Fair competition and striving for excellence were part of this family ideology, whereas cheating, doping, and indeed any unfairness were rejected totally. Such unethical behavior would undermine the family's life, to repeat the metaphor of the Olympic sporting family, by destroying mutual confidence. This strong belief in the validity of the Olympic ethos or religion can possibly be considered as a reason why some Olympic priests like Brundage were not ready to acknowledge the reality of cheating by doping in Olympic amateur sports.

This strong ethic or ideology of sport began to change through the process of "politicization of sport" at the beginning of the 1960s, or through the Cold War on the track.[27] As J. Hoberman has pointed out, the functionalization of sport by politicians for the apparent benefit of nation-states, a process he has referred to as "sportive nationalism," was regarded as a major cause of the spread of doping, at least according to documents from the 1950s and 1960s.[28] The Austrian sports doctor Ludwig Prokop, one of the first and most prominent critics of doping, spoke at the time of the "national factor" motivating athletes as well as coaches, doctors, and officials to take or support doping substances.[29]

The Cold War, which began no later than the 1950s, also took place "on the track" by representing the political as well as economic and even military power of nation-states.[30] This politically induced functionalization or instrumentalization of sport legitimized the increasing support of top-level sports with state finance and state power, as Barrie Houlihan has stated: "The most notable change in the relationship between government and sport over the last fifty years has been the shift away from occasional involvement by the former in sport, to a situation where governments are now an integral part of the sports infrastructure in almost all countries in Europe and throughout the world."[31] In precisely that context, the Olympic Games achieved outstanding significance,[32] as underlined and enforced by the participation of the USSR as an Olympic team and its acknowledgment as a member of the Olympic family starting with the Games of Helsinki in 1952. From then on, the Cold War on the track was in full swing, and the Olympic Games gained new political dimensions, as Allen Guttmann asserts.[33]

From that point onward, medal counts were listed and propagated by the various states and in the public media as a matter of course, although they were not reported in the Olympic Charter. Since the days of Pierre de Coubertin, the Olympic Games had been propagated as a nongovernmental international sporting power resting on the basis of strong nations, with the aim of spreading peace and understanding by means of sports and athletics. Nonetheless, the performance of athletes was intended to be regarded less as product of the nation-states from which they came, and more as expressions of the athletes' strength, will, and character. However, during the Cold War, the medal counts were in fact used to compare the states (overall) and their political systems in the East and in the West, between the United States and the USSR, as well as between the West German Federal Republic and the East German Socialist Republic. Sports constituted less a demonstration of the achievements of a single athlete, and were used rather as a symbol of political achievement. Successful athletes became heroic idols and symbols of the respective political system and nation.[34]

In West Germany, the paradigmatic change of recognizing sporting achievement and success as part of representing the nation-state occurred in relation to the development of the sports system of the East German GDR.[35] The increasing international success of East German athletes, resulting from systematic and indeed excessive support by the socialist state, provoked appropriate reactions from the West.[36] After the allocation of the 1972 Games to Munich during the 1960s, the West German Federal Republic decided on radical structural changes to the traditional sports system. The system became more centralized and concentrated, so as to support top-level athletes by various measures, beginning with the employment and education of professional coaches, and extending to the construction of central facilities and sports sites, as well as the provision of medical support. The Ministry of the Interior became a fundamental institution of the federal government to support top-level sports for the purpose of national representation. Its budget was increasing constantly, as we will see below.

The politicization of sports is often regarded as having caused the growing intensity of doping misuse since the 1960s, according to numerous contemporary documents.[37] The GDR regime had installed a consistent system of supporting top-level sports starting in the late 1950s.[38] GDR athletes were referred to as "diplomats in track suits." They were obliged to represent the GDR in international competitions and tournaments through their performances and success, as well as their reliable political and ideological opinions, of course strictly according to the socialist dogma of the GDR.[39]

Part of this sports system of the GDR was a consistent and sophisticated use of doping substances, in effect ordered by the state authorities. The existence of such a doping system, installed and prescribed by the state, was in fact the main difference between how doping worked in East as opposed to West Germany. In the Federal Republic, medical science for sports and for athletes was intensified as well, in order to support West German athletes. However, the presence of doctors was indeed not obligatory, except in cases of emergency at sporting events, and there were definitely no orders to administer doping substances to athletes. Even so, the success of East German athletes motivated athletes, coaches, and doctors in the West to dope as well. It was common knowledge in the West, at least in the communities of sporting experts, that the East German athletes were doped. This conviction was partly used to legitimize doping practices in the West as a means of ensuring equal conditions and fair play.[40] On the side of the East German sports regime, the same argument was used to legitimize its own doping system. However, the doped athletes of the West were in fact a reason to question sports and doping practices in top-level sports in general, as the initiatives of Brigitte Berendonk and Hansjörg Kofink since the late 1960s clearly exemplify.[41]

THE "MEDICALIZATION" OF SOCIETY AND SPORT, AND OTHER DOPING AND ANTI-DOPING ISSUES

The number of positive samples of forbidden doping substances taken from athletes in doping tests is declining, or at least has remained roughly at the same level for many years or even decades. However, researchers agree that the use or misuse of doping has in fact been increasing substantially.[42] Contemporary sources assume a consistently increasing use or misuse of various doping substances or doping methods since the 1960s.[43] In addition, a number of developments and circumstances within and beyond sporting contexts have favored the use of doping. These developments make the hypothesis of ever-increasing doping misuse more plausible. The German sociologists Werner Pitsch, Eike Emrich, and Michael Klein as well as Pitsch, Peter Maats, and Emrich have calculated the actual percentage of athletes using forbidden doping substances at 20–35 percent,[44] whereas the number of positively tested athletes by the NADA statistics has remained at about 2 percent since 2004.[45] The above researchers used modern statistical randomized-response techniques to establish this more realistic and alarming view of doping in top-level sports.

The intention to use drugs or doping substances to enhance physical performances is associated with the main characteristics of competitive and achievement-orientated sports. Therefore, numerous scholars are convinced that doping is mainly a problem of the system and characteristic of modern sport itself, and thus less a problem that has been transferred from society to sports. Doping is regarded as a structural phenomenon and a problem of modern sport.[46] The Olympic ideal of *citius, altius, fortius,* which largely parallels the ideal of achievement sports in general, has prevailed in the process of sportization since the late nineteenth century. It extended to less competitive or noncompetitive and achievement-orientated forms of physical exercise, training, German gymnastics, Swedish gymnastics, workers' sports and physical education, and, not least, the idea and concept of amateur sports. The latter was in fact a model of Olympic sports thirty or forty years ago, which contradicted central principles of progress, achievement, and success within the ambiguous and eclectic Olympic idea.[47] In consequence, steadily improving performance and records in sports, as well as a concentration or even fixation on these top achievements, imply the use of substances and various artificial methods for enhancing performance, although they are strictly forbidden by both the rules and norms of sport.

In addition to these conditions and structures of the sports system itself, there were and still are processes of medicalization in society in general that influence doping practices in sports. Numerous and varied reasons can be given as to why, in modern societies, the production of and need for pharmaceuticals and doctors is apparently increasing, with inevitable consequences for doping. Scientific and technical possibilities for producing such substances and their potential use by the masses have improved markedly. Analogous to this process of medicalization of modern society since the 1960s, the role and functions of medicine and doctors have been changing. This paradigmatic change can be regarded as a reinvention of modern preventive medicine. At the same time, the public demand for and the scientific, commercial, and even pragmatic interest in amphetamines, hormones, vitamins, and various enhancement products have accelerated. Both developments, the medicalization of society on the one hand and the reinvention of preventive medicine on the other, have led to the social phenomenon that the use of pharmaceuticals without clear medical indications is increasingly becoming recognized as usual or normal. "Everybody" did or does it, and everybody took or takes it.[48] In addition, the duty of sports medicine and sports doctors seems increasingly to be regarded less as healing injured athletes and more as enhancing their performance. Sports medicine has become part and parcel of producing high achievement in sports. Consequently, a new relationship between athlete and doctor has emerged. The sports doctor is now defined less as an expert who optimizes the health of athletes in a conventional sense and more as a central player in the top-level-sports figuration who actively produces sporting performance and success. In addition to the coach, the doctor has become the next most important partner of the athlete, and both unite to achieve the aim of maximized performance and sporting success.[49]

The commercialization and professionalization of sports are factors that are stronger than ever in motivating athletes to use doping, as numerous scholars argue.[50] Yet this popular hypothesis should also be established on the basis of empirical facts. Some sports at high levels of commercial and professional development, like cycling, football, and soccer, are associated particularly with doping. However, sports like weightlifting, which have low levels of commercialization and professionalization, are also affected. Sports like cycling and weightlifting have in fact cultivated certain doping practices for longer than more commercialized sports, especially the use of amphetamines in cycling and of anabolics in weightlifting and other heavy athletics. Independent of these specific doping practices in various sports, general developments and circumstances in top-level sports seem to be pervasively relevant for doping in top-level sports. Some result from the high intensity of training, need for medical support, and living conditions of top-level athletes, including eating, drinking, sleeping, resting, and further aspects that seem common to all top-level sporting achievements.[51]

Viewed in a historical perspective, the extent and intensity of doping depend on the specific sports and their culture or subcultures. In cycling, such practices of doping had clearly been cultivated for many years without conspicuous public resonance. The few available results of early doping tests from the 1960s yield a higher number of positive doping tests than today, but these facts probably do not reflect the reality of doping in current professional cycling. It seems unrealistic that current doping misuse is less than in the past, although the results of positive doping tests are actually lower today.

The first urine tests of cyclists took place in 1955 and 1962 in Italy. Of the cyclists tested, 20 percent in 1955 and 46.6 percent in 1962 tested positive for amphetamines.[52] When testing started again in 1966, the number of positive tests had decreased to less than 20 percent, and in 1967 it was down to 8 percent.[53] Tests in the Italian soccer league in the 1960s yielded similar results: 1961, 27 percent; 1962, 14 percent; and 1963/64, 0 percent.[54] All these tests were of course competition controls, and it seems clear that they were only of very limited relevance to the reality of doping in cycling and soccer at that time.

However, the determined controlling and sanctioning of athletes motivated them to make decisions concerning doping, either to stop doping or to do so in such a way that the forbidden practice would not be discovered. Both decisions could explain the reduction of positive doping tests.[55] The concealment of doping practices is in fact a relevant but unintended result of controls. The networks of top-level athletes learn quickly enough how to conceal doping practices. As a result, doping entails more than the use of performance-enhancing drugs. It provokes all manner of deviant, criminal behavior, and creates new criminal subcultures. Doping controls reveal an aspect of the civilizing process in general: practices that used to be unquestioned are suddenly forbidden, and finally criminalized, and regarded as immoral, unethical behavior. Former heroes of sports and society are ostracized from society when they test positively for doping and when these results are made public. There are numerous examples of this phenomenon, from Ben Johnson to Lance Armstrong, to name just two prominent individuals. Despite this process of criminalizing doping, some sports like cycling or weightlifting continue to cultivate their specific doping subcultures.

A new chapter in the history of doping in top-level sports was opened in the 1960s through the use of anabolics, at first mainly in heavy athletics like weightlifting, but also in field sports like javelin, discus, and shot put. From these sports, anabolics found their way into women's athletics and women's sports in general.[56] Doping with anabolics developed in a specific and inhuman matter, changing the traditional practice of doping with stimulants. Whereas stimulants were (and still are) taken immediately before competitions, anabolics are useful only when taken over longer periods before sporting events. The ability of anabolics to build muscles has to be combined with effective and systematic training. In consequence, and in addition to competition controls, doping tests were also undertaken before competitions and during training. However, this change in doping controls did not occur until the 1980s.

SPREAD AND DEVELOPMENT OF ANTI-DOPING IN THE 1950S AND 1960S

Doping and anti-doping are two sides of the same coin. Doping can be defined as part of a social process or social construction based on rules and norms about what is regarded as normal and what is deviant. If the use of certain substances to enhance achievement in sports is defined as forbidden, the question arises as to how to control and sanction this deviant behavior. It seems typical of doping history that athletes who have taken drugs did not recognize initially that this usage was not only morally wrong and unfair to others, but even socially deviant and criminal. The subcultures to which they belonged were stronger and more influential for their deviant but subculturally accepted doping behavior than the moral constraints of society.

Those groups in society with the power to define what is wrong and right are referred to by Howard Becker[57] as "moral entrepreneurs." In sports, it is difficult to clearly identify these moral entrepreneurs. They are in fact the sports organizations, including the IOC and the international federations, but with respect to questions of public morality, there are also other and more powerful elements of society than sports organizations, like the church, the media, and—not least—state politics, including the laws, all of which play a part. In the case of doping, many influences always were and still are responsible for doping being defined as deviant and criminal and for specifying how it could be controlled, sanctioned, and prevented. This process started in the 1950s and accelerated in the 1960s, when a specific "frame of reference" was developed through various "social, cultural as well as ethical and moral perspectives."[58] Theories of deviant behavior assume that doping is controlled mainly by rules, norms, and behavior in such subcultures like cyclists and heavy athletes. For extended periods, some sports have cultivated subcultures with a more or less close affinity to drug or doping usage. This behavior even became an essential element of high achievement in sports. Therefore, anti-doping in the context of codified rules for controlling and sanctioning doping contrasted in some respects with longer-term subcultural processes of high-achievement sports, at least in those with a close affinity to doping.[59]

This context should be borne in mind in explaining the fact that anti-doping actions that conflict with subcultural traditions have always been difficult to implement. Anti-doping policies, which were rather unorganized, rare, and sporadic in the 1950s, changed fundamentally during the 1960s on various levels. Doping issues no longer concerned only closed sporting circles and networks, but clearly affected broader constellations, including national and international sports agencies, policies, and politics.

Numerous international conferences concerning the efficiency as well as the risks of taking performance-enhancing substances or drugs in sports took place, mainly in Europe. Experts on sports and sports medicine also discussed the chances of containing the misuse of pharmaceuticals and drugs in top-level sports.[60] Particularly sports doctors initiated ideas on how to organize the fight against doping. The numerous meetings and conferences created international social networks of anti-doping and even influenced state politics.[61] Finally, the activities of the Council of Europe since 1963, especially its commission for physical education outside school, were crucial for the development of anti-doping policies by sports organizations, as well as the activities of national governments. All these activities flowed into the Resolution against Doping of the Minister Committee of the Council of Europe in 1967. Although this resolution was not legally binding for the national governments or other responsible authorities, its consequences for anti-doping activities cannot be underestimated.[62]

The IOC, as the most important umbrella organization for amateur sports in the world, became interested in and suspicious of doping, at least after the death of the Danish cyclist Knud Enemark Jensen at the Olympic Games of 1960 in Rome.[63] He apparently died as a result of taking performance-enhancing stimulants.[64] In consequence, the IOC installed its Medical Commission in 1967 to intensify efforts to curb doping. Additionally, the spectacular and extensively reported death of the professional cyclist Tom Simpson on Mont Ventoux at the 1967 Tour de France motivated the IOC to introduce the first anti-doping tests at the Olympic Games of 1968 in Grenoble and Mexico City.[65] The Olympic officials used to argue that doping in amateur sports was only an exception, whereas in professional sports, doping was a logical and inevitable consequence of the capitalist and commercial model of sports. Therefore, the case of Jensen was seen in public discussions as a freak accident, but also as a warning that Olympic amateur sports should be separated from professional sports. The case of Simpson and other doping cases in professional sports, like that of the German boxing champion Jupp Elze, were seen as affirmative answers to the question of just how corrupt and degenerate professional sports really were. However, doping events occurred during the processes of delegitimizing the traditional concept of amateur sports in the context of modern Olympism. For those in the IOC, apart from Avery Brundage, who were gradually realizing that the borders between amateur and professional sports were becoming increasingly blurred, the conviction arose that the IOC needed to become much more active in anti-doping.

Step by step, hard reality seemed to have prevailed over Olympic amateur ideology, even in the heads of Olympic enthusiasts in the IOC. The speaker of the Medical Commission of the IOC, Alexandre de Merode, may have helped with some serious efforts at persuasion. Finally, the doping tests in Grenoble and Mexico City signaled a change in the anti-doping policies of the IOC, although it could or should have been done far earlier. Furthermore, the tests were during competitions and mainly for amphetamines. However, at that time, doping with anabolic steroids was well established, but it was still impossible to verify conclusively whether athletes had taken them or not. In addition, the power of the IOC and the tests in Grenoble and Mexico City were limited to amateur sports. Doping in professional sports remained essentially uncontrolled.

Despite the above-mentioned initiative of the IOC, which was in fact an important step forward in establishing at least some international anti-doping policies, the world of sports in the 1960s was still a long way from having consistent anti-doping policies. Apart from equestrian sports and the doping of horses, anti-doping rules were unusual and unknown for most of the national and international sports organizations. The report from the conference of the International Organization of Sports Medicine (FIMS) in 1954 mentions that a few sports federations had introduced a doping ban into their statutes. Others had created commissions of sports doctors and and other scientists.[66] The first and unique international sports federation that had defined and banned doping in its statutes was the International Amateur Athletics Federation (IAAF) in 1928. The International Fencing Federation (FIE) had established anti-doping rules in 1950,[67] and the International Amateur Boxing Federation followed in 1951.[68]

In 1955, Italian sports doctors tested cyclists during various cycling races in an effort to conduct empirical research on doping. The alarming results motivated Italian sports doctors and the Italian Association of Cyclists (Unione Velocipedistra Italiana) to adopt the first anti-doping convention.[69] In Italy, the "law for protecting health and sports," passed by the parliament in 1950, transferred all public obligations for health prevention and protection to the Italian Federation of Sports Medicine (FMSI). According to this law, amateur athletes, as well as professional ones, were obliged to visit a doctor of the FMSI once a year. The results of these medical checks were registered in a Libretto di Valutazione, which was obligatory for athletes to be accepted for events and competitions.[70]

In Germany, cyclists were dealing with doping and anti-doping issues in the 1950s, motivated by repeated cases during the Tour de France and reactions from the International Cycling Association (UCI).[71] In 1956, the Bund Deutscher Radfahrer (German Cycling Federation) included anti-doping rules in the competition regulations.[72] The German Athletics Federation included a similar paragraph in 1959.

However, none of these initiatives dealt effectively with the reality of controlling and sanctioning doping, either in the national or international contexts of any sports. In spite of this deficiency, it can be asserted that at least in the 1960s, more or less consistent anti-doping policies were evident. The French and Belgian parliaments passed anti-doping laws in 1965. In Austria, the Ministry of Education adopted an edict in 1963 that opened up the possibility of persecuting doping.

However, all these initiatives, even those from the state, lacked any serious consequences for offenders.[73] Their main objective was to discourage doping rather than to control and sanction it. A common understanding of doping still had to be found. A major element of doping prevention was the education of the athletes, as practiced, for example, by the British Association of Sport and Medicine.[74] Additionally, and in contrast to the current understanding of education and enlightenment, an element of this educational strategy against doping was to keep athletes naive and ignorant of doping substances.[75] Another strategy was to deny or to trivialize the effects of various doping substances—that is, to imply that they did not really work. The Austrian anti-doping protagonist Ludwig Prokop often argued that the assumed impact of doping substances was just a placebo effect.[76] Whatever the case, both strategies failed. The main reason was the regrettably positive experiences of the athletes themselves, which contradicted these educational strategies of ignoring, denying, and trivializing.

In sum, doping had been accepted as a severe problem in sports since the 1950s, but tests, controls, prosecution, and sanctioning were minimal, if they prevailed at all. A fundamental change in anti-doping policies became evident in the 1960s however, when doping controls were introduced into important sporting events, at least in principle. This development can be interpreted as a change in anti-doping from recognizing and defining doping, to dealing with the practical problems of testing, controlling, and sanctioning. Modern strategies of doping controls like urine tests for amphetamines (and later blood tests) were first used in 1965 at the Tour of Britain and the Tour de France. Such tests also took place at the World Cup in England in 1966, where even German soccer players tested positively on ephedrine, a substance normally used to counter the common cold.[77]

SELF-CONCEPT AND FUNCTIONS OF GERMAN SPORTS MEDICINE

The German Association for Sports Medicine (Deutscher Sportärztebund, DSÄB) was founded in 1912 and still exists, without a break having ever occurred. Since its beginnings, sports medicine in Germany has been interpreted mainly as preventive medicine for health and fitness, and therefore closely connected to physical education, physical exercise, and training. After World War II and the Nazi regime, Dr. Alfred Koch became the first postwar president of the DSÄB. He lived his own life very successfully according to the principles of preventive medicine until the impressive age of 105. In the 1950s, he divided sports medicine into three main areas of interest, curative medicine, preventive medicine, and medicine for performance and physical achievement. He and the majority of German sports doctors emphasized preventive medicine.[78] Several conferences were held during the 1950s, dealing with self-perceptions of German sports medicine as the main focus. The congresses in 1953 on "Sport and Aging," in 1954 on "Physical Training and Health," and in 1955 on "Preventive Medicine and Physical Training for the Youth" focused clearly on prevention.

Then sports doctors considered this change from curative to preventive medicine in physical training and sports as a paradigm shift.[79] The idea of prevention was not new, but it received fresh impetus from the increasing number of so-called diseases of civilization, often caused by a lack of exercise combined with the physical demands of the workplace.[80] Since the nineteenth century, physical education and physical exercises had served to prevent the spread of infectious diseases through *Abhärtung*—that is, strengthening the body and mind—but since the 1950s, sports medicine has been dominated by the notion of preventing diseases of modern civilization, such as heart attacks. However, concerns about the health of the people (*Volksgesundheit*) in general were common. Finally, the German Association for Sports Medicine was not renamed until 1999 as the German Association for Sports Medicine and Prevention. The reason for this rather late renaming by adding the attribute of "prevention" is that the focus on achievement and performance through sports medicine had prevailed since the 1960s.

Initially, skepticism toward and criticism of the "excesses" of achievement in top-level sports had shaped the discourses of sports medicine in Germany. Even leading sports officials like Willi Daume and the former president (from 1951 to 1960) of the National Olympic Committee, Karl von Halt, a former Olympic athlete and Nazi official, had warned against a fixation on performance and success, which the old German Turners had criticized since the nineteenth century as *Rekordsport* (sport for records). This orientation (*Raubbau am Körper*, ruthless bodily exploitation) would destroy the human body. Sports medicine should help prevent athletes from these serious dangers, and doctors should encourage athletes to do sports healthily and fairly. A sports doctor should be a guardian of sports and their morality, functioning as the "biological conscience" of sports.[81]

A consequence of this moral and ethical prescription of sports medicine was its latter role as the most important protagonist of anti-doping policies, at least in the 1950s and 1960s. However, the public and the sports people themselves requested more effective support simultaneously for sports medicine to improve sporting performance and to attend to athletes during the process of training. In 1952, the popular athletics coach Woldemar Gerschler of Freiburg drew attention to the sciences in general and to sports medicine specifically to support sports and athletes in their quest for sporting excellence, even if this meant intervening in coaching.[82] Karl von Halt, simultaneously warning of the dangers of excessive sports, believed the sports doctor and medication to be the most important factors in improving performance

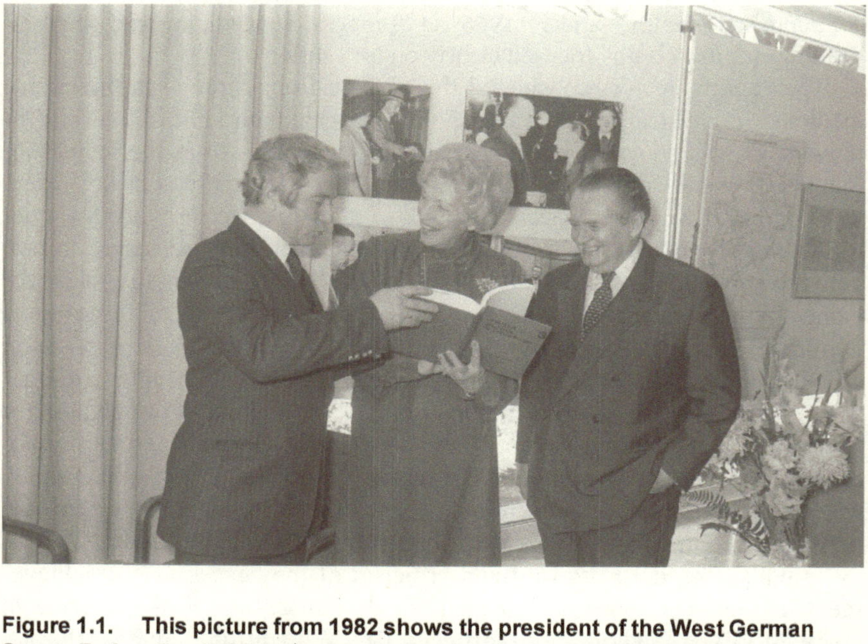

Figure 1.1. This picture from 1982 shows the president of the West German Sports Federation (DSB), Willi Daume, former chair of the DSB and NOK, as well as president of the Organizing Committee of the 1972 Munich Olympics. In the middle stands Annemarie Renger, leading member of the Social Democratic Party of the FRG and then president of the German Bundestag, with Professor Horst Ueberhorst (Bochum) presenting his voluminous work of the universal history of sports. Annemarie Renger was the daughter of Fritz Wildung, secretary of the Social Democratic Workers' Sports Association in the 1920s and 1930s. ***Source: Bundesarchiv/ B 145 Bild-F062233-0020/ Ludwig Wegmann***

and success in sports, apart from the coach.[83] Sports medicine, it was argued, should also pay attention to special diets for athletes. This opinion was not new, and most of the officials, coaches, and sports doctors at that time very distinctly remembered the Olympic Games of Berlin in 1936, when the teams from different countries brought their own cooks to the Olympic Village to provide special diets for their athletes.[84] Some sports doctors had been researching these specific diets during the Games.[85] After the war, the sports doctors Prokop and E. Engelhardt presented papers at the conference for German sports medicine in 1952 and discussed such diets, including how to live healthily by, for example, visiting a sauna that had been constructed in the Olympic Village of Berlin in 1952 or in Helsinki at the Olympic Games of 1952, and the need for calories, carbohydrates, proteins, vitamins, and minerals among Olympic athletes in different sports.[86] In contrast to Hoberman, who regarded German sports medicine as academic and far removed from the reality of sports, sports doctors in Germany were in fact familiar with the needs of top-level athletes, even in the 1950s.[87]

Finally, a large number of German sports doctors decided on a commitment to performance in top-level sports and *not* to preventive medicine. In order to understand this decision better, it should be borne in mind that sports doctors were outsiders to the elite class of doctors and medical scientists in Germany, the "demigods in white," as they are still commonly called. A tracksuit did not (sometimes even now) conform to this elevated social class. Sports medicine is not really accepted as academically sound, and the doctors themselves felt and still feel excluded from the exclusive circles of academic medicine.[88] This rather ostracized role of sports medicine may have been an important reason why many sports doctors sought other fields in which to achieve recognition in German society. The developing field of top-level sports seemed to offer such opportunities for public recognition, in addition to money and other profits.

In fact, the still-small group of German sports doctors divided into those working for preventive objectives, mainly in leisure sports for all, and the others working for elite, Olympic, and professional athletes. In principle, these differences did not necessarily conflict with one another. After all, health and fitness are necessary preconditions for high achievement. However, achievement and top-level sports may also harm or even destroy an athlete's health. Sports medicine is obliged by the Hippocratic oath to care for the health of humans, and not to enhance achievements at the cost of health. Therefore, the engagement of sports medicine in top-level sports could and still can create serious ethical dilemmas for sports doctors. A doctor who gives forbidden doping substances to athletes is undoubtedly breaching the ethical standards of his profession and the Hippocratic oath.

Apparently, the shift in sports medicine toward supporting top-level athletes applied not only to the increasing significance of the phenomenon of achievement and competitive sports in modern society, but accompanied a change in the hierarchy of ethical norms in medical care from prevention to enhancing fitness and achievement. Medical concerns about the health of athletes and their bodily integrity contrasted with the goals of better performance and greater success. Such conflicts can be regarded as part of the "sportization process," as Guttmann, Elias, and Eric Dunning have all pointed out, or, in the even stronger words of the Finnish sociologist Kalevi Heinilä, the "totalization" of sport.[89] Doping was and remains an example of how the traditional norms and moral standards of medical ethics conflict with the needs of modern top-level sports.

Some doctors of sports medicine were moving gradually closer to the world (or subculture) of top-level sports, and their distance from doping declined accordingly. Modern medical sciences believe in progress and in their contribution to human health through medication. Since the 1960s, biological, chemical, and pharmaceutical progress has been immense, and an increasing number of the resulting products have entered the markets. Initially, they were created and developed for the treatment of serious diseases. However, they could also be used to improve the performance of healthy and fit athletes. The ethical dilemma confronting doping doctors—namely, that of administering pharmaceuticals intended for sick, and mostly very sick, people to perfectly healthy athletes—could be resolved by arguing that athletes were not really healthy after all, but suffering from the consequences of their extremely demanding physical training. However, this argument was never more than a specious rationalization.

Whatever the case, the traditional configuration of top-level sports was being widened by medical science. One of the most crucial differences between modern top-level sports and doping configurations and earlier drug taking in sports is the nature of the networks involved. An increasing number of people, as well as institutions like sports organizations, administrations, and, not least, doctors and other experts in the various associated sciences, became part of the production process of high-performance sports. The athlete as a unique hero is a myth of modern sports and was probably never more than that. The athlete's performances were not possible without the team or network. In East Germany, this network was organized by the state, whereas in West Germany, it was based on private initiatives. A West German athlete willing to dope successfully—that is, effectively, secretly, and indeed economically—had to be advised and supervised by doping experts, mostly doctors. In fact, sports doctors developed a real affinity to doping. The case of Martin Brustmann, a pioneer of German sports medicine since the 1920s, exemplifies the close connection among the medical sciences, sports doctors, and top-level sports.

The other side of the coin is that the increasing need for sports medicine experts produced an interesting and sometimes profitable field of work. The use of substances to enhance sporting achievement ultimately exceeded the traditional limits of curative and preventive medicine for therapeutic needs. This development has been part of a massive process of legitimizing trans-therapeutic enhancement by medical means, including plastic surgery and many other techniques. In this manner, doping in sports is part of broader changes in bioethical paradigms of modern or postmodern societies.

The following chapters will demonstrate that German sports medicine was not limited to doping, but extended to anti-doping as well. Initially, sports doctors led the fight against doping, the more so as doping was initially regarded as a medical-care problem. The experts were discussing serious general issues of modern sports development, such as the differences between legitimate and illegitimate ways of enhancing performance, or the limits of human physical capacity and how to extend them. The basic issue in all these complicated sporting and general ethical debates was how to define doping. German sports doctors and, as an institution, the Deutscher Sportärztebund started with a definition in 1953 that was intended to remain relevant and applicable for many years.

ANTI-DOPING POLICIES IN THE 1950S AND 1960S

From Martin Brustmann to the Doping Definition of 1953

The first, and for a long time unique, case of doping in the young Bundesrepublik Deutschland was that of Martin Brustmann (1885–1964) and the eight of the rowing club Flörsheim-Rüsselsheim in 1952. Dr. Brustmann had been a well-known athlete, coach, and sports doctor since the 1920s, with a close affinity to performance sport and top-level athletes. In the 1920s and 1930s, he had been a medical coach for Otto Peltzer, German world-record runner over 1,500 meters in 1926 in Berlin (in 3:51), where he had defeated Paavo Nurmi.[90] Dr. Brustmann had been testing various means of enhancing sporting achievement since his long and colorful carrier in different political regimes in Germany. He did not stop even in the 1950s, when he was an old man and sports in West Germany were still young. Brustmann was the doctor for the German Rowing Federation (Deutscher Ruderverband, DRV) and administered drugs to the rowers of Flörsheim-Rüsselsheim, especially testoviron, a male-hormone substance, before the qualifying race for the Helsinki Olympics in 1952. However, the eight lost the race and accused Brustmann of "negative doping." He was blamed for having given them this substance in order to weaken the team as opposed to enhancing their performance. Although this accusation was not true, Brustmann was dismissed as doctor of the Rowing Federation and charged in the federation's court (a disciplinary commission), not an official state court. However, Brustmann was rehabilitated because it was not possible to prove that his behavior was intentional. So he was not guilty, in the opinion of the court.[91]

This case is typical of that period and interesting in various ways. First, the "Brustmann case" became public because of the participation of an additional prominent personality associated with the Flörsheim-Rüsselsheim eight. This person was Georg von Opel, car-company heir, businessman, active sportsman, president of the German Olympic Society, and favorite of the developing yellow press in West Germany. More than fifty articles were published on the Brustmann case alone in various papers of the young republic.[92] Second, Brustmann had not been charged for doping, but for negative doping, which was known from equestrian sports, in which horses from competitors had been "doped" with and weakened by arsenic.[93] Whether or not Brustmann was actually guilty of doping, including the intention to benefit a particular athlete or team, did not seem relevant to the public or the rowing community. Third, the doping substance was not an amphetamine (like pervitin), as was usual at that time in cycling and other endurance sports, but the hormone testoviron. The full effects and (negative) side effects of these substances were still unknown. However, there was one doping case involving hormones in 1950, when the Danish rowing team had doped with the hormone androstin and won the European championship.[94] At that time, hormone substances were not generally regarded as doping, in contrast to amphetamines and stimulants in general. In addition, it was not possible to prove decisively whether an athlete had taken such substances or not. Therefore, the Rowing Federation closed the file on this charge with no consequences for anyone.[95]

However, the Brustmann case did motivate some doctors in the Deutsche Sportärztebund to put the doping problem on the agenda of the association. During the debate about the Brustmann case, they had declared officially, in the name of the entire association, the following definition: "The German Association of Sports Medicine supports the view that any medication—whether effective or not, which is taken before a competition with the intention of enhancing performance, must be regarded as doping."[96]

This initiative is significant in demonstrating that the German sports doctors were in fact pioneers of anti-doping and not only of doping. They were among the "moral entrepreneurs" of that field,[97] in claiming that doping would become one of the major problems confronting sports medicine in the future. Resolving the issue of what exactly constituted doping was as necessary as it was urgent.

The sports organizations in Germany represented by the Deutsche Sportbund adopted the DSÄB's definition of doping immediately,[98] which shows how influential the doctors and their advice were in German sports organizations. In addition, the definition corresponded to the prevailing opinion that taking drugs to enhance performances was unfair, and as the definition ex-

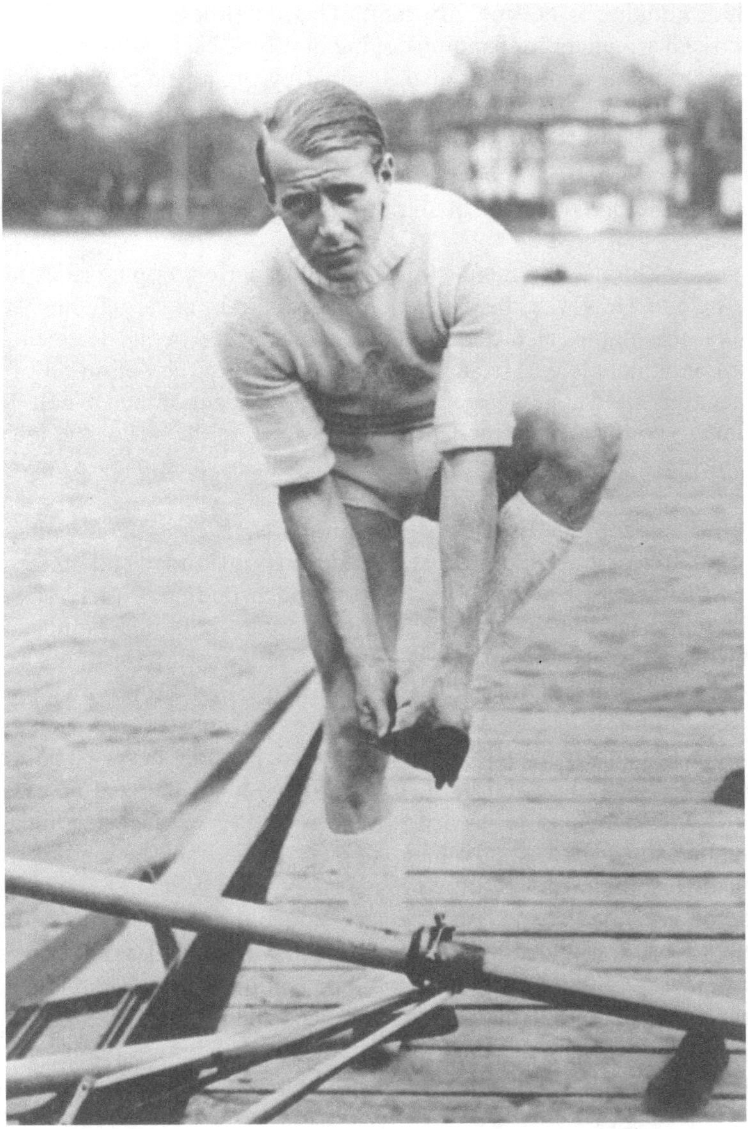

Figure 1.2. Georg von Opel (1912–1971), German businessman and one of the heirs of Opel car industries, which are today part of General Motors. Opel was also a sportsman, member of the IOC, and German sports official in numerous functions. In 1951, he became a German rowing champion as a member of the eight of Flörsheim-Rüsselsheim. The doping scandal involving Dr. Martin Brustmann became of public interest, not least due to the involvement of Georg von Opel. *Source: Picture Alliance/ Schirner Sportfoto*

pressed, even the intention to dope was unfair. This was fundamental to the definition: doping is not morally right! This unfairness was and still is the most crucial argument for banning doping in sports, besides the health issues. The unfairness of doping was also justified by the artificial nature of these performance-enhancing substances—that is, they are not produced by the athlete's own body, or through training and intrinsic strength. Typical of those substances at that time were amphetamines, stimulants, and other drugs that had to be taken before or during a competition in order to be really effective.

These traditional arguments are still used in current doping rules like the WADA Code. However, the difference is the focus of the arguments. Whereas today, the empirical fact of forbidden substances being detected in the body of an athlete is defined as doping, according to the definition of 1953, the intention of the athlete was crucial, as the president of the DSÄB, Werner Ruhemann, pointed out: "Fundamental, however, is the *dolus*, the intention, why and how the pharmaceutical is taken, not the pharmacy or substance itself."[99]

Already at that time, sports doctors and sports officials had also discussed the possibility of publishing a list including specific medications and substances that would be categorized as forbidden doping. Not least for our current understanding of doping and anti-doping, it is interesting that the responsible officials of sports and medicine refused to publish such a list. Two reasons were put forward: First, the list could be used as potential "recipes" to imitate or create new medications and substances to achieve the same object of enhancing performance. Second, it would never be possible to publish a complete list, and the list would have to be updated consistently. Finally, Dr. Ruhemann refused doping controls for ethical, technical, and practical reasons. He did not want a "doping police," and he did not want to take urine or blood tests of athletes, as if they were criminals or alcoholics. Instead of a doping list and doping controls, he preferred pedagogical means. Teachers, coaches, and doctors should teach the athletes not to use these unfair means. Doping, he argued, should be completely banned and tabooed, because it was unfair and dangerous, as well as undignified.[100]

As mentioned above, this initial attempt to define doping in fact contrasted completely with the current principle of "strict liability" on the basis of a clearly defined list of forbidden pharmacies or pharmaceutical substances.[101] The athlete alone is responsible for what happens to his body, with the burden of proof devolving on him. This principle of control and prosecution is unique to doping and does not apply to the rule of law in general.

The definition of doping of 1953 expressed a strictly moral understanding of deviant behavior (and its control) in sport. It was not intended to control and prosecute athletes or to criminalize them, whereas current doping definitions, based on lists of substances, were and still are regarded as more appropriate for controlling doping. However, one of the consequences of this approach is the criminalization of doping and of doped athletes. Whereas the doping definition of 1953 just implied a moral taboo on doping, doping definitions based on concrete doping lists include the consequence of controlling and sanctioning forbidden behavior. Dopers are therefore against a new law of sport, which entails the prohibition of drugs on a defined list. This approach was regarded as foul play.[102] The practical contribution of the doping definition of 1953 to solving the doping problem was small. The definition did not help create a consensual understanding of doping, nor was it possible to work out a common guideline for anti-doping among the various German sports organizations. The lowest common denominator was that everyone involved in sports and society as a whole was against doping and thought it unfair and dangerous. The situation could be compared on some levels with illegal work or tax fraud, which are also forbidden but difficult to control and prosecute.[103]

The lack of control and the consequences of doping had been discussed several times by various boards of German sports organizations. However, it took until 1966 before the umbrella organization DSB recommended to its member organizations—encouraged, by the way, by the DSÄB—to include anti-doping rules in their statutes.[104] A leaflet of the DSB in 1966 included detailed proposals on what to do against doping and how. This booklet, titled "Das Dopingproblem im internationalen Sport" (The Doping Problem in International Sports), was also related to the anti-doping activities of the German sports organizations, which were indeed the above-mentioned international conferences and initiatives of the European Council at the beginning of the 1960s.[105] Some German sports federations and associations followed these recommendations. In every case, German sports officials respected the initiatives of the European Council and formulated a list of forbidden doping substances, as well as stipulating urine controls and sanctions in the event of breaches. Urine tests seemed to be the most compelling and valid method for detecting doping offenses, at least for amphetamines taken before competitions. As mentioned above, stimulants and amphetamines still were used most.

DOPING RULES OF SOME SPORTS FEDERATIONS

However, when the DSB asked its members in 1969 about the status of the recommendations of 1966, only four of forty-two sports federations in Germany had indeed included specific anti-doping rules in their statutes, as recommended by the European Council and the DSB. These four were the German Boxing Federation, the Cycling Federation, the Athletics Federation,

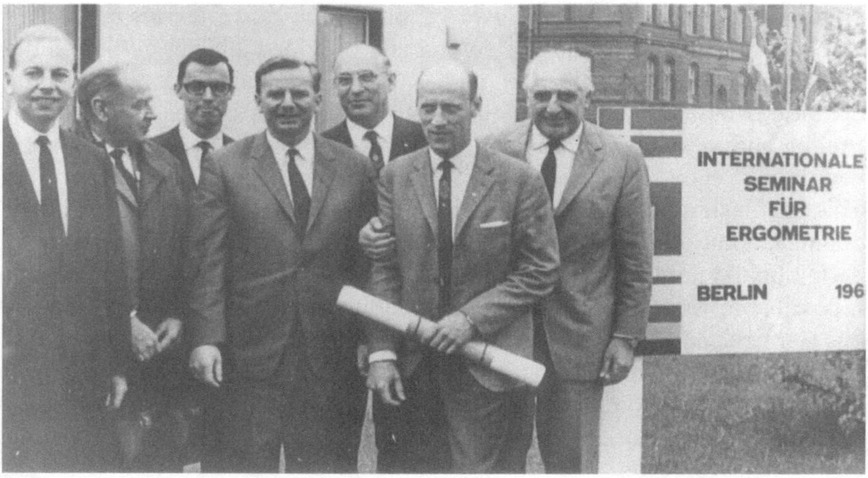

Figure 1.3. International meeting of sports doctors in Berlin, 1965. On the very left is Wildor Hollmann of Cologne, the most influential professor of sports medicine in West Germany, and on the very right is Herbert Reindell, founding professor of sports medicine at the University of Freiburg. In the middle (background), Ernst Jokl (1907–1997), one of the "fathers" of American sports science and sports medicine. Jokl was born in Breslau, Germany (now Wroclaw, Poland), where he became the first professor of sports medicine at the university in 1931. He was also a talented and successful athlete at the Jewish sports club Bar Kochba in Breslau. When Hitler and the Nazi regime rose to power in Germany, he immigrated to South Africa. He returned to Germany in 1950 to join his friend Carl Diem at the Cologne sports university. In 1952, he left West Germany for the United States, where he was one of the eleven founders of the American College of Sports Medicine (ACSM). ***Source: Carl-und-Liselott-Diem Archiv (CuLDA)***

and, finally, the Equestrian Federation. However, all of them had already included their own anti-doping rules in their statutes before the DSB recommendation of 1966.[106] It seems relevant that at that time, eight international sports federations—boxing, fencing, soccer, canoe, athletics, cycling, equestrian, rowing, and modern pentathlon—had already introduced anti-doping rules.

These facts demonstrate that on the one hand, most officials of sports clubs and sports federations were not really aware of the gravity of doping problems in sports, and were therefore not willing to act against a phenomenon of whose existence (and problematic nature) they were not at all convinced. On the contrary, most officials believed that doping may well occur in some sports and by some athletes, but not in "theirs," as the well-known German sports doctor Joseph Keul had written in a letter to the Ministry of the Interior.[107] However, these anti-doping rules were just a few sentences including some specification of what constitutes doping and listing potential sanctions, which were never enforced.[108] Doping controls were mentioned first in the statutes of the Athletics Federation (Deutscher Leichtathletik-Verband, DLV) in 1969. At the same time, the DLV implemented the first doping controls on the occasion of the German athletics championships.[109] The swimmers had done the same just one year before. However, neither the German nor the International Swimming Federation (FINA) took urine tests on the basis of rules in their statutes.[110] The German Federation for Modern Pentathlon followed the rules of its international federation, the Union Internationale de Pentathlon Moderne (UIPM).[111]

Common to all these sports is that they seemed to or were regarded as having an affinity to doping misuse. All were individual and summer sports. None of the winter sports federations had integrated any anti-doping rule into their statutes.

The Bund Deutscher Radfahrer (German Cycling Federation) had the most complex anti-doping rules at that time, including specific controls. Several times during the 1960s, this association had completed and elaborated its anti-doping rules. Whereas in 1956, only controls of food for cyclists had been announced, in the 1960s, controls of urine, blood, and saliva were provided for by the anti-doping rules: "medical tests" of body fluids should be allowed if there were any justifiable suspicions of doping misuse.[112] The selection of tested athletes was not only random, but also according to performance or ranking. In 1968, at first, athletes could be and were in fact sanctioned if they refused to be tested, a measure that was introduced because of the many deliberate doping violations.[113] In addition, the sanctions were defined more precisely. Whereas in the earlier regulations of 1956 and 1963 a general sanction by the association was the withdrawal of a license to participate, in 1968 the sanctions were differentiated, ranging from a ban of one month for the first doping offense up to a lifetime ban when an athlete tested positively four times.

The change from vague doping controls external to the athlete's body, like food and drink, to substances inside the body marks a paradigm shift. Controls no longer stop outside the body, so to speak. With some respect, controls of an athlete's body include the violation of his bodily integrity. This change is reminiscent of Michel Foucault's analysis of modern societies as superpowers of control, which even penetrate the body and the most intimate personal spheres. In sports and doping, this process began in the 1960s, supported by modern science and medicine. However, not only did the controls become more elaborate, but also the practical implementation of sanctions, as in the case of the famous Belgian cyclist Eddy Merckx and other champions. He had tested positively several times but consistently questioned the validity of the tests because of some negative results.[114] The difference from the current practice of doping tests becomes apparent by comparing the case of Merckx with that of the American athlete Marion Jones in 2004, during the Bay Area Laboratory Cooperative (BALCO) scandal. Her argument that she had been tested negatively 160 times had no consequence for her subsequent punishment.

The example of the irregularities of the cyclists reveals the dynamic process of doping and anti-doping in general. At first, when only a few vague anti-doping rules existed, the athletes had no problems avoiding detection. This became increasingly more difficult when the nature of misconduct was specified precisely. However, more detailed rules produced more complex methods of both testing and avoiding detection, in a vicious circle.[115] The change from simple and few anti-doping rules to complex, very specific anti-doping codes in long documents also took place internationally.

The International Cycling Union adopted its anti-irregularity measures in coordination with larger and relevant national cycling federations. In fact, the cyclists, including cycling clubs, managers, and others were concerned about the increasing number of doping controls. They protested and organized a cyclists' strike during the Tour de France in 1966.[116] The cyclists protested against the "criminalization" of behavior that had for so long been unquestioned in cycling sports.[117] In 1965, the sponsor of a cycling team, the German company Fichtel & Sachs, complained about the numerous doping tests during a race in Belgium. In a letter to the German Cycling Federation, Fichtel & Sachs criticized the controls by the Belgian police as an "unlawful attack."[118]

The difference between token, purely rhetorical anti-doping and real anti-doping has always been a substantial problem, reinforced by the lack of valid and objective methods for proving doping misuse. In 1969, Manfred Donike, later the head of the anti-doping laboratory in Cologne, reported initially about the new methods for proving doping by gas-liquid chromatography. According to medical publications in certain international journals, chemical and pharmaceutical methods of analysis were being adapted to doping tests. However, these tests were still not reliable or sufficiently sensitive by the end of the 1960s. Among others, gas-liquid chromatography seemed to be the best method and was ultimately used successfully to test for doping.[119] Nonetheless, doping tests were implemented neither consistently and in a standardized manner, nor reliably and validly. The managers of sports events used different medical institutes to test urine and blood. For example, in 1966, on the occasion of the cycling world championships in Germany, a member of the Medical Commission intentionally used doping substances in order to test the testing methods.[120] Difficulties in establishing reliable methods of testing doping were associated with problems in the installation of appropriate test equipment and their cost. The most important step toward solving these problems was the foundation of the doping-control laboratory in Cologne in 1974, as a consequence of the Munich Olympics of 1972 and the doping tests that had been organized and financed by the Munich Organizing Committee (see chapter 2).

The lack of regulation and standardization, as well as of transparency and coherency, of doping tests resulted in an increasing diversity of approaches in the different sports. Doping history after the 1960s was therefore also marked by attempts to provide more and better rules, standards, and methods to prove doping reliably in all sports and to ensure consistent sanctions by the sports authorities. However, this was then and still is a major problem confronting both doping and anti-doping. Who is really capable of and responsible for testing doping and sanctioning athletes who dope?

The sports organizations were undoubtedly regarded as the naturally competent and responsible institutions for reducing doping. All sports organizations agreed in this regard—that is, the IOC as well as the international sports federations, the national Olympic committees, and, finally, the national sports organizations. The majority of politicians in the European states and their governments shared this opinion. In Germany, the competence of the free and autonomous sports organizations responsible for anti-doping was defined explicitly by the DSB's "Rahmenrichtlinien gegen Doping" (General Guidelines against Doping) in 1970 (§9). These guidelines were a benchmark in anti-doping policies, insofar as they expressed the common-sense view of doping and anti-doping in German sports at that time. This means, first, that the definition of doping differed fundamentally from that in 1953. The intention of the doper was no longer central, but rather the "attempt to enhance the performance of athletes for competitions with non-physiological substances." Second, such "non-physiological substances" were specified precisely: "Derivatives of phenylethylamine (stimulants, amphetamines, ephedrine, adrenaline), narcotics, analeptics (derivatives of camphor and strychnine), sedatives, psychotropic drugs and alcohol." Third, forbidden behavior and actions in the context of doping were also defined: "Doping is the application of doping substances by athletes as well as by supporting persons (especially team mangers coaches, medicines, assistants, masseurs) before or during a competition." Fourth, the regulations and criteria for doping controls and sanctions were defined.[121] Notably, doping was still seen as a problem of competition itself, although hormone doping was being practiced during training and could barely be tested before or even during competition. In addition, the sports organizations alone felt responsible for and competent to manage doping controls, as well as sanctions against doped athletes and their supporters.

However, doubts were emerging as to whether the model of doping tests as the sole responsibility of sports organizations would really be sufficient to reduce doping sustainably and effectively.[122]

THE ROLE OF STATE AND GOVERNMENT IN ANTI-DOPING POLICIES

Whereas in the 1950s doping and anti-doping policies did not really interest the state or politicians, this changed in the later 1960s, not least because of various anti-doping initiatives of the European Council. When, in the summer of 1965, the European Council invited European governments to an anti-doping conference in Strasbourg, the West German government not only asked a sports official to attend the conference, but sent a senior civil servant (*Regierungsrat*) of the Ministry of the Interior for the first time. The sports doctor Dr. Joseph Keul, a junior colleague of Professor Herbert Reindell of Freiburg, was asked to send a "report on the need and viability, as well as the status of anti-doping activities in the Federal Republic." Apparently, the West German government was not well informed about what was going on in performance sports and whether the status of doping and anti-doping in Germany was comparable to that in other European countries. The DSÄB was expected to make appropriate recommendations to the government. However, the responsible civil servant insisted "on getting by with flexible and pragmatic regulations of the sports organizations themselves as long as possible" and, if possible, "avoiding a law against doping."[123]

At first glance, it seems remarkable that a representative of the government had indeed mentioned "law" or the legislature in the context of doping in sport, because, since the end of the war, all sporting issues had been the responsibility of the sports organizations and not of the state and its organs. Until that point, no discussion about sports law or specific regulations of the doping problem by the state had ever taken place. The remarks of the civil servant can therefore be understood only against the European background and in terms of the fact that Italy, Belgium, and France were discussing and introducing anti-doping laws.

Joseph Keul commented that in Germany, consistent actions against doping did not yet exist. The reasons were that "the majority of sports associations in the DSB were arguing [. . .] that specific actions against doping would not be necessary, because they did not observe a real danger of doping misuse. However, he would prefer the DSB to generally ban doping."[124] When the Strasburg conference on doping was over, the Ministry of the Interior initiated closer teamwork between sport and government to reduce doping. Although the sports organizations were at first obliged to combat doping, the Ministry argued that "actions to reduce doping had to be organized and coordinated right away between the sports organizations and the government."[125]

Some days after the Strasburg conference, Federal Public Prosecutor Max Kohlhaas gave a speech at a DSÄB symposium on "Legal Fundaments of a Prohibition of Doping." However, Kohlhaas warned the German parliament

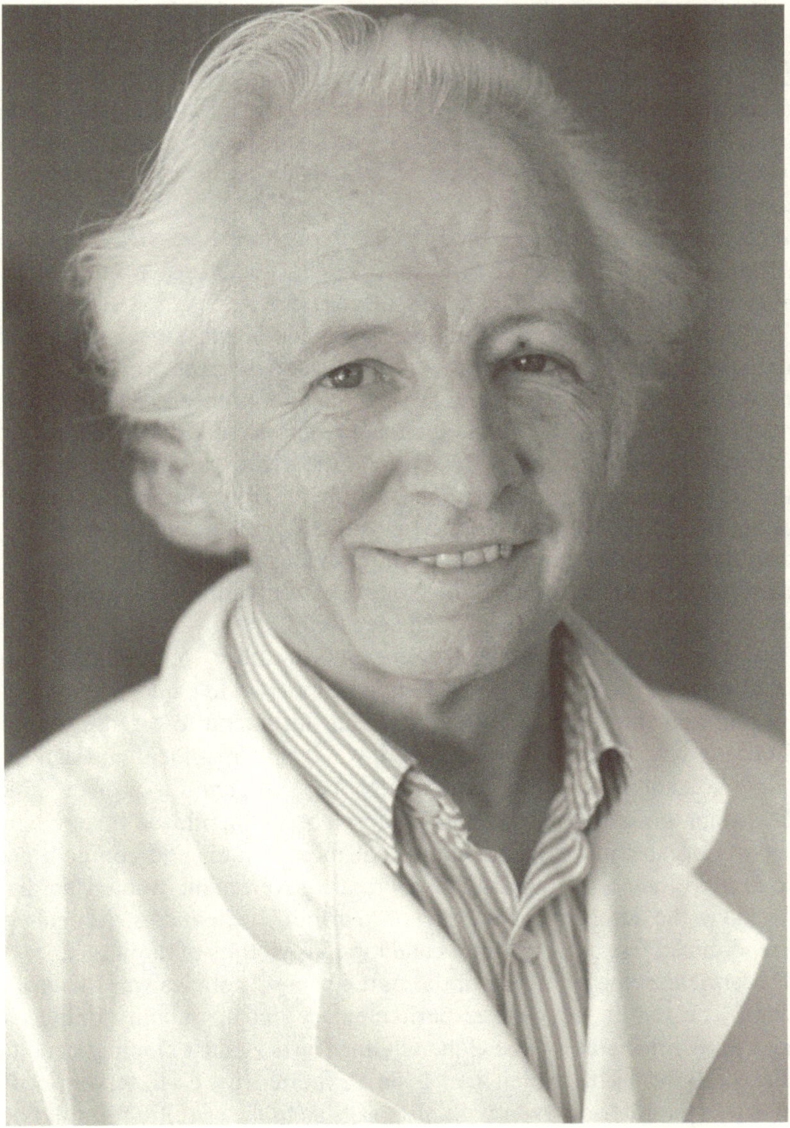

Figure 1.4. Dr. Joseph Keul (1932–2000), sports doctor and professor of sports science at the University of Freiburg. Keul was a key person in the history of doping and anti-doping in Germany, including scientific research about them. ***Source: Picture Alliance, dpa/ Rolf Haid***

and the government that they needed to discuss and decide on an anti-doping law. He in fact preferred solutions from the sports organizations. The existing laws would be sufficient to prosecute and sanction criminal behavior, but doping, as well as banning and reducing doping, was within the sphere not of state responsibility, but of sports organizations. For a long time, this opinion remained the ruling principle of the German state and government, and it still prevails, although the influence of the state in sports and in anti-doping actions was growing rapidly.

The German professional boxing champion Jupp Elze died from a cerebral hemorrhage during a match in June 1968. The autopsy revealed various doping stimulants. Elze's death was discussed extensively by the German public with respect to the risks of doping in general and especially in professional sport. The fact that Elze was a professional boxer provided the officials of amateur sports organizations with the opportunity to declare doping a problem of professional, but not amateur, sports. At that time, Olympic sports were exclusively amateur, although the dogma of amateur sports was losing legitimation. However, officials of the DSB became increasingly nervous and asked the Ministry of the Interior to consider legal steps to reduce doping in sports. The experiences of the previous few years had demonstrated that "no anti-doping rules in the context of competition regulations by the sports associations had not been at all successful."[126]

However, in the German parliament on November 15, 1968, the responsible Minster of the Interior, Ernst Benda, responded to a question on doping by saying that the German government did not intend to discuss a specific anti-doping law, "because the existing laws against negligent and dangerous criminal assault and killing would also be sufficient to protect athletes against doping. Additional actions against doping should be undertaken by the sports organizations in the context of their statutes and competition instructions."[127] In other words, the German government wanted neither to intervene in the autonomy of sports nor to criminalize athletes. Athletes were still recognized less as perpetrators and more as victims of doping.

Nevertheless, the influence of the state in sports policies was increasingly evident. The public, as well as parliamentary debates about doping, were crucial for the decision on the General Guidelines against Doping, concluded by the DSB in 1970, which had been supported by civil servants of the Ministry of the Interior, even with proposals as to the specific formulation. A further impulse for these actions against doping was certainly the spectacularly influential article about doping in German sports by Brigitte Berendonk in the journal *Die Zeit*, a paper that is read mainly by the educated classes in Germany. The headline was "Do We Feed Monsters?" Formerly a top East German shot-putter, Berendonk had fled from the GDR in 1958 and become the most popular and active critic of doping in German sports. She and her husband, the biochemist Werner Franke, fought against doping like no one else in Germany, and have continued to do so up to the present. They uncovered and published secret documents about doping in the GDR, and they denounced doping in the West as well.[128]

DOPING DURING THE 1950S AND 1960S—INTERMEDIATE RESULTS

During the postwar period of the 1950s, doping became evident in sports in Germany as well as internationally. Step by step, new stimulants and performance-enhancing drugs were used. Although valid empirical data about the use of such drugs is lacking, they were undoubtedly used and had become a real danger for athletes as well as for sports themselves. Various cases of athletes using such pharmaceuticals were reported. However, this behavior was not yet forbidden explicitly by most sports authorities. Therefore, sports doctors discussed this problem for two reasons. First, they worried about the health of the athletes; and second, they argued that fair play in sports was in danger if some athletes secured advantages in competition though such immoral means. In the background, they were indeed concerned about the general function of sports medicine in society and sports—the balance between prevention and performance enhancement, including the ethical dilemma. The German Sports Doctors Association (DSÄB) proposed defining doping and reducing it by declaring this behavior clearly as unfair and forbidden. The umbrella organization of all German sports associations accepted this definition of doping and tried to make the ban on doping in German sports public.

Various explanations of this reciprocal development of doping and anti-doping can be proposed. Top-level sports became a worldwide phenomenon of modern society, with respect to professional as well as amateur sports. The Olympic motto of *citius, altius, fortius* (faster, higher, stronger) applied to the principles of progress in modern societies, not only in the capitalist world of the West, but even in the socialist world of the East, which so desperately wanted to be better and more successful than the capitalist one. This notion of progress was certainly part of the background of doping in sports regarding the causes and the remedies. In the Cold War period, this general tendency of sports and society to strive for more and better achievement and progress was placed in a political context. The political and national functionalization or instrumentalization promoted more doping. In addition, the progress of science in medicine, biochemistry, and pharmaceuticals led to numerous new drugs appearing on the market, which were used not only by victims of severe diseases, but also by athletes who were basically healthy. Some doctors were torn between their obligation to help the sick and the demands of athletes to support their efforts at enhanced achievement. However, doctors violate their professional oath, then as today, by administering medications intended for sick people to healthy top-level athletes. Additionally, the ethos of sports and fair play is also violated. This simple fact was unmistakable, at least when the German Association for Sports Medicine first defined doping in 1953.

Apart from the political and national functionalization of sports, the process of medicalization of modern society in the context of economic progress was additionally responsible for the genesis of a doping helix, which implies an inevitable development and use of performance-enhancing drugs in sport. The sports organizations tried to stop this, but they did so slowly, hesitatingly, inconsistently, and with little real commitment. As a result, they failed miserably from the beginning to control the doping problem.

It should be stated that doping was practiced in sports in general, in the East as well as in the West, and not only in top-level sports, either. However, as we know today, in East Germany, a system of taking drugs in sports had been installed by the state. It was part of a systematic pushing of top-level sports and a clear breach of the Olympic ethos and principles. The officials of the GDR were indeed aware of this fact. Not so in West Germany, however, where doping was practiced as well. The difference was that neither state officials nor politicians nor sports officials had ordered anybody to dope. Many may have been aware of doping practices, but they started, at least in public, to reduce doping and not to enforce it, assuming we can believe the documents of the time.

However, the definition of doping in 1953 was the first step in reducing doping and in introducing serious anti-doping policies. Until the 1960s, doping was seen in German society, as well as in international sports and other societies, as morally wrong behavior on the part of athletes. Yet this behavior was not controlled or merely reduced by rules and sanctions. Step by step, in society and in sports, doping rules were introduced. There was growing awareness on the part of the public and the sporting community of doping as unethical, immoral, unfair, and unhealthy. Anti-doping gradually became a fundament of sports, society, and politics.

In West Germany, as in most countries in the Western world, sports and doping were regarded as a matter for sports organizations, and less as a problem of society in general and of state politics especially. The theory of autonomy of sport implied the obligation of sports organizations to deal appropriately with doping. However, the expectations of society, as well as of sports policies, were ambiguous. On the one hand, the athletes should be strong and successful in national and international events, but on the other hand, they were expected to be models of fair play and healthy living, and also amateurs without any earnings. Doping simply did not apply to these high moral expectations.

When the public and politicians became aware that the doping phenomenon could not be regulated away by the sports organizations, political actors started to play a major role in anti-doping. First the European Council intervened, followed by national initiatives of anti-doping. Germany, too, started various actions and made recommendations to curb doping. These international activities, mainly by the European Council, were very important and relevant for German politicians and political institutions, from the government and the Ministry of the Interior to the German parliament. They placed the doping phenomenon on the political agenda. Initially their interest in sports and actions against doping was rather reluctant. Neither sports as a whole nor individual athletes were to be sanctioned, but rather supported in their own efforts against doping. Politicians in Germany had believed too long in the willingness and ability of sports to prevail alone in the fight against doping. Gradually, however, politicians as well as sports officials became aware that another approach altogether was needed.

A new stage of dealing with doping and anti-doping in German sports was reached with the Olympic Games Munich of 1972, from the preparation for and allocation of these Games in 1965/66 to the consequences in the 1970s and 1980s. Munich was a benchmark on the long road of the major part of Germany to the West, as well as to the modern concept of Western sport, and it constituted a turning point in the Cold War. In terms of doping and anti-doping, the Munich Olympics marked the emergence of doping substances like hormones and anabolics, which entailed new challenges for the various aspects of doping and anti-doping.

NOTES

1. As introduction and overview, see Michael Krüger, *Leibesübungen im 20. Jahrhundert: Sport für alle*, 2nd ed., Sport und Sportunterricht 10 (Schorndorf: Hofmann, 2005), 164–99; and Michael Krüger, "60 Jahre Sport in Deutschland," *Sportwissenschaft* 39, no. 3 (2009): 237–50.

2. Michael Krüger, "The History of German Sports Clubs between Integration and Emigration," *International Journal of the History of Sport* 30, no. 14 (2013): 1586–1603, doi:10.1080/09523367.2013.822862; Michael Krüger, "The German Workers' Sport Movement between Socialism, Workers' Culture, Middle-Class Gymnastics and Sport for All," *International Journal of the History of Sport* 31, no. 9 (2014): 1098–1117, doi:10.1080/09523367.2014.882327.

3. Marcel Reinold and John Hoberman, "The Myth of the Nazi Steroid," *International Journal of the History of Sport* 31, no. 8 (2014): 871–83, doi:10.1080/09523367.2014.884563.

4. From another, Weberian perspective, see the fundamental contribution of Allen Guttmann, *From Ritual to Record: The Nature of Modern Sports*, updated, with a new afterword (1978; New York: Columbia University Press, 2004).

5. The German football (soccer) history is well researched mainly by Franz-Josef Brüggemeier, *Fußball—Mehr als ein Spiel,* Informationen zur politischen Bildung 290 (Munich: Franzis-Verlag, 2006); Franz-Josef Brüggemeier, *Das Wunder von Bern: The 1954 Football World Cup, the German Nation and Popular Histories,* and Nils Havemann, *Fußball unterm Hakenkreuz: Der DFB zwischen Sport, Politik und Kommerz* (Frankfurt: Campus-Verl,

2005); Nils Havemann, *Samstags um halb vier: Die Geschichte der Fußballbundesliga* (Berlin: Siedler, 2013).

6. Willi Daume, *Deutscher Sport, 1952–1972* (Munich: ProSport, 1973), 74.

7. Daume, *Deutscher Sport*, 23.

8. Carl Diem, *Weltgeschichte des Sports*, 2nd ed., 2 vols. (Stuttgart: Cotta, 1967). See also Frank Becker, *Den Sport gestalten: Carl Diems Leben (1882–1962)* (Duisburg: Universitätsverlag Rhein-Ruhr, 2009–2010), 4:91–94.

9. Hans-Heinrich Sievert, "Aufgaben und Grenzen staatlicher Hilfe für den Sport," *Die Leibeserziehung* 4 (1954): 73.

10. Quoted in Hartmut Becker et al., eds., *Die Gründerjahre des Deutschen Sportbundes: Wege aus der Not zur Einheit*, with the assistance of Ommo Grupe and Giselher Spitzer (Schorndorf: Karl Hofmann, 1990), 330.

11. Sievert, "Aufgaben und Grenzen staatlicher Hilfe für den Sport," 74.

12. Karlheinz Gieseler, ed., *Der Sport in der Bundesrepublik Deutschland*, Ämter und Organisationen der Bundesrepublik Deutschland 35 (Bonn: Boldt, 1972), 118.

13. In 1950, one US Dollar converted to four German Marks and twenty Pfennig, in 1960 to DM 4.17, and in 1970 to DM 3.65.

14. Quoted in Daume, *Deutscher Sport*, 94.

15. Uta Andrea Balbier, *Kalter Krieg auf der Aschenbahn: Der deutsch-deutsche Sport, 1950–1972. Eine politische Geschichte*, Sammlung Schöningh zur Geschichte und Gegenwart (Paderborn: F. Schöningh, 2007), 63.

16. Guido v. Mengden, "Beiträge zur Geschichte des Deutschen Sportbundes," *Jahrbuch des Sports, 1959–1962* (1962): 62.

17. Daume, *Deutscher Sport*, 93.

18. Guido von Mengden was not only an experienced sports manager and administrator, but also a former Nazi sports politician. See Hajo Bernett, *Guido von Mengden: "Generalstabschef" des deutschen Sports*, Turn- und Sportführer im Dritten Reich 5 (Berlin: Bartels & Wernitz, 1976).

19. Mengden, "Beiträge zur Geschichte des Deutschen Sportbundes," 60ff.

20. Ibid., 55.

21. Ibid.

22. Balbier, *Kalter Krieg auf der Aschenbahn*, 18.

23. Daume, *Deutscher Sport*, 101.

24. "Zone" refers to the territory of East Germany, occupied by the Red Army after 1945.

25. Daume, *Deutscher Sport*, 118.

26. The history and notion of German sports clubs is explained in detail by Krüger, "The History of German Sports Clubs between Integration and Emigration."

27. Ivan Waddington and Andy Smith, *An Introduction to Drugs in Sport: Addicted to Winning?* (London: Routledge, 2009), 70.

28. John Hoberman, "How Drug Testing Fails: The Politics of Doping Control," in *Doping in Elite Sport: The Politics of Drugs in the Olympic Movement*, ed. Wayne Wilson and Edward Derse (Champaign, Ill.: Human Kinetics, 2001), 241–74.

29. Ludwig Prokop, "Das Dopingproblem im Sport," *Leibesübungen/Leibeserziehung* 9, 5/6 (1955): 6.

30. Balbier, *Kalter Krieg auf der Aschenbahn*, 473.

31. Barrie Houlihan, *Dying to Win: Doping in Sport and the Development of Anti-Doping Policy*, 2nd ed. (Strasbourg: Council of Europe Publications, 2002), 19ff.

32. Rob Beamish and Ian Ritchie, "From Chivalrous 'Brothers in Arms' to the Eligible Athlete: Changed Principles and the IOC's Banned Substance List," *International Review for the Sociology of Sport* 39, no. 4 (2004): 259.

33. Allen Guttmann, *The Olympics: A History of the Modern Games*, Illinois History of Sport (Urbana: University of Illinois Press, 1992), 97.

34. Waddington and Smith, *An Introduction to Drugs in Sport*, 70ff.

35. Balbier, *Kalter Krieg auf der Aschenbahn*, 18, 131.

36. Ibid., 13.

37. Deutscher Ruder-Verband, supplement to the minutes of the conference of the *Verbandsausschuss* of the Rowing Federation, 18 October 1952, p. 4; Prokop, "Das Dopingproblem im Sport," 6; Council of Europe, *Doping of Athletes: Reports of the Special Working Parties, Strasbourg, January 1963, Madrid, November 1963* (Strasbourg, 1964), 4.

38. Balbier, *Kalter Krieg auf der Aschenbahn*, 57ff.

39. Giselher Spitzer has done extensive work on the GDR doping system. See *Doping in der DDR: Ein historischer Überblick zu einer konspirativen Praxis; Genese—Verantwortung—Gefahren* (Cologne: Sport und Buch Strauß, 1998).

40. B. Gilbert, "Drugs in Sport: Part 1: Problems in a Turned On World," *Sports Illustrated*, 23 June 1969, shows that this argument was used in the Western world of sports at all.

41. The article of Brigitte Berendonk in the high-quality journal *Die Zeit* (5 December 1969) and the demotion of the track-and-field coach Kofink were crucial steps in seriously questioning doping in the West.

42. Waddington and Smith, *An Introduction to Drugs in Sport*, 48, 64, 205.

43. E. J. Ariens, "Organisation et résultatsdu contrôle antidoping," in *Doping: Proceedings of an International Seminar Organized at the Universities of Ghent and Brussels, May 1964, by the Research Committee of the International Council of Sport and Physical Education (U.N.E.S.C.O.)*, ed. A. F de Schaepdryver (Oxford: Pergamon Press, 1965), 27–50, esp. 47; Deutscher Olympischer Sportbund (DOSB), minutes of the meeting of the DSB, 11 October 1969, p. 8ff., in folder Protokolle DSB-Bundestage, DOSB Archive.

44. Werner Pitsch, Eike Emrich, and Michael Klein, "Doping in Elite Sports in Germany: Results of a www-survey," *European Journal of Sports and Society* 4, no. 2 (2007): 89–102; Werner Pitsch, Peter Maats, and Eike Emrich, "Zur Häufigkeit des Dopings im deutschen Spitzensport: Eine Replikationsstudie," in *Sport und Doping: Zur Analyse einer antagonistischen Symbiose*, ed. Eike Emrich and Werner Pitsch (Frankfurt am Main: Lang, 2009), 19–36.

45. Werner Pitsch, "Dopingkontrollen zwischen Testtheorie und Moral: Nicht intendierte Folgen prinzipiell nicht perfekter Dopingtests," in *Sport und Doping: Zur Analyse einer antagonistischen Symbiose*, ed. Eike Emrich and Werner Pitsch (Frankfurt am Main: Lang, 2009), 95–110, esp. 97.

46. Rob Beamish and Ian Ritchie, *Fastest, Highest, Strongest: A Critique of High-Performance Sport,* Routledge Critical Studies in Sport (New York: Routledge, 2006), 6; Karl-Heinrich Bette and Uwe Schimank, *Doping im Hochleistungssport: Anpassung durch Abweichung,* Edition Suhrkamp 1957 (Frankfurt am Main: Suhrkamp, 2006), 35ff.; Paul Dimeo, *A History of Drug Use in Sport, 1876–1976: Beyond Good and Evil* (New York and London: Routledge, 2007), 312.

47. Hans Lenk, *Werte, Ziele, Wirklichkeit der modernen Olympischen Spiele*, 2nd ed., Beiträge zur Lehre und Forschung der Leibeserziehung 17/18 (Schorndorf bei Stuttgart: Hofmann, 1972).

48. Waddington and Smith, *An Introduction to Drugs in Sport*, 65.

49. Ibid., 81.

50. Houlihan, *Dying to Win*, 27ff.; John Milton Hoberman, *Testosterone Dreams: Rejuvenation, Aphrodisia, Doping* (Berkeley: University of California Press, 2005), 182ff.; Daniel M. Rosen, *Dope: A History of Performance Enhancement in Sports from the Nineteenth Century to Today* (Westport, Conn. and London: Praeger, 2008), 3.

51. Ibid.

52. Antonio Venerando, "Patalogia del doping e mezzi di controllo," *Medicina dello sport* 3, no. 9 (1963): 32, 38; A. Venerando and F. de Sio, "Organisation et résultats du control antidoping," in *Doping: Proceedings of an International Seminar Organized at the Universities of Ghent and Brussels, May 1964*, ed. A. F. de Schaepdryver and Marcel Hebbelinck (Oxford: Pergamon Press, 1965), 133–45.

53. Ludwig Prokop, "Zur Geschichte des Dopings und seiner Bekämpfung," *Sportarzt und Sportmedizin* 21, no. 6 (1970): 130; Rüdiger Rabenstein, "Some Facts about the History of Doping in Cycling History Competition," in *Proceedings 8th International Cycle History Conference, 1997*, 124.

54. Venerando and de Sio, "Organisation et résultats du control antidoping," 133–45.

55. Rabenstein, "Some Facts about the History of Doping in Cycling History Competition," 124.

56. Andreas Singler and Gerhard Treutlein, *Doping im Spitzensport: Sportwissenschaftliche Analysen zur nationalen und internationalen Leistungsentwicklung (Teil 1)*, 6th ed., Sportentwicklungen in Deutschland 12 (Aachen: Meyer & Meyer, 2012); Martin Lames, "Leistungsentwicklung in der Leichtathletik: Ist Doping als leistungsfördernder Effekt identifizierbar?" *dvs-informationen* 17, no. 4 (2002): 15–22.

57. Howard Saul Becker, *Outsiders: Studies in the Sociology of Deviance* (1963; New York: Free Press, 1997), 147.

58. Dimeo, *A History of Drug Use in Sport, 1876–1976*, 93.

59. Rob Beamish and Ian Ritchie, *Fastest, Highest, Strongest*, 117ff.

60. See among others Venerando, "Patalogia del doping e mezzi di controllo"; Arthur Porrit, "Doping in Sport: Chairman's Opening Remarks," *British Journal of Sports Medicine* 4, no. 2 (1969); Gilbert, "Drugs in Sport"; Prokop, "Zur Geschichte des Dopings und seiner Bekämpfung," 128ff.; Dimeo, *A History of Drug Use in Sport, 1876–1976*, 101.

61. Ibid., Dimeo, *A History of Drug Use in Sport, 1876–1976*, 93, 103, 128.

62. Council of Europe, *Doping of Athletes*; Resolution on the Doping of Athletes, adopted by the Ministers' Deputies on 29 June 1967, Committee of Ministers of the Council of Europe (1967); Judith Amelie Schmidt, *Internationale Dopingbekämpfung: Grundlagen und nationalstaatliche Umsetzung,* Schriftenreihe Causa Sport 1 (Stuttgart, Zurich: Boorberg; Schulthess, 2009), 24.

63. Dimeo, *A History of Drug Use in Sport, 1876–1976*, 95. IOC policies are well researched and discussed by Thomas M. Hunt, *Drug Games: The International Olympic Committee and the Politics of Doping, 1960–2008*, Terry and Jan Todd Series on Physical Culture and Sports (Austin: University of Texas Press, 2011); and S. Boyes, "The International Olympic Committee, Transnational Doping Policy and Globalisation," in *Drugs & Doping in Sports*, ed. John O'Leary (London: Routledge-Cavendish, 2001), 167–79.

64. Verner Møller, "Knud Enemark Jensen's Death during the 1960 Rome Olympics: A Search for the Truth?" *Sport in History* 25 (2005): 452–71, is critical of that hypothesis. In fact, the reasons for his death have never been resolved definitively.

65. A. Wrynn, "The Human Factor: Science, Medicine and the International Olympic Committee, 1900–1970," *Sport in Society* 7, no. 2 (2004): 211–31; Hunt, *Drug Games*, 27ff.

66. *Zeitschrift Sportmedizin*, 9 (1954), 149.

67. Deutscher Fechterbund (F.I.E.), *Kampfregeln des Internationalen Fechterbundes (F.I.E.)* (Krefeld: Verlag van Acken, 1950), 51ff.

68. Patrick Laure, *Le dopage: Pratiques corporelles* (Paris: Presses Universitaires de France, 1995); E. Vettenie, "Runners, Rumors, and Dreams of Representations: An Inquiry into Drug Use by Athletes in the 1920s," *Journal of Sport History* 37, no. 3 (2010): 405ff.

69. Dimeo, *A History of Drug Use in Sport, 1876–1976*, 13, 90.

70. J. Bliesener, "Zur Frage des Doping: Mit Hilfe von Umfragen und zum Teil eigenen Beobachtungen im Radsport" (Thesis, Sporthochschule Cologne, 1959), 47ff.

71. Michael Krüger, "Doping im Radsport—Zivilisationstheoretische Anmerkungen zu einer langen Geschichte," *Sport und Gesellschaft*, no. 3 (2006): 324–52. The German press as well as cycling journals had always reported regularly on doping cases, as early as in the 1950s, for example: *Illustrierter Sport-Kurier*, 8 August 1955; *Welt*, 21 July 1955; *Kölnische Rundschau*, 21 July 1955; *Spiegel*, 3 August 1955; *Radsport*, 30 August 1955, 2; 29 November 1955, 9.

72. Bund Deutscher Radfahrer (BDR), Sportordnungen, Ziffer 243 of the Wettfahrbestimmungen (competition rules) of 1956.

73. Council of Europe, *Doping of Athletes*, 35–37; M. Kohlhaas, "Gesetzliche Grundlagen für ein Verbot von 'Doping,'" *Sportarzt und Sportmedizin* 17, no. 2 (1966), 83; Ludwig Prokop, "Praktische Erfahrungen mit dem Doping in Österreich," *Sportarzt und Sportmedizin* 17, no. 2 (1966), 59.

74. W. Ruhemann, "Einführung," in *Sportmedizin und Gesundheitserziehung*, ed. Deutscher Sportbund (DSB), Schriftenreihe des DSB 4 (Frankfurt am Main: Limpert, 1954), 7–12, esp. 12; W. Kleffel, "Wunderpillen endgültig verboten," *Die Zeit*, no. 47 (1952); E. J. Klaus,

"Sporthygienische Fragen," in *Sportmedizin und Gesundheitserziehung*, ed. Deutscher Sportbund (DSB), Schriftenreihe des DSB 4 (Frankfurt am Main: Limpert, 1954), 31–41, esp. 36.

75. Franz Friedrich, *Sport und Körper: Die biologischen Grundlagen der Leibeserziehung*, 4th ed. (Munich: Ehrenwirth, 1950), 312; W. Ruhemann, "Einführung," 7–12, esp. 12.

76. Prokop, "Zur Geschichte des Dopings und seiner Bekämpfung," 130; Prokop, L. & Radbauer, F., "Die Placebowirkung der Injektion beim Doping," in *XVI. Weltkongress für Sportmedizin 1966 in Hannover 12. bis 16. Juni 1966: Kongressbericht: Generalthema: Funktionsminderung und Funktionsertüchtigung im modernen Leben*, ed. Günter Hanekopf (Cologne: Deutscher Ärzte Verlag, 1966), 635–37, esp. 637.

77. Dimeo, *A History of Drug Use in Sport, 1876–1976*, 14, 61, 105, 119; Robert Jütte, "Zur Geschichte des Dopings," *Geschichte in Wissenschaft und Unterricht*, 5/6 (2008), 321; Patrick Laure, "Zur Entwicklung von Dopingregeln und Antidoping-Gesetzen," in *Dopingprävention in Europa: Grundlagen und Modelle; Erstes internationales Expertengespräch 2005 in Heidelberg*, ed. Wolfgang Knörzer, G. Spitzer, and G. Treutlein (Aachen and Graz: Meyer & Meyer, 2006), 121–32, esp. 122.

78. Alfred Koch, "Der Präsident des Deutschen Sportärztebundes zum Kongreß 1954," *Sportmedizin*, no. 9 (1954): 258; Alfred Koch, ed., *Präventive Medizin und Leibesübungen in der Jugend: Vorträge und Referate anläßlich des Deutschen Sportärztekongresses 1955 in Augsburg* (Freiburg im Breisgau: Tries, 1956), 10ff.

79. Alfred Koch, Hanns Hoske, and J. M. Hammacher, "Vom Wirken des Sportarztes," in *Sportmedizin und Gesundheitserziehung*, ed. Deutscher Sportbund (DSB), Schriftenreihe des DSB 4 (Frankfurt am Main: Limpert, 1954), 15–29; Koch, *Präventive Medizin und Leibesübungen in der Jugend*, 14.

80. Jörg Vögele, "Zur Entwicklung der Gesundheitsverhältnisse im 19. und 20. Jahrhundert.," in *Geschichte, Theorie und Ethik der Medizin: Eine Einführung*, ed. Stefan Schulz et al., Orig.-Ausg., 1. Aufl, Suhrkamp-Taschenbuch Wissenschaft 1791 (Frankfurt am Main: Suhrkamp, 2006), 166ff.

81. Typical are contributions like that of Ommo Grupe, "Was erwartet der Sport von der Sportmedizin: Sonderdruck aus der Zeitschrift 'Der Sportarzt,'" *Der Sportarzt* (1959); or Willi Daume, *Deutscher Sport* (1973/1953), pp. 23–27 about the relationship between sports doctors and practical sports. See also Karl Ritter von Halt, "Olympia," *Leibesübungen-Sportarzt-Erziehung* 4, no. 6 (1952), 34.

82. Woldemar Gerschler, "Diskussionsbemerkungen eines erfahrenen Trainers," in *Training, Leistung, Gesundheit: Vorträge und Referate anlässlich des Sportärztekongreses Berlin 1952*, ed. Deutscher Sportbund et al. (Frankfurt am Main: Limpert, 1953), 182.

83. Ritter von Halt, "Olympia," 34; also Alfred Koch, *Sportmedizin*, Therapie und Praxis H. 17 (Vienna and Innsbruck: Urban & Schwarzenberg, 1958), 18.

84. Emanuel Hübner, *Planung, Bau und Nutzung des Olympischen Dorfes von 1936* (Paderborn: Schöningh, 2015), forthcoming.

85. Martin Brustmann, "Erfahrungen mit der Verabreichung von Zellaufbaustoffen beim Körpertraining," *Arzt und Sport: Mitteilungen des deutschen Sportärzte-Bundes* 12, no. 23 (1936): 94; P. Schenk, "Bericht über die Verpflegung der im Olympischen Dorf untergebrachten Teilnehmer an den XI. Olympischen Spielen 1936 zu Berlin," *Die Ernährung* 2, no. 1 (1937); A. Bickel, *Die Ernährung der olympischen Kämpfer in Vergangenheit und Gegenwart* (Berlin, 1936).

86. E. Engelhardt, "Ernährungsprobleme im Sport," in *Training, Leistung, Gesundheit: Vorträge und Referate anlässlich des Sportärztekongreses Berlin 1952*, ed. Deutscher Sportbund et al. (Frankfurt am Main: Limpert, 1953), 103–5, esp. 104; Ludwig Prokop, "Sport und Sauna," in *Training, Leistung, Gesundheit: Vorträge und Referate anlässlich des Sportärztekongreses Berlin 1952*, ed. Deutscher Sportbund et al. (Frankfurt am Main: Limpert, 1953), 37–40.

87. John Hoberman, "The Early Development of Sports Medicine in Germany," in *Sport and Exercise Science: Essays in the History of Sports Medicine*, ed. Jack W. Berryman and Roberta J. Park, Sport and Society (Urbana: University of Illinois Press, 1992), 233–82, esp. 239.

88. Alfred Koch, Hanns Hoske, and J. M. Hammacher, "Vom Wirken des Sportarztes," 15–29, esp. 19ff. Even today sports medicine cannot be studied as a specialist discipline of medicine in Germany.

89. Allen Guttmann, *From Ritual to Record: The Nature of Modern Sports*, updated, with a new afterword (New York: Columbia University Press, 2004); Norbert Elias and Eric Dunning, *Quest for Excitement: Sport and Leisure in the Civilizing Process* (Oxford: Basil Blackwell, 1993); Kalevi Heinilä, *The Totalization Process in International Sport: Toward a Theory of the Totalization of Competition in Top-Level Sport,* Tutkimuksia / Jyväskylän yliopisto. Liikuntasuunnittelun laitos 23 (Jyväskylä: University of Jyväskylä, 1982).

90. See the biographical draft of Erik Eggers, "Der Sportarzt Martin Brustmann, das Rudern und das Testoviron—Über die Anfänge des Hormondopings im deutschen Leistungssport vor den Olympischen Spielen 1952 in Helsinki," in *Jahrbuch 2011 der Deutschen Gesellschaft für Geschichte der Sportwissenschaft e.V*, ed. Jürgen Court, Studien zur Geschichte des Sports 14 (Berlin: Lit, 2012), 227–44; also Vettenie, "Runners, Rumors, and Dreams of Representations," 411.

91. The proceedings are documented in the archive of the DRV. See Verbandsausschuss des DRV, 1952.

92. For example, *Frankfurter Allgemeine Zeitung*, 07/07/1952, 14/07/1952, 15/08/1952, 23/08/1952; *Spiegel*, 23/07/1952, 30/07/1952, 13/08/1952; *Stern*, 20/07/1952; *Süddeutsche Zeitung*, 21/07/1952; *Welt*, 15/07/1952, 31/07/1952, 30/09/1952; *Zeit*, 20/11/1952.

93. Doping was familiar to equestrianism. John Gleaves, "'Enhancing the Odds': Horse Racing, Gambling and the First Anti-Doping Movement in Sport, 1889–1911," *Sport in History* 32, no. 1 (2012): 26–52. Some of the works of the novelist Dick Francis deal with doping in equestrian sports, such as Dick Francis, *For Kicks*, large print ([S.l.]: Ulverscroft, 1973); the title of the German translation is Dick Francis, *Doping: Roman*, new trans. by Malte Krutzsch, De te be 23254 (Zurich: Diogenes, 2000).

94. Hoberman, *Testosterone Dreams*, 189; Bulletin officiel du Comité International Olympique No. 28, July 1951, 25ff.

95. Verbandsausschuss des DRV, 1953.

96. "Der Deutsche Sportärztebund steht auf dem Standpunkt, dass jedes Medikament—ob es wirksam ist oder nicht—mit der Absicht der Leistungssteigerung vor Wettkämpfen gegeben als Doping zu betrachten ist." W. Ruhemann, "Doping," *Sportmedizin*, no. 2 (1953): 26.

97. Becker, *Outsiders*.

98. See the correspondence between Daume and Ruhemann in Deutscher Olympischer Sportbund (DOSB) Archives, folder 193; and *Sportmedizin* 4 (1953), 64.

99. Ruhemann, "Doping," 26.

100. W. Ruhemann, "Einführung," 7–12, esp. 12.

101. Tanja Haug, *Doping: Dilemma des Leistungssports* (Hamburg: Merus-Verlag, 2006), 159; Horst Hilpert, *Sportrecht und Sportrechtsprechung im In- und Ausland* (Berlin: de Gruyter Recht, 2007), 312ff.

102. The ethical and moral implications of the criminalization of doping behavior are discussed in numerous current doping discourses, for example by Christoph Asmuth, "Dopingdefinitionen—Von der Moral zum Recht," in *Was ist Doping? Fakten und Probleme der aktuellen Diskussion*, ed. Christoph Asmuth, Brennpunkt Doping 1 (Bielefeld: transcript, 2010), 13–32; Bette and Schimank, *Doping im Hochleistungssport*, 167ff.

103. This lack of consequences was also observed by contemporaries, see, for example *Die Zeit*, 20 November 1952, 47; *Frankfurter Allgemeine Zeitung*, 10 March 1953, 5; also in the journal *Sportmedizin,* for example L. Lendle, "Stimulantio—Excitantia (Dopingmittel)," *Sportmedizin*, no. 1 (1957): 22–26; E. Fischbach, "Zum Kapitel 'Doping,'" *Sportmedizin* 9 (1955): 145–46.

104. The debates on doping were intensified in 1965/66. See correspondence archived in the Bundesarchiv Koblenz (BA Koblenz), B 322/9, and the Deutscher Olympischer Sportbund (DOSB) Archive, esp. folder minutes of the main assemblies.

105. Bundesarchiv Koblenz (BA Koblenz), B 322/9: "Das Dopingproblem im internationalen Sport" (report about "the doping problem in international sports") .

106. Ibid., B 322/9.

107. Ibid., Keul to the BMI, 16 August 1965.

108. For example Deutscher Leichtathletik-Verband (DLV), Amtliche Leichtathletik Bestimmungen 1968, Regel 16; Deutscher Boxsport Verband (DBV/DABV), Wettkampf-Bestimmungen 1967, § 38.

109. Deutscher Leichtathletik-Verband (DLV), Amtliche Leichtathletik Bestimmungen 1969, Regel 16, Unterpunkt 3; *Leichtathletik* 13 (1969), 431.

110. Bundesarchiv Koblenz (BA Koblenz), B 322/9: Deutscher Schwimm-Verband to DSB, 9 June 1969.

111. Bundesarchiv Koblenz (BA Koblenz), B 322/9: Deutscher Verband für Modernen Fünfkampf to DSB, 3 June 1969.

112. Bundesarchiv Koblenz (BA Koblenz), B 106/158217, § 29 of the cycling rules (Wettfahrbestimmungen) of the BDR 1963.

113. See many reports in the journal *Radsport*, 10 May 1966, 2; 9 August 1966, 2; 6 September 1966, 16; 3 October 1967, 2; 28 November 1967, 3, 8; 28 May 1968, 14, 17; 12 August 1969, 14, 22.

114. *Radsport*, 17 June 1969, 5.

115. The process of regulation in cycling sports and by the UCI is considered in Krüger, "Doping im Radsport—Zivilisationstheoretische Anmerkungen zu einer langen Geschichte," 336ff.

116. Reports of the strike in *Radsport*, 5 July 1966, 2, 11; 12 July 1966, 14; Bulletin officiel du Comité International Olympique No. 95 (August 1966): 61; Christopher Thompson, *The Tour de France: A Cultural History*, new ed. (Berkeley: University of California Press, 2008), 233.

117. *Radsport*, 5 July 1966, 11.

118. Fichtel & Sachs to BDR, 24 March 1965, in Deutsche Sporthochschule Köln (DSHS Köln), Deutsche Sporthochschule, inheritage Gronen, folder 11.

119. Manfred Donike, "Der Dopingnachweis mit Hilfe chromatographischer Methoden," *Sportarzt und Sportmedizin*, no. 2 (1966): 84; H. Alfes, J. C. D. Reisch, and H. Möllmann, "Der Nachweis von zentralstimulierenden Arzneimitteln (Dopingmitteln) durch die Gaschromatographie," *Sportarzt und Sportmedizin*, no. 11 (1968): 495ff.

120. The problems of doping tests have frequently been described, for example with respect to Germany, by ibid.; Donike, "Der Dopingnachweis mit Hilfe chromatographischer Methoden,"; internationally by Venerando, "Patalogia del doping e mezzi di controllo"; Venerando and de Sio, "Organisation et résultats du control antidoping," 133–45; A. H. Beckett, G. T. Tucker, and A. C. Moffat, "Routine Detection and Identification in Urine of Stimulants and Other Drugs, Some of Which May Be Used to Modify Performance in Sport," *Journal of Pharmacy and Pharmacology* 19 (1967): 273–94.

121. Deutscher Sportbund (DSB), Rahmen-Richtlinien zur Bekämpfung des Dopings. Beschlossen am 26. September 1970 durch den Hauptausschuss des DSB in Mannheim, 1970.

122. See, for example, the opinion of anti-doping experts like Venerando, "Patalogia del doping e mezzi di controllo," 975ff.; and Prokop, "Zur Geschichte des Dopings und seiner Bekämpfung," 126, 130.

123. Bundesarchiv Koblenz (BA Koblenz), B 322/9: BMI to Reindell, 10 August 1965.

124. Bundesarchiv Koblenz (BA Koblenz), B 322/9: Keul to BMI, 16 August 1965.

125. Bundesarchiv Koblenz (BA Koblenz), B 322/9: BMI to Reindell, 27 September 1965; H. Weidemann, "Internationale Konferenz über Doping bei Sportlern vom 23.–25. September in Straßburg," *Sportarzt und Sportmedizin* 17, no. 2 (1966): 49ff.; Herbert Reindell, "Begrüßung durch den Präsidenten des Deutschen Sportbundes," *Sportarzt und Sportmedizin*, 17, no. 2 (1966): 45ff.

126. Deutscher Olympischer Sportbund (DOSB), letter of the DSB to BMI, 11 July 1968. Regrettably the response of the Ministry to this letter could not be found in the archives.

127. Parlamentsarchiv (PA), Bundestagsdrucksache, 5. WP, 196. Meeting 15 November 1968, p. 10556.

128. *Die Zeit*, 5 December 1969, 73.

Chapter Two

Cold War and the Climax of Doping in Germany

From the Munich Olympics of 1972 via Montreal 1976 to the Introduction of Out-of-Competition Controls in the 1980s

In contrast to nineteenth- and early twentieth-century sports, Cold War–era sports were regarded as a symbol not only of the power and strength of a nation-state, but of certain ideological systems of politics, economy, and society, in particular capitalism and socialism. The Olympic Games became one of the most important "battlefields" of this Cold War, since the Soviet Union had decided to take part in these major events of bourgeois body culture after World War II.[1] The IOC, as a nonpolitical institution of worldwide Olympic sports, invited the Soviets to join the Olympic family.[2] From then on, just as after the Helsinki Olympics of 1952, the Games ceased to be merely an exciting event for athletes from all over the world. Sporting contests seemed to replace wars, at least in some instances and to some extent. They compensated for the ideological and political conflict between the superpowers and their satellites.[3] Concerning sport, the GDR was by far the most successful younger brother in the socialist or communist "family" behind the Iron Curtain. The East German athletes were so successful that they gradually threatened the sporting dominance of big brother Soviet Union.

Beyond doubt, the Cold War between East and West Germany played a major role in the development of doping and anti-doping. Given East Germany's small population of just eighteen million people, as well as the small area of the country, the only explanation for the *Sportwunder DDR* (GDR sports miracle) seemed to be the its "system" of sport. The success of GDR athletes in international contests, especially in sports that had been selected specifically as likely to yield Olympic medals, was indeed founded on a perfectly organized Prussian system of managing and supporting sport. However, doping, and not anti-doping, was a fundamental part of this system.

How did the West Germans react to that challenge? On the one hand, they (along with other sporting nations in the Western world)[4] tried to imitate the successful East German sporting system (including doping) with respect to the systematic promotion of sporting talent and scientific methods of training, other means of support, and institutional effectiveness. Medical support had a particularly high priority. West German athletes, coaches, sports representatives, and (sports) politicians did not want to surrender the sporting field to the GDR and tried to beat them at their own game by adopting essential elements of their successful sporting system. But on the other hand, the Federal Republic of Germany fully embraced the Western world of free and democratic societies, and accordingly wanted to become a role model of the Olympic movement. This meant that the sporting system ought to be free and independent of the state, in order to develop fair sport without doping, as stipulated in the Olympic Charter. Freedom, autonomy, and independence from politics are among the most important ideals of the Olympic movement.

For West German sports politicians and officials, this dilemma seemed impossible to resolve. One solution was for the state to support top-level sports by spending more money but taking no responsibility for the consequences. The politicians simply expected success in return for the money and did not ask how it was spent, thus neglecting their duty to control the tax-financed support of top-level sports.

The Cold War period can be considered as shaping both modern doping and anti-doping in West Germany. First, potential performance-enhancing substances had flooded the market since the postwar period, because of scientific progress in pharmacology, biology, chemistry, medicine, and the associated industrial production. As a result, doping became a somewhat rubbery and vague concept, again raising the central issue of how to define doping precisely, so as to separate legal dietary supplements from illegal doping substances. Second, the development of sports medicine as a specialized discipline produced a new group of scientific experts who were highly involved in doping prevention and control—and, regrettably, some who were doing the diametrical opposite and administering illegal substances in high-performance sports. Together with trainers and sports officials, they played a key role in athlete networks. Third, the increasing use of anabolic steroids in sports since the 1960s changed doping fundamentally. Their use, effects, and side effects differed significantly from the *purely* stimulatory doping substances used earlier. Dealing appropriately with highly controversial anabolic steroids was a major issue in West Germany. The year 1977 marked an important step in this process because the German Sports Federation adopted a Grundsatzerklärung für den Spitzensport (Declaration of Principles for Top Sport) and parliament discussed the issue of doping. Fourth, these processes took place within the context of the increasing commercialization, professionalization, and politicization of sport. When doping spread rapidly in the 1960s, the policy of anti-doping was born and developed in the international sporting world, as well as in Germany. In West Germany, the Cold War "on the track" between East and West Germany was an important instigator of both doping and anti-doping policies. Compared to the international situation, the German-German relationship was unique. On the one hand, the German sports experts and representatives on the two sides of the wall were grim enemies, but on the other hand, they were very familiar with and jealous of each other. After all, they were all Germans.

In the 1970s, the structure and concept of sport in West Germany changed. This became obvious in connection with the organization of the Munich Olympic Games of 1972, with regard not only to Germany, but also to the international development of sports and doping, which were becoming increasingly intertwined. For the first time since the Berlin Games of 1936, the Olympic Games were taking place in Germany, and the new and modern Federal Republic was keen to present itself as especially progressive, creative, and innovative, precisely the opposite of what the world still remembered from the prewar games of Berlin. The organizers wanted to demonstrate in particular that sport in West Germany was free and independent of politics and not exploited in this or any other context.

In their book *The 1972 Munich Olympics and the Making of Modern Germany*,[5] the British historians Kay Schiller and Christopher Young reflect on the epochal changes introduced in the context of this event for sports, politics, and society in Germany, and internationally. Schiller and Young emphasize the political aspect of the Games and omit the question of doping, which they seem to regard as relevant only to the narrower context of sport itself. This is in accordance with the official West German standpoint, that doping was of concern only within the world of sports and had nothing to do with either national and international politics or sports politics. Indeed, doping was not regarded as any broader interest.

Today, we claim to know better; doping is not just a sporting issue, but also affects politics and society. "The Making of Modern Germany," which is the second part of the book title of Schiller and Young, also implies that German sports had become truly international, which therefore included both doping and anti-doping. East and West Germany even played a pioneering role in doping, and partly in anti-doping as well. The prevailing configuration of doping in the elite sports of the 1970s extended increasingly to the political arena. In the 1980s, sports finally crossed the borders of the economy and labor market. This pioneering role applied particularly to the clandestine, systematic doping by the GDR government, which was not yet widely known throughout the field of contemporary sports.

THE 1972 OLYMPIC GAMES OF MUNICH AND THEIR IMPORTANCE FOR THE DEVELOPMENT OF DOPING AND ANTI-DOPING IN GERMANY[6]

In the 1970s and in particular through the Munich Games in 1972, the Olympic Games developed into an internationally preeminent sports event. This was also accompanied by an increased politicization, in the sense of international competition beyond sports. Not least, the prominent position of the Olympic Games led the IOC—intentionally or unintentionally—to become the central stakeholder of anti-doping. The IOC's anti-doping politics left their mark throughout the anti-doping scene of the 1970s. Nevertheless, errors and mistakes also played a major role, as Thomas Hunt and Paul Dimeo have pointed out in recent publications.[7] Most of the international sports associations began to adjust their anti-doping actions to those of the IOC. While some associations simply left it to the IOC, others felt more or less obliged to conform to these arrangements themselves. This process dragged on through the 1970s, as well as for part of the 1980s, accompanied by various conflicts and controversy.

During the 1970s and especially the 1980s, the field of anti-doping underwent a profound shift regarding its protagonists. While in the 1950s it was mainly sports physicians who tried to deal with the various doping issues, as medical, ethical, and pedagogical arguments emerged during the 1970s and 1980s, more and more politicians and officials appeared on the scene. In 1973, the American hammer thrower Harold Connolly remarked that athletes would do anything to reach the top, even risking severe health damage or death.[8] This statement, which research has confirmed as representative of prevailing opinions at the time, revealed a process in international elite sports that the Finnish sociologist Kalevi Heinilä referred to in Munich in 1972 as the "totalization" of sport.[9]

Although it seemed obvious that the various sports organizations, the IOC included, were unable to cope with the doping problem, most Western governments retained the principle of the autonomy of sports organizations, as the IOC demands in its charter up to the present. At first glance and to the public at large, it appeared that they were leaving the resolution of the doping problem to the mostly voluntary sports officials. In this context, France constituted an exception by attempting to control doping in elite sports centrally, and with close government supervision.[10] Other examples revealed that doping was knowingly supported, or at least tolerated, by Eastern and Western sports associations, such as the International Association of Athletics Federations (IAAF).[11] Accordingly, the chief physician of the United States Olympic Committee, Robert Voy, compared the anti-doping policy to a fox being employed to guard a chicken coop.[12]

On April 25, 1966, Munich was elected by the IOC to be the site of the twentieth Summer Olympic Games at the second ballot. The election, as well as the subsequent preparation and organization of the Summer Olympic Games, including the attack by Arab terrorists, changed the Federal Republic of Germany politically, socially, and culturally, as Schiller and Young have argued.[13] The consequences of the successful Olympic application were naturally most obvious within the field of sports and sports policy, although Schiller and Young mention only marginally the consequences of modernism for sports. Nonetheless, their thesis that the Olympic Games in 1972 served as a catalyst for West German modernization can be applied to sport itself. However, in this connection, modernism means not only westernization, opening, democratization, sport for everyone, economization and rationalization, rest and recreation, but also those aspects of modern sports that are commonly regarded as negative or problematic: politicization, commercialization, gigantism, bigger events, totalization, and, last but not least, doping.

"The Making of Modern Germany," in terms of sports development, can be summed up in the following three parameters: (1) the political enhancement of sports, (2) the specification of elite sports, and (3) the scientification of sports. These parameters are assimilated in international sports development as a whole.

1. Political Enhancement of Sports

The political interest, in the sense of federal governmental politics, along with the responsible ministers, parliament, and parties, in sports and especially in elite Olympic sports, grew considerably over the period 1965 until 1972. Even in the Federal Republic, *elite sports* became a means of national representation and constituted criteria for governmental power and performance. As a result, elite sports in West Germany received stronger governmental support, whereas in the early years, it was considered as merely a private pleasure of the Federal Republic.

Some figures demonstrate the enormous development. The government publication "Core Activities in the Field of Sport and Physical Education" from the Bundesministerium des Inneren (Home Office) amounted to a modest DM 2 million in 1960. In 1965, it had already mounted to DM 4.6 million, and by 1970, it had increased threefold to DM 17.4 million. In the year of the Olympic Games, it was DM 23.5 million.[14] This money was spent primarily by the German sports associations and the National Olympic Committee on the support of elite sports. Neither the building of sports facilities, nor the Organizing Committee of the Olympic Games, nor school sports was financed in this manner. However, with this money, the government directly and indirectly paid the salaries of full-time officials and coaches.

It is obvious that the massive increase in financial support on the part of the government consistently raised political or state influence in sports. On the one hand, this contrasts with the model of autonomous sport that was postulated by the state as well as private sports organizations since the founding of the Nationales Olympisches Komitee für Deutschland (NOK, National Olympic Committee for Germany) in 1949 and the Deutscher Sportbund (DSB, German Sports Federation) in 1950 as umbrella organizations of all German sports associations and federations.[15] On the other hand, this principle of autonomy was partly abandoned by the policy of sports subsidies, since it was out of the question for sports organizations to be led and organized on a voluntary basis. Nonetheless, in West Germany, elite sports were simply not competitive in international Olympic events without the financial and material support of the political system. Elite sports had a unique relevance for national pride. For this reason, essential elements of monetary and administrative responsibility for elite sports were assigned to the German Home Office (BMI).

Since then, the BMI has negotiated annual allocations of funds for the various elite sports with the German sports associations and umbrella organizations. Inside the DSB, a specific and powerful committee was installed in 1965 to deal with the state subsidies and to find appropriate criteria for allocating this money to athletes. This committee was called the Bundesausschuss zur Förderung des Leistungssports (BA-L, Federal Committee for Achievement Sport). At this point, there would at least have been a hypothetical opportunity for the government to arrange anti-doping measures by spending tax money on elite sports, even if only for specific applications like anti-doping.

Uta Andrea Balbier, a sports historian, has noted that sports in West Germany became progressively more part of the responsibility of government, rather than of society. Accordingly, the German sports associations, represented by the NOK and the powerful BA-L in the DSB, degenerated into an instrument for organizing governmental allocations of funds, but without any efficient, democratic parliamentary control. The political desire for political-governmental participation became apparent with the founding of the Special Committee of Sport and the Olympic Games in the Bundestag in 1969. After the Olympic Games, this committee was renamed the Sports Commission in 1973 and became a regular Bundestag committee.[16]

This growing political and governmental influence on sports was partly the result of awarding the Games to Munich. However, it was also a reaction to the GDR and its sports policy, which firmly established sports in its constitution in 1968. The GDR served as an example for West Germany with regard to its sports system, support of athletes and talent, and talent scouting.

The GDR's sports policies served in many respects as a model for West Germany, as the exhibition "We Against Us," in the House of History in Bonn and Leipzig in 2009/10, clearly demonstrated.[17] All responsible, "modern"-thinking sports officials and politicians were aware of the fact that the old and essentially voluntary sports system needed to be reformed if they wanted to keep up with East Germany. This also meant that the democratic West Germany had to support sports mainly through tax revenue, but somehow without endangering its freedom and independence. Indeed, this turned out to be an idealistic and purely rhetorical strategy, which did not work in reality.

2. Specification of Elite Sports

Parallel with increasing governmental support, the field of elite sports and sports self-administration was centralized and professionalized in the run-up to the Olympic Games in 1972. This development was initiated partly by the sports organizations and their officials, but also partly from outside. With regard to this development, crucial steps entailed employing full-time national coaches and sports officials in the different sports associations, preparing medium-term benefits (mostly salary increases) and financial plans for sporting success, establishing and enhancing the Federal Committee for Achievement Sport as a central control and planning instrument, founding the German Sports Aid Foundation, establishing elite sports centers, forming A-, B-, and C-squads, establishing high schools with an emphasis on sports, and developing the competition *Jugend trainiert für Olympia* (Youth Training for Olympia).[18]

Many elements were based on the institutions and methods of the GDR, which seemed distinctly superior to West Germany regarding its preparation for the Olympic Games in Munich. However, because of the federal structure and democratic laws of West Germany, these measures could not be replicated precisely. Even so, they gathered a momentum of their own, which reduced their efficiency. A good example was the attempt to exploit "science" for elite sports, as was so commonplace in the GDR. However, this was impossible to replicate fully in West Germany, given the constitution and the freedom accorded to science and the universities.

3. Scientification of Sports

The sports sciences enhanced their status at the national and international levels in the course of preparing for the Olympic Games and through the associated increase in emphasis on elite sports.[19] The Olympic Congress of Science in Munich in 1972, which was organized by sports pedagogues and sports scientists, reflected the importance and advancement of these new sports sciences.[20] It is noteworthy that this was the only major international scientific congress in modern Olympic history to this day that formed part of the Games themselves.[21]

Governmental support for sports science was also noticeable in budgets. In 1960, the Federal Republic funded sports science with DM 70,000, and by 1965, with DM 560,000. Since 1970, financial support increased threefold within five years, excluding personnel expenses for professors and lecturers of sports science, who had been employed at universities, financed by the federal states, since the end of the 1960s.[22]

This development culminated in the foundation of the Bundestinstitut für Sportwissenschaft (BISp, Federal Institute of Sports Science) in October 1970. The German Home Office was and still is superior to the BISp. The support of science in the field of sports had been an activity that the DSB and the NOK, the umbrella organizations of federations and clubs in Germany, had been planning to conduct on their own since their founding. This changed with the establishment of the BISp as a department of the Home Office of the FRG. The support of the DSB for science and education became more theoretical than real. However, the structure of the former Central Committee for Scientific Research in the Field of Sport[23] of the DSB was essentially taken over from the BISp. From then on, the science of sports, developed mainly by scientists and physical educators at universities, was administered and financed through taxes and thus directly by the government. The initiation, support, and documentation of sports science and the building of sports facilities were established as a specific responsibility of the BISp. In the fiscal year 1972, the newly founded federal institution was already entitled to DM 5 million, of which DM 2 million was allocated to sports science research.[24]

Sports science entailed, first, sports medicine research and development. However, this all provoked an ongoing conflict between sports medicine and sports pedagogy or physical education, a dilemma that even increased subsequently in the course of the debate on the Grundsatzerklärung für den Spitzensport (Declaration of Principles for Top Sport) in 1977. While all questions concerning elite sports and the support of athletes were firmly located within the sports medicine sphere during the 1960s, and sports educators were responsible only for gymnastics at school, sports physicians lost their credibility and influence, not least because of doping problems that came to light step by step after the Games of 1972 and 1976. Not one sports physician was involved in preparing the Declaration of Principles for Top Sport in 1977. It was formulated by sports pedagogues and sports officials under the direction of Ommo Grupe, a leading professor of physical education and sports science, and was intended to place sports in the Federal Republic on a sounder ethical basis.

In the first two decades after the Second World War, it was unclear what direction the German sports model would take. Some debates took place between popular gymnastic sports (*Turnen*) on the one hand and the advocates of other elite sports on the other hand. However, after the award of the Olympic Games to Munich, all forces were concentrated on elite sports. In a sense, the Munich Games resolved the competition between gymnastics and sports in Germany in favor of the latter. From this perspective, the Munich Games decided the competition between gymnastics and sports in Germany. This could also be interpreted as a modernizing consequence of Munich. The orientation toward objective criteria and the expectations of athletic and sporting performance led to the fact that "the nomination of national teams [. . .] not only resulted from calculated figures according to the entry conditions of Olympic Games, but moreover, performance norms were taken into consideration," as a statement of the BA-L announced.[25]

The BA-L voted at the "allocation of public funds and private donation (German Sports Aid Foundation) in September to give priority to promising disciplines and athletes."[26] This was the decisive step toward the criterion of the *Endkampfchance* (finals opportunity) as a guideline of nomination, which has remained valid until today.

The public condemnation of doping through politics and sports officials, on the one hand, and the support criterion of the *Endkampfchance* that they required, on the other, led to structural support for hidden doping practices in both German and international sports.[27] The athletes and representatives of German sports in the government, clubs, and sports federations were divided between the expected striving for excellence—*citius, altius, fortius*—on the one hand and their commitment to a fair and doping-free sport on the other.

Therefore, while it appears quite obvious how the structure as well as the ideals and norms of sport changed in the Federal Republic over the course of the Olympic Games in 1972, the role of the Munich Games in the development of doping and anti-doping in the Federal Republic of Germany has barely been researched. This is even more surprising, since the parameters considered with respect to the political enhancement of conventional sports, elite sports, and sports science relate precisely to those fields that are fundamental to doping and anti-doping.

Below, the consequences of the allocation, preparation, and implementation of the Games for doping and anti-doping in the Federal Republic of Germany are examined. This is based on the doping controls at the Olympic Games of 1972 in Munich and the almost parallel establishment of a central department for doping analysis. To understand this process, it is necessary to outline the anti-doping policies of the International Olympic Committee, which is in charge of the Olympic Games.

ANTI-DOPING POLITICS OF THE IOC IN THE 1970S

A general problem of the IOC anti-doping politics had always been indecision about anti-doping measures. This was reflected especially in the IOC's way of dealing with anabolic steroids, which became more and more prominent from the late 1960s. At this time, sports physicians and IOC members such as Arthur Porritt and Arnold Beckett were already drawing attention to the fundamental problem of controlling the use of anabolic steroids:[28] Their long-term effectiveness made it possible to stop taking the steroids just before competing. This way, the doping tests could not prove the intake of steroids, but the athletes still gained the desired performance-enhancing effect.

This circumstance had a major effect on the previously used methods for controlling doping. It called for a new procedure that included, in particular, the establishment of all-year and unannounced "out-of-competition controls." However, it took thirty years for these controls to be converted into action. It was C. E. Yesalis and M. S. Bahrke who referred to this scenario in 2002 as the "IOC's Loss of Credibility," which the Canadian Dubin Commission had already criticized in 1990; the IOC had failed to counteract the spread of anabolic steroids in time and did not react to the shifting dimensions of doping, in comparison to previously used substances.[29]

The very late and hesitant attitude of the IOC had also been a result of its president's attitude. For a long time, Avery Brundage, the IOC president, misunderstood doping as an exclusive problem of professional sports and often came into conflict with the chairman of the Medical Commission, Alexandre de Merode (1934–2002).[30] In 1968, for the first time, the IOC conducted tests under the supervision of the Medical Commission during the Games of Grenoble and Mexico City. The tests were based on a list of prohibited substances and measures,[31] but they mostly tested for stimulants.[32]

The attitude of Avery Brundage was not only a result of his unbending attitude toward tradition, but was ultimately also caused by the financial and other options open to the IOC at the time. When the supervisor of IOC public relations work, Monique Berlioux, informed Brundage that the commission planned two conferences about doping before the Olympic Games in Munich started, Brundage responded that he did not see any need to spend time or money on such a redundant conference.[33]

After Brundage was informed that the Munich Organizing Committee was willing to pay the cost of those conferences, he clearly appreciated this offer but still emphasized that the IOC should delegate the responsibility. He wrote to de Merode that it would be "a little embarrassing" to let others settle the bill, "but probably in this instance it is not out of order, seeing that it is one of the obligations of the Organizing Committee to prepare for the medical tests."[34] In terms of the IOC's financial problems, it might also have had an effect on their members' perceptions of the forecasted cost of $1.5 million for the laboratory experiments.[35]

Looking at it from this aspect, financial considerations might have played an important role in the moderate approach to anti-doping activities in the environment of the Munich Games. The administration was left to the German Organizing Committee. The IOC published a doping brochure that reported on the meeting of the Medical Commission on July 29, 1971. A total of four thousand copies were sent to all members of the "Olympic establishments." Paul Dimeo has referred to this action as a "little gesture,"[36] which nonetheless raised anxiety among the IOC members with regard to the expected cost of doping tests. The brochure outlined the regulations of the Games of Sapporo and Munich, and distinguished clearly between the responsibilities of the IOC commission and the international associations of the different sports disciplines. The associations were in charge of technical issues, such as the amount of samples and the choice of participants and subjects for testing doping. The commission had the moral responsibility for the different kinds of controls and the supervision of the organization. Moreover, the commission suggested the exclusion of convicted athletes from the Olympic Games by the international associations.[37]

In the end, the IOC doping regulations were reformulated in the form of Rule 26, the so-called Eligibility Code, in April 1971.[38] However, the new version did not have any important differences in comparison to the old Games regulations of 1968. For that reason Dimeo has questioned its significance as a huge step toward the formalization of anti-doping rules.[39] In reality, the traditionalist Brundage was retaining his view that athletes had to be amateurs who committed themselves to the spirit and ethics of the Games: "The use of drugs or artificial stimulants of any kind is condemned."[40] But that was as far as he went, and he was not in favor of any concerted action.

SPORT POLITICS, DOPING, AND ANTI-DOPING IN WEST GERMANY

During the 1960s, the West German public took doping more and more seriously.[41] One of the most compelling cases was the death of the professional boxer Jupp Elze, which captured the attention of the German public in 1968. Elze died of cerebral bleeding, which he suffered during a boxing match. A postmortem revealed the use of various doping substances, such as amphetamines. As a result, an official anti-doping law, parallel to those in force in France and Belgium, was extensively discussed. Even the German Sports Federation (DSB) asked the Home Office (BMI) to consider to what extent legislation against doping could be implemented, especially given that previous and well-intentioned competition rules had proved ineffective.[42] However, the German government clung to its opinion that "the existing criminal law about negligent bodily injury and murder offered enough protection against doping, and further actions should be carried out by the sports associations themselves."[43]

One year after Jupp Elze's death, in 1969, the German public was confronted with a *Zeit* article called "Züchten wir Monstren?" (Are We Breeding Monsters?). The article in the highly regarded German weekly referred to the shot-putter and discus thrower Brigitte Berendonk, who fled the GDR in 1958. Berendonk served as an excellent example of the phenomenon of escalating anabolic steroid use in the GDR, as well as in the Federal Republic. Berendonk, who became one of the most famous critics of doping in Germany (and worldwide), claimed:

> Almost all world-class decathletes are on the pill, 90 percent of the throwers, putters and weightlifters, about half of the jumpers and sprinters, and also the oarsmen, swimmers and team players are becoming more and more in favor of it.[44]

Although Berendonk could not prove her figures empirically, the article still caused a sensation. Interestingly, copies of this article were found in the files of the BMI. Yet there was no reaction whatsoever, not even the briefest note in the files or an internal memorandum.

In spite of this article, the government maintained its position. This becomes quite clear with its response to the inquiry of the Christian Social Union politician Erich Riedl as to whether the federal government considered an anti-doping law to be necessary. The reply was that there were no indications that "sports in the Federal Republic were endangered by doping,"[45] that specific information about the use of doping substances was not available, and that the existing criminal law offered "extensive protection against doping."[46]

Instead, an attempt was made to control the use of doping substances with amendments of the statutes, controls, and sanctions that were internal to sports. Consequently, in May 1969, the BMI asked the German Sports Federation, the NOK, and the German Association for Sports Medicine and Prevention (Deutsche Gesellschaft für Sportmedizin und Prävention, DGSP) for information about previous steps against doping.[47] This led to the "General Guidelines for Doping Control," which were passed by the German Sports Federation in autumn 1970. It is interesting to note that the BMI was not only the catalyst for the development of the general guidelines, but also was actively involved in its formulation. As an example, a list of various medicines that contain prohibited substances can be traced back to a suggestion by the BMI. For the first time, a third, neutral opinion was brought into play in the course of the guideline formulation. This position was responsible for doping controls and analysis.

Unfortunately, the guidelines turned out to be worthless in terms of the anti-doping fight. This was caused by their separation from implementation and by the lack of interest on the part of the sports associations. Until 1977, only four associations, the Bund Deutscher Radfahrer (BDR, German Cycling Federation), the Deutsche Leichtathletik-Verband (DLV, German Athletics Federation), the Deutsche Reiterliche Vereinigung (German Federation of Equestrian Sports), and the Deutsche Tischtennis Bund (German Association of Table Tennis) had accepted the anti-doping regulation, which was actually expected of all the associations.[48] Furthermore, the doping reality had already superseded the guidelines before they were accepted. In conformity with IOC regulations, they prohibited only the use of soothing and stimulating substances, although at that point the anabolic period had already dawned.[49]

The German associations of elite sports, as well as other national associations, simply did not do enough to improve doping controls. In the course of the Winter Olympics of 1972 and during the preparations for the Munich Games, it was especially embarrassing for Germany, or rather for the German Association of Ice Hockey, that the one athlete out of 211 who tested positively for doping happened to be a West German ice-hockey player.[50] This occurred six months before the Summer Olympics started in Munich. On the occasion of the Munich Games, the German Organizing Committee offered to carry out tests itself. However, for the BA-L, this one case turned out just to be an unpleasant mishap, which was caused by individual misconduct of the team physician.[51]

Although the Deutscher Leichtathletik-Verband had signed the guidelines and also carried out tests, it did not enforce any consistent sanctions against positively tested athletes, as demonstrated by the case of the shot-putter H. B.,[52] who tested positively for stimulants (leptazol) in 1971. As a result, he was banned from the German athletics indoor championship, but was nominated again for the European athletics championship in Helsinki in the same year, owing to extenuating circumstances—the athlete had taken the medicine to treat influenza. This procedure provoked controversy with the IAAF, which had again demanded strict sanctions of doping cases prior to the championship.[53]

Both politicians and the public of the Federal Republic had the opportunity to gain information about anabolic doping before the Munich Games had started. Hansjörg Kofink, former track-and-field coach and representative of physical educators at schools, complained in an open letter to the German NOK that the female DLV shot-putters were not nominated in Munich "because of a lack of athletic performance." The West German female athletes had no chance against the doped athletes of East Germany, he complained.

This was also demonstrated by the remarkable sports performance in shot put of the latter since the mid-1960s. Kofink wrote in his letter to the NOK on August 5, 1972:

> Based on the experiences that I had during my time as a DLV coach since 1970 and the international contacts I made during that time, it is absolutely clear to me that such development without anabolic steroids or similar substances is inconceivable! It is surely a fact that the GDR and the USSR have passed the experimental stage with those substances and probably work with better (tolerable) substances. By the way, the experimental stage in Eastern Europe has apparently been stimulated by the pending Munich Summer Olympics. I can provide further information.[54]

DOPING CONTROLS AT THE MUNICH OLYMPIC GAMES OF 1972 AND THE ESTABLISHMENT OF A CENTRAL DOPING-ANALYSIS INSTITUTION IN COLOGNE

Before it became clear to what extent, which substances, and which testing procedure the IOC would use to control doping during the Olympic Games of 1972, the BMI had already been concerned with this issue. In May 1969, the BMI asked the NOK about the "1. latest regulations of the IOC with respect to doping, including a doping list; 2. work of the medical commission and 3. appropriate implementation and effectiveness of doping controls during the Olympic Games."[55]

On May 12, 1969, Manfred Donike sent a list to Herbert Reindell, president of the German Sports Doctors Association, about the time they would require to prepare the doping controls in Munich. Moreover, he promised to be "available for the doping examinations and their preparation in Munich."[56] Donike had a doctorate in biochemistry and had worked under Wildor Hollmann at the Institute for Sport Medicine and Circulation Research at the Sports University of Cologne since the mid-1960s. Here, he specialized in biochemical-detection methodology. The fact that Donike himself had been a professional cyclist was an asset to his doping research.[57]

However, Donike had a fellow applicant for the job of implementing controls and analysis during the Olympic Games. The Institute of Medicine Law and Insurance Medicine at the University of Munich applied as well and was initially preferred by the Organizing Committee (OC). Even at this early point in time, the Olympic Games in Munich acted as a motor for the further development of doping controls and analysis, at least at the level of science and research. The opportunity to conduct the controls in Munich was quite tempting for scientific institutes, since, apart from the scientific laurels and public attention, this project promised new jobs and modern equipment.

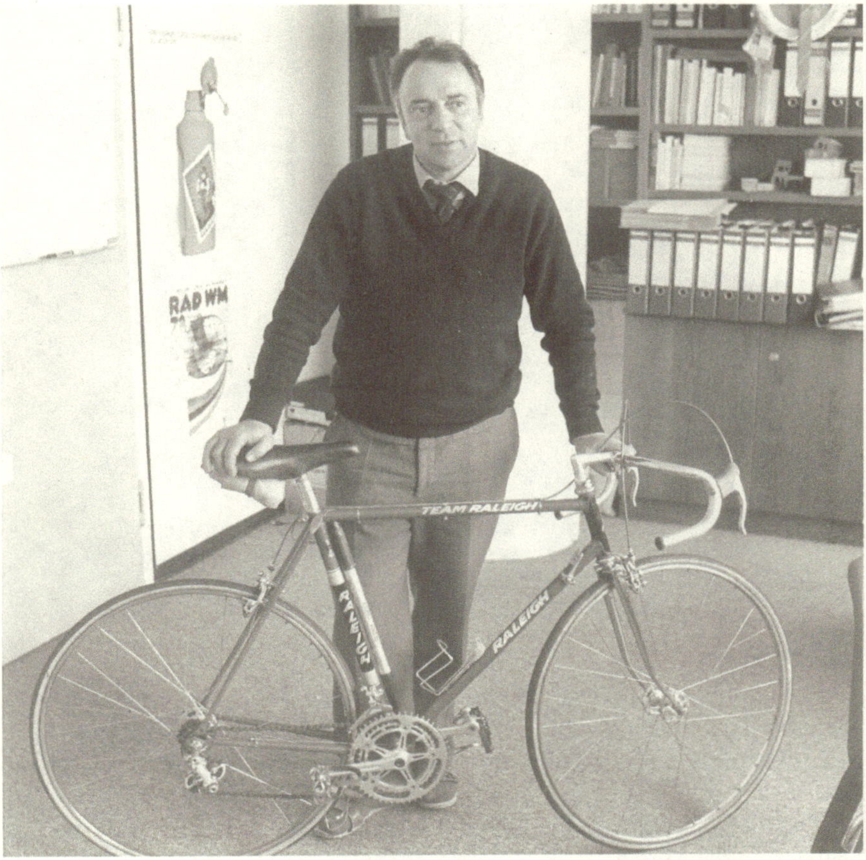

Figure 2.1. Professor Dr. Manfred Donike (1933–1995), founder and head of the Doping-Control Laboratory in Cologne (1974–1995). As a young man, Donike was a well-known and successful German cyclist. He participated twice in the Tour de France (1960 and 1961). After studying chemistry in Cologne, he became a scientist and was responsible for the doping controls of the IOC at the Olympic Games in Munich. After the Games, he became head of the German Doping-Control Laboratory and one of the most famous doping controllers in the world, a pioneer of doping analysis. ***Source: DSHS Köln***

This was all the more appealing as the Medical Commission of the IOC decided, together with the OC, to carry out doping controls in all sports disciplines for the first time in June 1970. The selection of the tested athletes, however, was still up to the various international associations.[58]The large scale of planned doping controls surprised the OC of the Games, which had not discussed any budgetary fund allocations for doping controls, at least not until May 1970.[59]

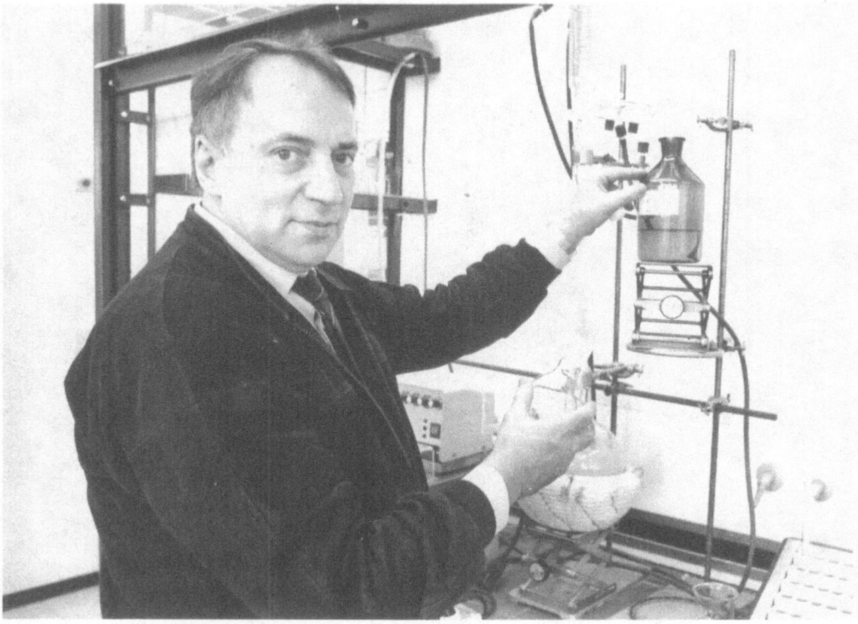

Figure 2.2.

Both applicants for the job of conducting the doping controls met once again during a meeting with the OC on October 16, 1970. The BMI was keen to ensure the establishment of an examination institution for the Olympic Games.

The Institute of Medicine Law in Munich offered to carry out the doping analysis on their premises. Professor Reindell rejected that offer. In his opinion, the responsibility should rest with a doping specialist, such as Dr. Donike of Cologne. Dr. Keul supported Professor Reindell, as well as Dr. Donike. The representatives of the Institute of Judicial Medicine intimated that they were not willing simply to offer their premises. If the leader of the doping analysis was not from the Institute of Judicial Medicine, another laboratory would have to be used.[60]

Apparently, the representatives of German sports medicine were quite determined to keep the nomination of doping controls and analysis inside the sports system—especially because this nomination would be a decision with an impact extending beyond the Games.

It was in fact about a major research resource in an area of general medicine and sports medicine, which was increasing in significance. At the same time, it was also about reputation, retaining participation in international congresses, and protecting the work that German sports medicine had already performed in this field since the mid-1960s.

Donike had never regarded himself as a sports physician, but always emphasized the fact that he was an independent biochemist and tied to the University of Cologne. Even though Donike was obviously not a sports physician, he was still respected by Hollmann, Keul, and Reindell as one of them. Subsequent discord between Donike and other specialists in sports medicine could also be understood in the context of Donike's increasing emancipation from his previous "fellow travelers."

The interference of the opinion leaders of German sports medicine was successful in the end. In early December 1970, the OC of the 1972 Olympic Games nominated Manfred Donike to head the Commission for Doping Analysis, and the sports physician Dr. Armin Klümper (Freiburg) for the Commission of the Sampling Procedure. During the Games, the doping analysis was to be performed in the Institute of Physiologic Chemistry and Physical Biochemistry at the University of Munich.

The decision for Donike and against the Institute of Judicial Medicine of the University of Munich, which extended beyond the Olympic Games, could be traced back to the advocacy of Hollmann, Keul, and Reindell. They had been the representatives of the Sports Doctors Association and original contacts of the BMI on questions of doping and anti-doping since the mid-1960s. For that reason, they had already gained the appropriate influence, and in addition, Donike had established a name for himself as a doping expert.

Along with the acknowledged doping experts Ludwig Prokop and Arnold Beckett, Manfred Donike was also actively involved in writing the twenty-four-page brochure of the IOC Medical Commission for the Games of Sapporo and Munich, as mentioned above. The brochure included a doping list (mainly stimulants, no anabolic steroids) and described the planned controlling procedure in detail. The criteria and number of tested athletes, as well as the implementation of sanctions, were up to the various associations.

Donike and his team were then allowed to try out the procedure and the instruments they would use for Munich during various German championships and international events.[61] During the Games in Munich, Donike and his team took samples in "all in all 282 assignments [. . .] 2079 urine samples and 65 blood samples."[62] The blood samples were taken at the shooting competition (pistol and rifle) in order to examine the blood-alcohol level. In the end, seven positive doping tests were officially confirmed and another fourteen tests were positive for sedatives. All fourteen were tested at the shooting competitions of the modern pentathletes and marksmen. Yet the perpetrators were not punished, because the responsible associations argued that the regulations were not provided on time.

Nonetheless, Manfred Donike and his colleagues Armin Klümper and Dirk Clasing regarded their doping controls and analysis as a complete success. The procedure of athlete selection was *allegedly* an optimal compromise between the laboratory capacity and the desire to test as many athletes as possible. "A sufficient spread" was assured.[63] The equipment used and the methods had proven successful. The only critique expressed by the three German specialists in sports medicine was the fact that the Medical Commission of the IOC did not allow accompanying interviews with athletes on their medication before the competition days commenced. Donike, Klümper, and Clasing held "national status-consciousness, mystification of the national performance, and concerns about discrimination" responsible for this shortcoming.[64]

More detailed information with regard to the substances contained is not listed in the report. Certainly, Donike and his team might also have found anabolic steroids. The American discus thrower Jay Silvester conducted an informal survey of athletes (apart from long-distance runners). Sixty-eight percent admitted taking anabolic steroids prior to the Games and 61 percent even within the previous six months.[65] Nevertheless Clasing maintained that the doping controls in Munich had set "internationally accepted standards."[66]

An important and sustainable result of the "successful" tests in Munich was the establishment of a central doping-analysis institution (*Dopingzentrallabor*) for the Federal Republic in Cologne in 1974 under the leadership of Manfred Donike. This doping laboratory was officially acknowledged by the IOC, as was its East German counterpart in Kreischa (near Dresden).[67] The laboratory in Cologne was established mainly with the equipment used for the doping tests in Munich. Related to its political meaning, it is remarkable that this analytical institution was installed mainly by the BMI and counseled by the Deutscher Sportärztebund (German Sports Doctors Association), whereas the German Sports Federation at best only accompanied this process. Nonetheless, the acceptance, utilization, and success of the new institution depended on the various sports associations, which still showed a lack of interest in doping controls.

INTERIM RESULTS

The preparation for and implementation of the 1972 Olympic Games in Munich entailed a drive for modernization of German sports, which included the role of doping and anti-doping. The social configuration of sports changed in that it became more complex and sophisticated. New national and international protagonists appeared on the scene and left their mark. Sports, government and policy, medicine and science, economy, and the media were all affected fundamentally. The doping issue, as a familiar and genuine problem, seemed to disappear behind new political and social sports challenges. The various sports associations, especially in West Germany, were not willing to accept that doping posed a serious threat to their sports. Considering this scenario, Munich served as a distinctive example of this public opinion. These Games were intended to show the world a new, modern, positive, colorful, and optimistic view of Germany and West German sports. The terrorist act on September 5, 1972, shattered this dream and pushed the doping issue even more into the background. Moreover, the volunteers working in the sports associations in Germany were overworked anyway.

The Games of Munich, their preparation, implementation, and consequences showed that the state itself, or rather the federal government and parliament, not only became the central financier of German elite sports, but also began to play an active role in sports policy. On the one hand, this affected the political expectations of sports association performance. On the other hand, it also affected the athletes who participated in international competitions and championships, as well as political engagement in and commitment to doping control. The establishment of the Federal Institute of Sports Science and the Doping-Control Laboratory in Cologne represented this political involvement in sports. Another crucial motivation was the rivalry with GDR sports or rather the "example of the GDR."

In a popular speech at the Protestant Academy of Tutzing, the parliamentary secretary of the BMI, Kurt Jung, defined the "norms, objectives and priorities of sports policy" to the federal government in September 1973:

> In terms of sport support, the federal government was guided by the independence of sports, based on a partnership which has to be protected. The federal government regards its main role as supporting the plans and visions of sports, giving advice and being flexible in the event of change. This does not mean that the control function, which is necessarily connected with the allocation of public funds, cannot be limited.[68]

In terms of the support of elite sports, Jung explained:

> We do not want to make robots, we just want to help optimize the present natural abilities. We are fully aware of the danger that during a competition in elite sports, the individuals involved may now and then attempt to find ways and means to extend human performance with inappropriate substances. That is why we are setting up a tight connection between the Federal Institute and a doping-analysis institution this year to counteract such dangers.[69]

The establishment of a central institution to analyze urine and blood samples was an important step for the anti-doping policy of the Federal Republic. For the first time, it was possible to examine a larger number of samples—up to two hundred per week—in a universal and standardized procedure. The examination was state of the art. At the same time, it was possible to research potential improvements to detection methodology. The

Federal Republic played a significant role in this development, through its financial funding of the "Donike Institute."

The creation of a central institution was closely connected with the doping controls carried out during the 1972 Olympic Games in Munich, which were also supervised by Manfred Donike. In a way, these activities can be viewed as a test run for the doping analysis in Cologne from 1974 onward. Therefore, the Olympic Games served, as mentioned before, as a catalyst for the development of systematic doping controls in the Federal Republic.

The doping-analysis institution involved the Federal Republic actively in anti-doping control, and the laboratory became a protagonist in this field. The fact that the Federal Republic also played an active part, or at least the role of a mediator, in doping matters, based on its increasing support of elite sports with a policy of not listening and turning a blind eye to problematic issues, was barely addressed by contemporaries at that time. Within the examined period, the Federal Republic did not do justice to its above-mentioned "control function" with regard to doping. Neither were the serious indications of the spread of anabolic steroid use investigated, nor were associations sanctioned that had not accepted the guidelines and did not conduct doping controls. It remains unclear whether this problem can be attributed to national-prestige thinking or to the postulated "independence of sports."

Furthermore, the belief was widespread that doping could be controlled with improved controls and analytical procedures alone, as expressed in a quotation from Donike before the Munich Olympics: "After all previous experiences, you can say that doping controls, when properly carried out, reduce the misuse of drugs in sports and with regular repetition, stop it almost completely."[70]

In conclusion, the will of sports associations, federal offices, politicians, and parliamentarians was not strong enough to impose effective anti-doping measures. The expectation of solving the doping problem solely with scientific methods simultaneously reflected the planning euphoria, excessively scientific orientation, and belief in the organizational power of the Federal Republic at that time. It was not until the so-called oil shock, first economic downturns, and terrorism that these expectations were permanently shaken. According to Dimeo: "The task of anti-doping was handed over to scientists who viewed the problem in a modernist rational-bureaucratic way, assuming that better science and more testing would solve the problem."[71]

The 1976 Olympic Games in Montreal and the great doping hearing of the Sports Commission of the German Bundestag constituted just such a shake-up to sports in the Federal Republic and the doping issue.

DOPING AND ANTI-DOPING UP TO THE OLYMPIC GAMES OF MONTREAL IN 1976

Initially, anti-doping policies since the 1960s were intended (only) to reduce the use of stimulants in top-level sports. Stimulants continued to be used, but new substances, especially hormones and anabolic steroids (anabolics), became popular in the 1970s and beyond. Whereas stimulants were used mainly in endurance sports like running, distance rowing, or cycling, anabolics had initially been developed to treat people with serious diseases, in order to prevent muscle atrophy and to enhance muscle growth during recuperation. Yet, not surprisingly, anabolic hormones like testosterone and artificially produced steroids such as, for example, the well-known drug Oral Turinabol ("blue pills"), found their way into top-level athletics. The pharmaceutical company Jenapharm in the city of Jena in the GDR produced these drugs specifically for use in sports. Anabolic steroids became a major phenomenon of top-level sports.[72] These drugs were highly attractive to athletes in sports that depended on muscular strength, like heavy athletics and bodybuilding, which is in some respects a unique sport or arguably no sport at all. One could argue that the only aim of bodybuilding is to show off one's overdeveloped muscles.

PROBLEMS IN PREVENTING ANABOLIC-STEROID ABUSES IN SPORTS

Sports physicians, sports doctors, and officials did not agree for a long time on whether or not certain medications like anabolic steroids should be declared as doping and thus put on the doping list. In 1970, the International Amateur Athletic Federation (IAAF) was the first international sports organization to ban anabolic steroids.[73] The West German Athletics Federation (DLV) adapted its competition rules quickly, but decided one year later to withdraw this decision. A year later, anabolic steroids could be seen yet again on the doping list of the DLV.[74]

Anabolic steroids particularly affected heavy athletics, namely the weightlifters. Whereas the DLV had declared anabolic steroids as doping, the Federal Association of German Weightlifters (BVDG) reported in 1972, "according to the medical commission of the European Weightlifting Federation [. . .] the use of anabolic steroids was not regarded as doping."[75] This message was published before the German championships of 1972 and before the Munich Olympics, for which doping controls had been planned.

The doping list of the Deutsche Sportbund (DSB) of 1970 in the "Rahmen-Richtlinien zur Bekämpfung des Dopings" (Guidelines for Combating Doping), intended to be an orientation for the national sports associations, which would specify their own anti-doping rules, did not include or even mention anabolic steroids until 1977. The anti-doping tests of Mexico City 1968 and Munich 1972, which were the responsibility of the IOC, also did not consider anabolic steroids. In 1974, the IOC Medical Commission and its spokesman, Alexandre de Merode, announced that in Montreal 1976, anabolic steroids would be tested for the first time in sports and Olympic history, given that scientists had succeeded in developing reliable tests to detect artificially produced steroids.[76]

The hesitance of the sports organizations to test and control the misuse of anabolic steroids cannot be explained only by a lack of interest or even attempts to conceal or neglect the fundamental problems caused by this new phase of doping. The documents show clearly that there are at least four more reasons why reducing anabolic doping was complicated, inconsistent, and controversial among the various actors attempting to reduce doping, or claiming to do so.

First, anabolic steroids seemed to be less relevant than stimulants. Fatal doping cases had been caused by stimulants and, therefore, the focus was still on them. Scientific discussions as well as political debates and proposals, for example, for the European Council and the IOC, but also from within the international and national sports federations, merely mentioned anabolic steroids in the 1960s and early 1970s, but anabolics had not yet been regarded as relevant doping.

Second, the traditional definition of doping referred to those stimulants that could be tested before and after competitions, but not to hormones and anabolics that could be tested effectively and sustainably only in out-of-competition controls. Numerous experts like the Austrian scientist and sports doctor Prokop were not even sure of the effects and side effects of anabolic steroids with respect to the performance and health of athletes. In 1970, Prokop spoke of an "unresolved problem" without "consistent opinions and therefore without general regulations and prescriptions."[77]

Third, sports physicians and sports officials assumed that anabolic steroids could be included in doping lists only to the extent to which clear testing methods were available. In 1965, the International Anti-Doping Conference, which had formulated some basics for the convention against doping of the European Council, had argued that the criterion of incontestable evidence was a precondition for including a substance or medication in a doping list. This argument had been repeated in the German directives of 1970. The IOC had classified anabolic steroids as doping after an intensive discussion during the IOC session in Tehran in 1967, but it had not listed them for the same reason that the use of these substances could not yet be proved conclusively: "There had been considerable progress in the field of hormones and steroids, but it was not possible at this point to control these substances. As the

Commission had to be certain before carrying out tests, these products were not on the list of prohibited substances."[78]

Fourth, the scientific community had not yet reached a consensus on the effects and side effects of anabolic steroids. The verdicts of experts ranged from highly effective to ineffective to placebo effects only, from harmless side effects for health to highly dangerous long-term damage, which indeed happened, as we know today. The final statement of an international conference on doping of the British Association of Sports Doctors in 1975 argued as follows: "The actions of anabolic steroids in healthy, training athletes are not fully understood. Studies show conflicting results in respect of increases in body size, measures of strength and improvement of performance."[79] While the experts did not agree, the athletes themselves were convinced that anabolic steroids enhanced performance enormously. Indeed, some athletes stated this openly and there was apparently an increasing prevalence of their use.

Compared to the deadly doping disasters caused by stimulants, the negative effects of anabolic steroids were regarded as fairly harmless. Scientists and pharmacists promised to enhance performance and at the same time to diminish the negative side effects. An important argument emerged, namely that anabolic hormones or steroids were actually "natural." Every human body produces these hormones all the time and athletes have to cope with extraordinary physical demands. Therefore, they need more calories, vitamins, minerals, and other substances than those who are physically less challenged. If the athletic body was not able to produce enough anabolic steroids by itself to perform at high levels, these hormones should be applied externally. This argument could even be used to legitimize anabolics according to the ethical principles of medicine, as well as of sports, because from this perspective, an athlete is not then a "normal," natural and healthy human being.[80] By contrast, he is a special human being supposed to deliver extraordinary achievements that are not possible without external support. It could even be regarded as unethical if an athlete were *not* supported in this manner and left alone with his deficient physical potential, given the expected performance. A doctor who supports an athlete by providing anabolic steroids in order to substitute expended natural resources does not act immorally or unethically, according to this philosophy, but fully in conformity with his oath as a doctor. French doctors spoke of "reéquilibrage hormonal," using the same argument to legitimize the administration of hormones for top-level athletes.[81] GDR sports doctors referred to "unterstützende Mittel"—supporting means, including not only anabolics, but everything they could come up with to enhance the performance of their athletes.

Arguing in this manner was intended to put doping on the same plane as other therapeutic means. This strategy may have helped to overcome the moral reservations of numerous medical scientists and doctors who wished to support top-level athletes without acting against the ethos of medicine and of sport. The view prevailed that the mere use of anabolic steroids or drugs in general was not illegal or nonlegitimized doping, but only their *uncontrolled* use. In contrast, top-level sports without medical expertise seemed to be impossible or even wrong. This discourse on anabolic steroids marked a point of no return with respect to the medical support of top-level sports. Sports doctors became major players in both contexts of top-level sports in general, and doping and anti-doping especially. Top-level sports had clearly ceased to be a leisure-time activity for amateurs.

ANABOLIC STEROIDS, THEIR PREVALENCE IN TOP-LEVEL SPORTS, AND DOPING CONTROLS

As mentioned above, proving the use of doping and especially of anabolic steroids has always been difficult, and this remains the case today. The estimated number of undetected cases of doping is probably much higher than detected ones. The official statistics of doping controls by the sports federations and their results are certainly not valid, and even less so with respect to anabolic steroids. Crucial to this problem are the technical, organizational, and logistical difficulties of proving the presence of doping substances by valid scientific methods, as well as the handling of doping controls. It is not sufficient merely to prove the use of artificial hormones; this must be tested before competitions and not on the occasion of competitions, as is the case for stimulants. However, out-of-competition controls were not introduced until the end of the 1980s.

Apart from doping practices in the former GDR, those in Western sports have not been well documented, if at all. As we know from the research of Giselher Spitzer and Brigitte Berendonk, based on documents in the archives, the "central anabolic period" in the GDR began in 1974 with the overall, systematic support and supervision of East German athletic use of anabolic steroids.[82] In West Germany, the situation was unclear. An essential indicator of the spread of anabolics in certain sports is the development of extreme achievements, especially in those sports measuring achievement in centimeters, grams, and seconds, the so-called cgs sports.[83] A survey of German top-level athletes in the 1980s, published by the journal *Sports International*, showed the widespread use of anabolic steroids in most German sports and by most athletes.[84]

In fact, athletes were able to dope with anabolic steroids until at least 1976 without any testing, controlling, or sanctioning by sports organizations. The first controls of anabolics took place at the Olympic Games of Montreal in 1976, when the doping tests seemed to be sufficiently valid. In general, the specific doping controls by the various federations differed, as the documents verify. The cyclists—Bund Deutscher Radfahrer (BDR)—and the track-and-field athletes—Deutscher Leichtathletik-Verband (DLV)—were the federations most actively controlling their athletes, but only at competitions and only for stimulant drugs, at least until the end of the 1970s. Further large and important federations—swimmers, boxers, equestrians, modern pentathletes, ice skaters, skiers, rowers, and weightlifters—were hesitant, testing or being tested rather unsystematically and mostly at larger international events only.[85]

Doping controls soon provoked various awkward questions with respect to ethical or moral as well as legal aspects. One issue was whether the tested and detected substances had in fact been used intentionally to enhance competitive performance. Most positively tested athletes argued that the doping substances had entered their bodies unintentionally, either by accident or as a side effect of dietary supplements. This serious regulatory problem has in fact never been resolved. The case of the German cycling champion of 1971, Dieter Leitner, who had tested positively for amphetamines, is typical. However, he was not sanctioned, because his explanation that he had drunk from the possibly drug-laden bottle of another cyclist could not be disproved.[86]

A second issue concerned athletes who really did need medical, therapeutic help (or who were declared as such by a doctor). This problem does not refer exclusively to anabolic steroids, but to the use of drugs in general. The myth of pervasively healthy top athletes is indeed not true, at least not across the board. In fact, many suffer some degree of ill health, which may be more or less relevant to their sport. In addition, diseases can also be alleged, in order to legitimize the application of certain drugs, which is of course doping. Numerous cases are reported of amphetamine and ephedrine dopers who attempt to explain or excuse their behavior on the grounds of medical, therapeutic necessity, and who are supported by their medical advisers or doctors. However, it seems strange indeed that numerous top-level cyclists suffer from asthma and therefore, say their doctors, desperately need ephedrine. A typical case was that of the German decathlete Erich Klamma. At the German championship of 1970, he had tested positive for Captagon, a popular stimulant drug of the 1970s and 1980s that included the stimulant substance fenethylline. There is some evidence that Captagon was also used in football and soccer. Klamma argued that he needed this drug to treat pyelitis, which had also been confirmed formally in a medical report from his doctor.[87]

Such arguments have often been used by athletes, coaches, supporters, officials, and doctors. On the one hand, these arguments can be seen as simple self-defense, but on the other hand, they concern serious and fundamental ethical, legal, and structural questions of doping control and sanctions. In fact, the difference between the doping-related misuse of drugs and therapeutic use has never been quite clear. The ongoing problems with doping controls and sanctions have led to more elaborate regulations, with the rules or regulations increasing from small brochures to entire volumes.

However, at that time, these fundamental problems had not yet been considered in the regulations of the sports federations, neither by cyclists nor by track-and-field athletes. According to the guidelines of the DSB of 1970, as well as the official competition regulations of the track-and-field or athletic federation (DLV), the application of listed substances was forbidden in general. However, such a solution is neither appropriate nor fair with respect to athletes who really need these substances because of specific and genuine health problems. On the other hand, medically indicated exceptions to the general rule could be and were undoubtedly misused.[88]

Beyond the question of what to do with positively testing and duly doped athletes who plausibly denied any intention to dope, further aspects can be identified concerning these basic and fundamental problems of testing and controlling doping.

First, the question of how valid the tests really were was a subject of ongoing debate. The above-mentioned athlete Klamma, for example, tested positive a second time in 1971 for amphetamines, one year after his positive Captagon doping test. He and his lawyer challenged the validity of the new method of gas chromatography, after which the sport tribunal of the DLV decided that Klamma could not be sanctioned after all because of the possible bias of various experts. It could not be stated categorically that Klamma had doped, so that "in dubio pro reo" applied, that is, when in doubt, (decide) for the accused.[89]

Second, the question of how to deal with the different doping lists from various national as well as international federations could not be answered satisfactorily. For example, a female high jumper tested positive for the amphetamine norfenefrine in 1975. The athlete could not be sanctioned and was merely reprimanded "because the detected substance was not listed by the IAAF but only by the German athletics federation DLV."[90]

Third, what was to be done with athletes who did not appear at doping controls or who refused to be tested? A typical case is that of a hurdle sprinter in 1974 who did not appear at the controls. The DLV chair again decided not to sanction, but only to admonish him. The chairman stated that the legal situation is "not sufficiently clear" if an athlete has missed testing or refuses to be tested.[91]

Fourth, evidence of whether and to what extent coaches and doctors were involved in doping cases was always difficult to provide. A good example was the case of a coach for the cycling team of Lower Saxony in 1973, who had been accused by a cyclist of encouraging athletes to take forbidden substances. However, the board decided to close the proceedings because of a lack of evidence.[92]

These cases show in general that the associations and federations of West German sports were controlling and sanctioning doping rather timidly. This behavior may, however, have been caused less by moral indifference than by technical and practical problems. What could one really do with positive tests when the intention of the athlete to dope was unclear or unproved? The athletes themselves were not used to being controlled and tested. Athletes who really had to take medically indicated pharmaceuticals did not care about these tests. Therefore, Manfred Donike claimed, with respect to the doping tests in Munich in 1972, that positive tests would be more the result of "misunderstandings than intended and conscious attempts at doping."[93]

In principal, the federations had little interest in controlling and sanctioning doping consistently, for two simple reasons. First, some successful (and honest) athletes would be excluded from competing, and second, doping cases damage the public image of sports. However, sports organizations wish to be successful with strong and healthy athletes, and they want to look after their public image. Therefore, sports organizations must always deal with fundamental conflicts of interest if they really wish to reduce doping consistently and sustainably.

THE DOPING GAMES OF MONTREAL 1976: "KOLBE INJECTION" AND "AIR CLYSTER SCANDAL"—AND THEIR POLITICAL CONSEQUENCES

The Olympic Games of Montreal 1976 and their aftermath marked a fundamental shift in international sports politics as well as national and international anti-doping policies. The Games had signaled clearly that the Olympic movement and especially the IOC had to change their policies and ideological basics if the Olympic Games were to have a bright future. The international Olympic movement had to become more independent of state politics, as well as more independent financially. Step by step, the IOC deviated from its dogma of amateurism and finally abandoned it in 1981 with the Olympic Congress of Baden-Baden.[94] This development was crucial. The first and most important Olympic principle had now been realized, that the truly best athletes from all over the world would participate at the Games. In fact, at that time, pure amateurs simply did not exist in top-level sports, and the best athletes were indeed professionals who worked hard at and for their sport. However, the departure from amateurism and its spirit also implied departing from the basic sense of Olympic amateur sports to be played for their own sake and not functionalized by economic and related motivations.

If sports and games simply become jobs and a way to earn a living and sometimes to become really rich, the temptation to dope increases commensurately. However, the—officially—amateur games of Montreal had already in fact been an arena for doping. For everyone willing to look, the Games had revealed the considerable prevalence of doping in specific sports and disciplines, especially swimming and track and field, mainly with anabolic steroids.

The history of the West German team and its preparation for the Montreal Games exemplified the general moral crisis of top-level sports, which can also be regarded as a result of defining doping merely in terms of a list of forbidden methods and substances. The Germans respected the doping list of the IOC. However, some of the representatives, athletes, and coaches tried everything else to enhance the performance of West German athletes at the Games, including means that cannot be regarded as a legitimate part of regular training or coaching, but that did not formally breach the anti-doping regulations. Vitamin pills or various dietary supplements seemed to offer an ideal means of enhancing physical performance without breaking the rules. In anticipation of the Montreal Games, West German athletes, some coaches, and doctors were thinking about creative solutions. They found at least two, the "Kolbe injection" and the "air clyster method" intended to improve swimming conditions and, ultimately, performance. Both were intensively and controversially discussed in the sports context, as well as in public, including the consequences for sports and anti-doping policies in Germany.[95]

The "Kolbe injection" became part of the German doping and anti-doping history because of the top-level rower Peter Michael Kolbe, odds-on favorite for the gold medal of the single final in Montreal. He had received such an injection before the race and failed disappointingly. The collapse of Kolbe was scandalized in the German media and by Kolbe himself, who justified his failure in terms of this injection. Kolbe had been rowing clearly ahead of the competition when he surprisingly broke down shortly before the end of the race. He was overtaken by his Finnish colleague Pertti Karppinen, who won the gold medal.[96]

The Kolbe injection was in fact not really doping, but included the substances cocarboxylase and thioctic acid, neither listed by the IOC anti-doping rules. However, this mixture had been created especially by West German scientists according to the pattern of a special drug for top athletes in the GDR. The secret behind these substances had been revealed by Alois Mader, a scientist and sports doctor of the former GDR who fled to the West in 1974. Immediately upon his arrival, Mader had been hired by the Centre of West German Sports Doctors in Cologne, where he worked at the institute of Wildor Hollmann, head of West German Sports Medicine. In spring 1976, the West German sports scientists started tests on these substances, based on Mader's revelations. The tests were successful and demonstrated impressive performance-enhancing effects.[97] "According to responsible officials of the German Sports Federation," reported Herbert Reindell, president of the German Sports Doctors Association, specific injections were produced for the use of the West German athletes in Montreal. More than 1,200 ampules were allegedly sent to Montreal.[98]

In sum, the Kolbe injection was indeed formally not doping, because the injection did not violate any doping rules. However, the whole story illustrated the will of athletes as well as of doctors and officials to enhance performance by all possible means beyond physical training, but without contravening the prevailing anti-doping rules and anti-doping lists. Compared to similar attempts in the early days of doping, the production of such performance-enhancing drugs was the result of scientific support, research, and testing. The athlete himself became part of a "system," dependent on support from his network. In this case, the Kolbe injection had additionally been imitated by the obviously successful model of top-level sports in the GDR, which was regarded by West German scientists, doctors, officials, and even politicians as a model of best practice. However, the experiment failed in reality, with Kolbe losing the race. He in fact became a victim of the development of modernization and *totalization* of top-level sports. However, there is no definite proof that Kolbe failed because of this injection or if there were other relevant reasons for the loss. But the principle of maximizing sporting achievement and success by all permitted (and sometimes not permitted) means had survived intact.

THE AIR CLYSTER SCANDAL

High-speed swimming depends essentially on the position of the body in the water. Therefore, tests were made to improve the positioning by means beyond the usual training of bodily, (natural) technical, and coordinative abilities. Experiments were conducted by putting air into the bowel, to put it bluntly. When these questionable experiments became public in the media, they caused a further scandal of West German sports in the context of the Montreal Olympics. This scandal is important in that not only sport officials and sports doctors fostered these experiments, but also the state and responsible politicians spent money testing these dubious practices.

The then chairman of the Bundesausschuss Leistungssport (BA-L, Federal Committee for Achievement Sport)[99] in the German Sports Federation (DSB), Helmut Meyer, described the unique history as follows. Some athletes had reported new methods of enhancing performance in swimming. The national handball goalkeeper Hans-Jürgen Bode, spokesman of the athletes in the BA-L board, had finally admitted knowing about such "special" methods of enhancing performance in swimming, and in some detail, which had already been tested successfully by top-level swimmers. He demanded DM 1 million to reveal his knowledge and announced that he would sell all that he knew to other national teams if the German sports officials did not accept his offer.[100] Clearly, this request could also be seen as a kind of blackmail, and because it came from an athlete representing all others in the BA-L board, it was more than unusual and demonstrated the moral change, even deterioration, as top-level athletes adapted their views of sports and games. They no longer saw themselves as amateurs playing for fun and for the sake of sports itself, but as businessmen. That the officials of the German sports organizations, as well as politicians, responded positively to this blackmail was more than just a sign of moral confusion as to the ethical fundaments of top-level sports and games. Sports had now very definitely departed the sphere of a harmless and innocent amateur activity to become part of business and politics.

As a result, the German Swimming Federation agreed to further negotiations with Bode on three conditions. First, the fee had to be reduced. Second, the methods or substances should not jeopardize the health of the athletes. Third, they should not contravene the competition and anti-doping rules of the international federation and the IOC.

The BA-L, led by chairman Helmut Meyer, arranged the negotiations between the German Swimming Federation and Bode. The contract with the latter included a fee of DM 150,000 if the performance enhancement amounted to more than 1 percent, and an incentive payment of DM 250,000 for more than 1.5 percent. At the same time, the BA-L and the Swimming Federation submitted an application to the Ministry of the Interior (BMI) to "support performance-enhancing methods" for swimmers to the amount of DM 250,000.[101] Whether the BMI knew about the arrangement with Bode remains unclear.

The BMI allocated the money to the Swimming Federation subject to the conditions that (first) Professor Keul would ensure that the methods did not jeopardize the health of the athletes, that (second) Dr. Donike had to ensure that the methods did not contravene to the rules of the IOC and the International Swimming Federation (FINA), and that (third) the methods would only be used at the Olympic Games in Montreal in accordance with the National Olympic Committee.[102] All of these conditions were duly fulfilled. The air clyster method was tested during the training camp in Calgary before the Games. Finally, all representatives of the BA-L, as well as the Swimming Federation and the doctors and athletes themselves, agreed to use the method in Montreal—with only one vote against. However, when the competition in Montreal had started, the tests had to be completed during the prelims, because of "the lack of technical preconditions." Finally, the new method was not even applied at all—DM 250,000, or about EUR 120,000, of tax money for nothing, and for a morally questionable method of enhancing performance that was based on a strange, blackmail-like business process.[103]

This second example, apart from the Kolbe injection, showed once again that German athletes, as well as officials, were looking for and testing all conceivable means of enhancing performance. However, all actors were eager to claim that what they were doing was neither illegal nor dangerous. In contrast to the case of the Kolbe injection, the state authorities were involved in this publicly scandalized air clyster project. However, although the politicians and state officials had provided money, they shifted the responsibility to the sports authorities. This dubious division of roles between state and sport had long been used in West Germany. The state sponsored top-level sports, but the sports officials decided how the (tax) money was to be spent. They were responsible for the "content," although politicians and administrators should have the political responsibility to ensure that tax revenue is spent appropriately and according to the law. Elected politicians and ministers are obliged to protect people from damage, according to the oath sworn by ministers. These public representatives are thus supposed to prevent and control doping, which is a danger not only to the ethos of sport in general, but in very real terms, to the health and bodily integrity of individual athletes, and in the longer run, also to those playing games and sports at a lower level. Regarded from a current perspective, it would seem that the state function of controlling doping and generally spending tax money suitably on top-level sports was not fulfilled. This failure can be explained by the historical and political context of the Cold War.

POLITICAL CONTEXTUALIZATION OF DOPING AND ANTI-DOPING IN THE 1970S AND 1980S

The leading politicians of the West German Bundesrepublik during the Cold War had to deal with conflicting objectives with respect to sports, the "benefits" of doping, and doping control. On the one hand, the autonomy of sport was to be maintained according to the principles of the relationship between state authorities and private clubs, as organized after 1945, based on dealing with the experiences of the totalitarian Nazi regime. This relationship rested on the mutual reliance that sport organizations would respect the laws of the Federal Republic, as well as those of fair play in sports and games and the applicable rules. On the other hand, top-level sports had become a respectable component of international and therefore national politics. The nation intended to become visibly successful at international sporting events like the Olympic Games and world championships. This became quite dominant over the course of the Cold War confrontation between top athletes of the capitalist West and the socialist East—and nowhere more so than in divided Germany. The East German politicians did literally everything possible to ensure that "their" athletes won or at least performed better than "their" West German competitors. The West German politicians recognized that their own athletes could keep up with those of the East only if they were better supported—with money as well as more effective institutions, professional coaches, medical aid, and so on. They were also aware of the fact that forbidden means like doping were used to win the Cold War on the track, relying not least on the knowledge provided by the secret services of both sides, as well as information from athletes, coaches, and doctors who had fled from the East.[104]

As mentioned above, the GDR athletes scored third on the medal count at the Munich Olympics of 1972, and second at the Montreal Games of 1976, immediately after their socialist "brothers and sisters" of the Soviet Union. For Moscow 1980 and, definitely, Los Angeles 1984, the GDR sports officials planned to beat the Soviet Union on the track.[105] Montreal was intended to demonstrate the superiority of the socialist world in top-level sports. However, it was common knowledge that this superiority was the result not only of consistent, systematic, and legitimate scientific support of all kinds, but of illegal doping as well. The swimmers of the GDR established seventeen world records at the twenty-seventh national swimming championships of the GDR in 1976, which were also used as qualifications for the Montreal Olympics. The female GDR swimmers set thirteen world records in the fourteen world-championship disciplines. At the world championships of Belgrade in 1973, the female GDR swimmers had already set seven world records and won ten of fourteen races, whereas one year before, at the Olympics in Munich, these swimmers had not succeeded in winning even one gold medal. When GDR coach Rolf Gläser was asked about the unusually deep voices of the female swimmers of the GDR, he gave the following cynical answer: "They are not here to sing."[106] Everybody knew that the deep voices were the result of long-term doping with anabolic steroids.

When the West German Bundesausschuss Leistungssport (BA-L) had asked for money to finance the air clyster project, it had argued that "there are rumors that various methods are being tested internationally to enhance swimming performance." Of course, these methods were mainly anabolic steroids. The Sportausschuss (Sports Commission) of the German parliament became aware of these issues and questioned Wildor Hollmann, professor of sports medicine at the Sports University of Cologne. As mentioned above, Hollmann had employed Dr. Alois Mader, a sports doctor who had fled from the GDR in 1974. In a meeting of the parliamentary committee, Hollmann reported what the West German sports scientists knew about the East German secrets of sports doctors and sports science, and how these secrets were handled:

> For the GDR, the highest priorities are military and nuclear secrets and scientific research on top-level sports. Revealing these secrets is punished severely. [. . .] One of the most important scientists in sports medicine in the GDR, Dr. Mader, fled from the GDR to the West one and a half years ago. He is now

> employed as a scientific researcher at my institute in Cologne. He told us every detail. [. . .] We also know about other researchers of the GDR in that field, and about the secret research institute in Leipzig, which is even closed to colleagues from the Soviet Union. When guests visit this institute, they can visit the first floor freely. But downstairs, there are special laboratories which can be entered only with special cards. Not even colleagues from the Soviet Union and Poland are allowed to see these laboratories. But we know what is going on there. We know the equipment, the number of staff members and their qualifications, and we know what research they are working on.[107]

GERMAN SECRET SERVICES ON DOPING

Alois Mader was asked about his experiences in the GDR not only by Wildor Hollmann, but undoubtedly by the West German secret service, the Bundesnachrichtendienst (BND). However, the archived documents of the BND could be cited with special permission and did not reveal actual names of informants. Nevertheless, they clearly disclose that both the East and the West German secret services were very interested in information about each other's sports and doping practices.[108] Refugees from the GDR who reached the free part of Germany were interrogated in order to determine whether they were in fact spies sent by the other side. Usually, the refugees were so ecstatic that they had succeeded in fleeing the tyranny of the GDR that they were only too happy to reveal what they knew. They were the most important source for the West German secret service and the political authorities about the GDR, about its political, social, and economic standards, about its everyday cultural and social life, about its opposition movements as well as their oppression, and, finally, about its sports. Along with Alois Mader, many athletes and other experts of the GDR sports system, including the female track-and-field athlete Renate Neufeld, told their stories to the West. She had fled in 1977 and reported in detail about her experiences, even writing a book on the subject.[109]

The number of athletes, coaches, doctors, and other secret carriers in the field of sports was increasing year by year. The Stasi, the world's largest secret service (measured by the number of inhabitants), was particularly concerned about the flight of people who knew state secrets, including those relating to top-level sports. With respect to sports, the political leaders of the GDR and the Stasi faced a dilemma. International top-level athletes had to be allowed out of the GDR to win international events for the glory of the socialist "workers' and farmers' state." The opportunity to travel from the small GDR, which was perceived by many inhabitants more as a prison than a homeland, was one of the strongest motives for young athletes to become top-level athletes. Yet these athletes and their entourage were inevitably tempted to abandon the GDR during contests abroad. They or their teams often found supporters in the West and could be sure of getting good jobs after leaving the GDR. Therefore, all athletes as well as their supporters, coaches, doctors, officials, and others were checked extensively for their political loyalty. The SED state party, as well as the Stasi, was supposed to investigate, check, and know "every important connection of top-level athletes."[110] The Stasi referred to these actions as "operative Personenkontrolle" (operational personnel control) and explicitly ordered their staff and instructed them how to work politically and operationally in the field of "body culture and sports."[111] If there were any doubts about someone's loyalty, he or she was to be refused permission to leave the GDR to take part at an international competition abroad, irrespective of the chances of winning. The same applied to the official tourist delegations, which comprised selected GDR fans for the Olympic Games. The distrust of GDR politicians and secret-service staff was painfully evident. GDR teams, as well as those of other communist states, were to be insulated strictly from contact with other teams and athletes of the West during international sporting events, like a flock of sheep being herded by their sheep dogs. However, many top athletes were clever and careful enough to flee successfully. The GDR called them *Sportverräter* (sports traitors).[112]

Alois Mader was one of the most important GDR refugees for West German sport, given his extensive knowledge of sports science, sports medicine, and doping. His flight to the West was seriously disturbing for the East German sports politicians as well as for the Stasi. He knew many secrets of GDR top-level sports and was familiar with the system in detail because of his employment at the Sportärztlichen Hauptberatungsstelle (Central Advisory Board of Sports Medicine) in Halle, where he had supervised coaches, doctors, and athletes, including the official and mandatory doping program. Anabolic steroids, as well as other medical services, were provided in the context of the hierarchical system of sports by order of the responsible doctors of the various federations and the medical services. Mader was indeed a central component part of this system. The effects of anabolic steroids were carefully researched in the GDR and applied systematically. The GDR sports doctors were aware relatively early of the fact that anabolic steroids were very effective in enhancing athletic performance, provided the athletes were carefully supervised and the medication was related precisely to the training process. They were also aware of the dangerous side effects of these doping substances. In addition, Mader had practiced and knew about special injections leading to better and faster regeneration of the athletes. Such injections served as a basis for the so-called Kolbe injection of 1976.

After his move to the West, the Stasi even planned to kidnap Mader and return him to the GDR, as had actually happened in various other cases. However, the plan was terminated because Mader was already integrated into the West German sports and medical communities, making this plan seem rather risky. Instead, the Stasi tried to discredit Mader by denouncing him as a GDR spy. As documents in the Stasi archive reveal, Mader was observed by GDR agents until the late 1980s.

The Stasi then tried to find out exactly what kind of knowledge of the GDR sports and doping system Mader could have indeed revealed to the Western secret service and sports officials. Concerning doping secrets, the Hauptabteilung XX/3 (Department XX/3) of the Stasi stated after the flight of Mader as follows:

> The application of anabolic steroids is not only used in the GDR but also in other countries. However, the performance-enhancement results were not as substantial as for top GDR athletes, because the optimal relationship between the application of anabolic steroids and training intensity is not yet known elsewhere. The application of Mader`s knowledge in this research field could provoke similar performance enhancement, if combined with sufficient support of sports medical research.[113]

The Stasi was right and the prediction became reality. The Stasi officers were highly concerned about the disclosure of sports and doping secrets of the GDR. Several copies of a typical document were found in the Stasi archive, namely a report of the West German Bundesnachrichtendienst (BND) on the "Application of anabolic steroids to top-level athletes of the GDR," dated June 1974. This report could also be found in the BND archives. Apparently, a Stasi agent or a double agent succeeded in obtaining this report, which was then transferred to the Stasi and delivered to several departments. This paper included details of the doping and anabolics program of GDR top-level sports. It seems likely that this information had been handed over by former sports doctors of the GDR who had fled. Mader himself was probably the main source. This essential report was found not only in the Stasi and BND archives, but also in the archive of the German Sports Federation (DSB). This proves additionally that West German sports officials had indeed been informed earlier and were more aware of the misuse of doping and anabolic steroids in the GDR than they conceded before this document was found. Another important issue is what German sports officials did with this and other information from the BND. In fact, West German sports officials and sports politicians did not openly and formally accuse the GDR of doping or foul play. Rather, they preferred to adopt the GDR sports system, including its forbidden doping methods.[114]

One possible answer to the critical question of why the international sports movement, especially the Olympic movement, did not protest more vigorously against the apparent and obvious systematic violation of anti-doping rules by the GDR can be found in the fact that Stasi spies and GDR sports officials were very familiar with the sports organizations, as well as the international conferences on sports medicine. The relationship between

East and West German sports doctors and medical researchers was also close. It seemed to be common sense that doping was in fact accepted as part of modern top-level sports by both East and West, and in the Olympic family as a whole.

Dr. Manfred Höppner was one of the leading internationally acknowledged sports scientists and doctors as well as one of the most important Stasi spies in the field of sports and sports science. He was one of the more than 150,000 so-called unofficial assistants (*Inoffizieller Mitarbeiter*, IM) of the Stasi. His secret name was "IM Technik." He provided the secret service with authentic and valuable information about international sports and current developments on doping and anti-doping. Höppner attended every important meeting on doping and anti-doping, including in June 1974, when the British professor Raymond V. Brooks presented his research on new methods for detecting anabolic steroids at a conference of the IAAF in Frankfurt am Main. Anabolics were on the doping list of the IAAF but could not yet be tested conclusively. Nonetheless, the conference decided to introduce this method at the European championship in Rome in August 1974. In addition, the IOC was advised to put anabolic steroids on the IOC doping list and to use the Brooks method to test athletes for these substances. When Höppner returned to East Berlin, he immediately stopped administering anabolic steroids to GDR athletes at least three or four weeks before a competition. Because out-of-competition controls did not yet exist, this was a simple and effective strategy for preventing GDR athletes from being detected. In his report, Höppner demanded a complete change in the training and supervision of athletes. In addition, he worried about physiological as well as psychological problems, as he believed that "many athletes are now convinced they cannot provide top performances without anabolic steroids."[115]

When Höppner (alias IM Technik) attended a conference of the Medical Commission of the IAAF in Amsterdam in November 1976, the West German president of the track-and-field athletes, Dr. Max Danz, proposed urine as well as blood tests to control athletes in order to determine whether they had received forbidden blood transfusions. Until then, only urine tests had been administered. Dr. Donike of Cologne had a new and reliable method for testing blood for hormone and blood doping. Although the majority of sports scientists accepted this proposal, Höppner opposed it and argued that an athlete could refuse the test for legal reasons. He gave the real motive behind his refusal in his report to the Stasi: "The extension of these tests would include the possibility to prove the presence of the hormone *testosterone,* which is used in the GDR by top athletes."[116]

Höppner influenced the attempts of international federations and organizations of sports to implement effective anti-doping tests. He was even chosen to work on the implementation of anti-doping tests in cooperation with his West German colleague Manfred Donike. This brings to mind the idiom of the fox looking after the chickens. Höppner travelled to Cologne several times to visit Donike and the anti-doping laboratory of the German sports university, which was situated in the same building as the institute of Wildor Hollmann, where Höppner's former colleague Alois Mader was working. Both men, if not all members of this scientific community during the Cold War, should have been aware that top-level sports were not only rife with doping, but infiltrated with spies.

The documents about Dr. Höppner in the Stasi archives reveal the loyalty and cooperation between East and West German sports scientists and sports doctors. When Höppner visited Donike on March 1, 1977, Donike showed and explained "voluntarily and unselfishly," as Höppner wrote in his report to the Stasi, all his research on current methods of anabolic steroids by means of modern mass spectroscopy. Donike even offered Höppner a test of these methods in the "anti-doping laboratory" of the GDR in Kreischa. However, Höppner added that a visit by Donike to Kreischa would not actually be possible because of the difficult political situation and because of the "relationship with Dr. Hollmann." A visit by Donike to Kreischa was planned for 1978.[117] Kreischa was in fact not an *anti*-doping laboratory, but a *doping* laboratory to prevent GDR athletes from being detected by international doping controls. In other words, it was an anti-doping-detection laboratory. In general, the sports doctors and scientists of both East and West, behind and beyond the Iron Curtain, met regularly at international conferences and meetings of experts, where they got to know each other personally, communicated about scientific objects, and probably also spied on each other.

The GDR doctors took great care to minimize the risk that athletes would be discovered by doping controls abroad. All top-level athletes were examined before leaving the GDR for international competitions outside the GDR. There is only one case of a GDR athlete testing positive for anabolic steroids, that of the female athlete Ilona Slupianek in 1977. She had been junior champion in shot put for 1973. Höppner was again involved in covering up this case and preventing an embarrassing international incident for the GDR. Slupianek had tested positive for nandrolon, an anabolic that used to be taken by GDR athletes. Höppner himself took the evidence and sealed the bottle. Later, when this bottle in reserve—the so-called B test—was opened, he insisted that *this* bottle was one he had sealed and therefore not the urine sample from Slupianek, but from someone else. He had marked this sample with a special sign that was missing now, and Höppner then declared that something was wrong. The background to this strange story was that Höppner had quite simply been ordered by the head of GDR sports, Manfred Ewald, to lie. Ewald demanded that Höppner demonstrate "whether he would really back the GDR and understand what the *Klassenkampf* [class struggle] means."[118] The GDR sports officials denied all responsibility or even guilt for this cheating and claimed that Ilona Slupianek was innocent.

Inside the Stasi world, Höppner was on the one hand praised by his superior officers for uncovering some details of West German sports and sports medicine development. But on the other hand, he was criticized sharply for not revealing the activities of people who were allegedly opposed to the GDR and its sports system. An internal dossier described Höppner's behavior as "extremely concerning and worrying, given his international reputation as a scientist." The allegation of behaving *kleinbürgerlich* (in a bourgeois behavior) was indeed a typical communist criticism of the values and norms of a civil society. He was labelled *kleinbürgerlich*, in reality, because he had fostered good and loyal relationships as well as scientific communication with his international colleagues, and thus was accused of disregarding the class interests of socialism and of the GDR as a socialist German nation-state.[119]

In sum, both sides of German sports were being informed mutually by their secret services. However, the information obtained by the West German BND was in fact rather basic and could be gathered from interviews with GDR refugees, as well as from articles in the press. The BND documents also included reports from other sources. It is no longer possible to determine whether and which parts were provided by special agents operating in the GDR and which were collected from the more or less routine questioning of refugees. In fact, the relationship between East and West German sports doctors seems to have been cooperative and respectful. Apparently, nobody in Cologne seems to have distrusted Dr. Höppner or suspected him of spying for the other side. At first, he was simply a competent colleague. Although West German sports officials, sports politicians, and coaches knew many of their East German competitors, they were apparently not well informed of the GDR sports system as a whole. What had really happened in Kreischa and at the Institute for Research on Body Culture and Sport (FKS) in Leipzig was not even clear to the West German secret service, as far as we know today and according to relevant documents in the archives. The FKS was the heart of scientific research on top-level sports in the GDR, including on doping.

There is also no concrete evidence on whether and to what extent communication between the BND and West German sports officials took place. The BND is considered to have been more interested in political than sporting aspects of GDR politics. They did not realize that top-level sports was on top of the political agenda of the GDR. The naïveté of the West German secret service, as well as of politicians in general, concerning sport at that time is easier to understand if one considers that the GDR succeeded in placing a top spy close to the chancellor, Willi Brandt, who finally resigned his office in 1974 because the West German secret service had failed to expose the spy Günter Guillaume.[120]

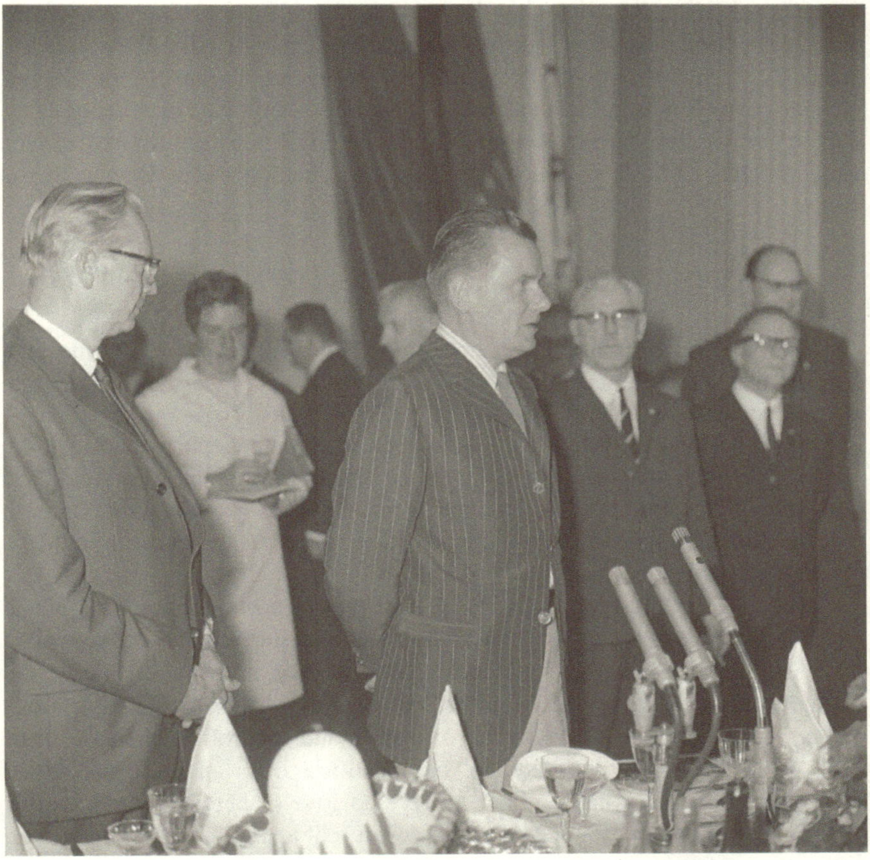

Figure 2.3. Welcome of the government of the GDR for participants in the Olympic Games of Mexico in 1968. The head of the GDR Olympic team, Manfred Ewald, gives a speech. This official picture from the GDR press agency ADN from 1968 shows the political elite of the GDR, including its leading sports politicians. From left: Dr. Heinz Schöbel, member of the IOC and president of the National Olympic Committee of the GDR; Margitta Gummel, winner of the gold medal in Mexico in shot put, and later proved by Brigitte Berendonk to have doped with anabolic steroids; Manfred Ewald, president of the East German Turn- and Sport Federation (DTSB) and member of the Central Committee of the state party SED; Willi Stoph, member of the politburo of the SED and head of the Council of the Ministers of the GDR; Erich Honecker and Alfred Neumann, both members of the politburo of the GDR at that time. In 1971, Honecker became general secretary of the SED, which was the highest position in the communist state. *Source: Bundesarchiv/ Bild 183-G1101-1001-002/ Felix Sturm*

On the other side of the Iron Curtain, the Stasi was evidently working much more professionally. They had two main objectives. The first was to learn everything possible about sports and sports science in the West, and the second was to keep the GDR sports system secret, including the doping program, which was in fact systematic state dishonesty. Part of this objective was to control the sporting community of the GDR consistently and to prevent athletes, as well as coaches and sports scientists, from fleeing to the West.

DOPING AND WEST GERMAN SPORTS MEDICINE

Competitive and internationally successful top-level sports without massive support from the sciences and especially sports doctors were unimaginable, at least since the Munich Olympics of 1972. The East Germans set the pace of scientification of sport, and all developed nation-states participating at the Olympic Games attempted to follow suit. Sports physicians were active on both sides of the Iron Curtain, but sports physicians were also active on both sides of the metaphorical coin—namely, doping as well as anti-doping. In a sense, they were double agents.

Inside the community of sports scientists and sports doctors, the debate had raged for years as to whether or not anabolic steroids should be recognized as doping. When the decision was finally made, and anabolics were put on the doping list after the Montreal Olympics of 1976, further questions arose. First, there was the question of testing and controlling the misuse of anabolic steroids. Although athletes had been tested for anabolic steroids at the Montreal Games, only eight tests were positive (3 percent).[121] However, everyone who had eyes and ears could detect that anabolic steroids were the rule and not the exception for athletes, certainly for top sports. Apparently, and almost everybody was aware of this, the misuse of anabolics could not be detected except for eight athletes because all others had stopped their doping program in time. Therefore, further issues were discussed among sports medicine experts. One was the introduction of out-of-competition controls, which could not, however, be introduced before the end of the 1980s. The other was the acceptance of anabolic steroids, but only under control of doctors. This was the apparent practice of GDR sports and sports medicine. Doctors were ordered to support athletes to enhance their performance by doping.

In West Germany, this practice was not allowed formally, but some doctors like Armin Klümper of Freiburg did so and argued strongly in its favor. The journalist Robert Hartmann of the German track-and-field magazine *Leichtathletik* had interviewed Klümper in 1973 about this problem. Klümper stated that doctors and athletes should cooperate freely with one another. The athlete should not be anxious of being detected by the doctor, but confident of his support. Instead of an uncontrolled, uninhibited injection or the like, the controlled application of drugs should be practiced—as far as they did not entail dangerous side effects, as Klümper added.[122] At that time, some doctors and scientists like Klümper were convinced that anabolic steroids had no dangerous side effects for athletes, which was certainly not true, as we now know, and which was certainly known at least by experts of the GDR at that time. For Klümper, the doping practices of GDR sports doctors were a model for the sporting world. The colleagues in the GDR knew exactly which athlete in which sport could use drugs and anabolics without health risks and when, how much, and with which possible and positive effects. To put this into practice successfully and secretly was the objective of sports doctors in the West as well, according to Armin Klümper.

It should be mentioned that Armin Klümper was a major personality in the community of German and international sports doctors at that time. He was considered a medical guru for top-level sports in West Germany, not only by athletes, but even by coaches and officials. All went on "pilgrimages" to his surgery in Freiburg, the same university town where one of the most influential sports scientists in Germany, Joseph Keul, worked, researched, and supported top-level sports medicine. Viewed against this background, it seems plausible that even in the Federal Republic of Germany, doping with anabolics had been practiced, not systematically, but at least by a number of athletes, training groups, and doctors, since the early 1970s. As Brigitte Berendonk reported in her book, and as reflected in various documents on doping, statements from athletes, and other documents, it is quite clear that before the Montreal Olympics, anabolic steroids had been administered to numerous athletes by West German sports doctors.[123]

The affinity of doctors to drugs may be a characteristic of the profession itself. However, at that time, a strong belief in scientific and medical progress prevailed generally in sports and society. With respect to this ideology of scientific progress, a process of medicalization in society can be observed, not only in Germany, but worldwide, in all modern, developed societies.[124] The overwhelming success of birth-control pills ("the pill") exemplifies this development, enabling originally natural processes to be manipulated very effectively by the medical profession.[125] Medical experts or doctors no longer provided assistance only in the event of diseases or injuries, but to improve the quality of life (at any rate, what some people regard as a good life) or for enhancing performance. Both anabolic steroids for enhancing physical performance and oral contraceptives are inventions of modern science in the field of hormones. Thus, doping in sport is related to wider-ranging developments in modern society and to paradigmatic changes to life in modern societies. Given this scenario, people may feel compelled or motivated to push their physical performance beyond natural limits. Whereas outstanding achievement in sports had always demonstrated human potential for physical

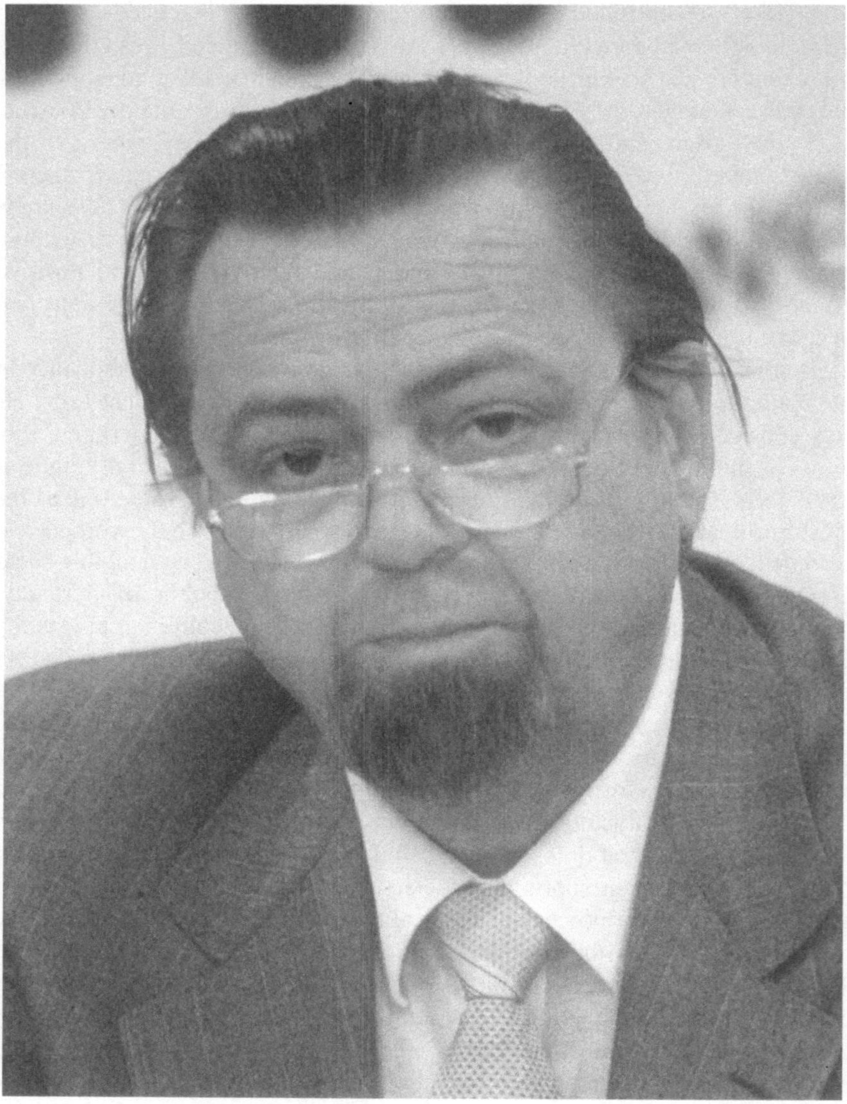

Figure 2.4. Dr. Armin Klümper (b. 1935), sports doctor and professor of sports science at the University of Freiburg. He was the best-known West German sports doctor in the 1970s and 1980s and became famous among athlete, thanks to his so-called Klümper cocktails, mixtures of various drugs for enhancing performance, consisting in part of dietary supplements, drugs for suppressing pain, or even anabolic steroids. He also medicated Birgit Dressel, the West German heptathlete who died in 1987 after a toxic shock, due to the hundreds of drugs found in her body. *Source: Picture Alliance/ Sven Simon*

performance by natural means, a doped athlete is in danger of being regarded as demonstrating little more than the quality of medical support and progress.

The status of sports doctors as indispensable elements in producing high achievement in top-level sports became manifest. Medical experts attended to, supported, and controlled the process of training top-level athletes. This development can even be confirmed by the amount of money spent on the medical support of top-level athletes. Whereas in 1971, the Federal Republic had spent, for the first time, the sum of DM 100,000 for the medical care of top-level athletes, these costs escalated to more than DM 1 million two years later. After 1978, every West German top athlete was obliged to visit a doctor twice a year.[126]

The Bund Deutscher Radfahrer (BDR, German Cycling Federation) provides another example of the increasing medical network that promoted sports performance step by step. Documents of the BDR reveal that in 1972, a standardized medical suitcase had been created, including medication as well as various materials such as dressings, in order to provide better medical care for the cyclists. "Never before has there been such intensive medical care and support," was one comment at the time. The BDR also introduced a central register of all cyclists in 1974. The cyclists were informed that "all athletes would receive vitamins, drugs and dressing material, as well as prescriptions for massages."[127]

These improvements in the medical care of athletes, which were in fact an imitation of the East German model of so-called *Sportmedizinischer Dienst* (sports medical service), did not necessarily imply the violation of anti-doping rules or of the spirit of fair sport. However, many doctors apparently felt confronted with serious ethical problems and by the practical and ethical limits of top-level sports. The temptation to exceed these limits was high. Sports doctors and the community of sports medicine as a whole felt the external pressure to enhance athletic performance.

The above-mentioned Armin Klümper was the official doctor for the West German cyclists. He was asked critically by officials and coaches in 1971 to explain "why the cyclists of France, Belgium and the Netherlands were racing one or two levels higher than our cyclists, [. . .] although you have for many years especially looked after the (German) road racing cyclists."[128] In other words, he was criticized for the insufficient achievement of the young German cyclists and indirectly supposed to deliver them with adequate (doping) means. The dynamics of top-level sports were crucial for the changing self-concepts and corporate identity of the sports federations themselves, as well as the expectations from their supporting partners, like sports doctors or sponsors, including the federal state. Concerning sports doctors, this development generated a new type of sports doctor or sports physician, who was in the first instance interested in and motivated by the needs of top-level sports and only secondly in the health of athletes. Thus the usual obligation of a mainstream doctor took a back seat.

ADAPTATIONS BY WEST GERMAN SPORTS ORGANIZATIONS

Beside the sports doctors, the coaches were crucial elements of the network of people and organizations participating in the doping process. At the core were the *Bundestrainer*, the coaches of the Federal Republic, who were responsible for the top-level athletes representing the federal state. These top coaches were paid by the state from the budget of the Ministry of the Interior. However, their employers were and still are the individual federations. This division is in accordance with the traditional model of the relationship between state and sport in the Federal Republic. However, the question arose as to what to do about, or rather how to sanction, coaches who were involved in forbidden doping practices. For example, in April 1975, two doctors wrote a letter to the president of the German Athletics Federation (DLV), August Kirsch, accusing a coach named Eberhard Gaede of having given anabolic steroids to a nineteen-year-old hammer thrower. This accusation was part of a trial of the President Kirsch of the DLV, as well as other DLV officials, which had been initiated by the pharmacist Horst Klehr of Mainz in 1978. Klehr was one of the main protagonists of anti-doping, apart from Brigitte Berendonk, Werner Franke, and Hansjörg Kofink. He intended to prove that the DLV officials knew about the involvement of federal coaches in doping. In the end, the hammer thrower denied that Gaede had given him any anabolics, and Klehr failed. The trial ended without a prosecution.[129]

Another example is the sprinter Manfred Ommer, one of the best German athletes of the 1970s. He had accused numerous federal coaches of administering anabolics to athletes. Women's coach Wolfgang Thiele had delivered injections to the female sprint-relay team at the Montreal Olympics. Women's shot-put coach Christian Gehrmann, whom Berendonk called "the worst German hormone coach," was nominated as federal track-and-field coach in 1976.[130] Gehrmann took on the job of the doping critic Hansjörg Kofink, who had resigned his employment as federal coach because his criticisms of doping were rejected by the officials. Kofink's and Gehrmann's stories are examples of the fact that doping with anabolic steroids was tolerated in West German sports by sports officials as well as politicians.[131] However, critics like Kofink and Klehr did not succeed in influencing public opinion in West Germany. The ruling officials were able to ignore, cover up, and trivialize doping. The German public obviously wanted victorious athletes and did not care whether they doped or not. In a meeting of the parliamentary Sports Commission in 1977, after the anabolics-laden Games of Montreal, the above-mentioned Manfred Ommer declared: "A lot of coaches—this fact can be proved—do not reject anabolics at all. Athletes then talk with officials about supporting doping by various means [. . .]. That even officials of the federations advised athletes to take anabolics is quite evident, even according to witness statements from athletes of the national team."[132]

Some top officials were aware of the responsibility of sports physicians, coaches, and officials, and concerned about moral legitimation in public. Willi Weyer, president of the Deutscher Sportbund (DSB) in 1974, and honorary president of the DLV, declared openly in an interview in 1977 that "[e]lements of German sport leadership, as well as some supporters of top athletes [. . .] are under pressure to neglect their obligation to monitor, either deliberately or by turning a blind eye. By so doing, they enhance the process of manipulation through pharmacological and medical means for an unknown number of athletes."[133] Incidentally, after this interview, the DLV asked the DSB president to communicate such problems inside the sports family in the future, rather than in public.

During the Cold War period, the West German sports model had changed fundamentally. Whereas in the past, individual athletes and clubs had tried to promote the Olympic ideal of faster, higher, and stronger under the political and social conditions of the 1960s and 1970s, networks of sports experts and organizations were actually striving for gold by all means, fair or foul. The model for sporting success was the GDR. Rather ironically, the West German sports system changed just when, as Willi Daume, then president of the DSB as well as the West German NOK, stated, "the decision was made inside the DSB officials in 1965 to pick up the 'gauntlet' of the GDR and to radically change the support system of top-level sport in West Germany."[134]

This radical change implied the massive growth of tax-financed support of top-level sports in West Germany according to the GDR model of state sports. Step by step, the West German sports concept came close to that of the GDR, whereas the official and ideological rhetoric of politicians as well as officials asserted the contrary.[135]

More state money corresponded with more effective structures of top-level sports. These included so-called *Bundesleistungszentren* (centers for sports achievement of the Federal Republic) since 1964; the employment of professional coaches financed by the Federal Republic, the opening of a foundation to support German sports and top athletes in 1967, chaired by Josef Neckermann, a famous businessman and Olympic equestrian; the opening of the Federal Institute of Sports Science (BISp) as an administration to support sports science within the Ministry of the Interior; the introduction of systematic medical treatment; the diagnosis and therapy of top athletes since 1971; and last but not least, the new Federal Committee for Achievement Sport (BA-L) within the DSB. Whereas the DSB had initially been an umbrella sports organization for all in Germany, this mass organization was in fact split into two sections, one truly for sports for all, and the other only for top-level sports. Actually, the BA-L became the most powerful organization inside the DSB because it had the power as well as the obligation to allocate large sums of tax money among the federations and associations of sports that had decided to participate in top-level Olympic sports. Additionally, the German parliament had created a Special Commission for Sport in 1969, initially because of the 1972 Olympic Games in Munich and the state responsibility for these Games. However, this commission became a permanent forum for discussion and action.[136] Its existence more than anything else symbolized the fact that sports had ceased to be a private affair just for fun, but was a factor of public and political interest and commitment.[137]

West German sports officials as well as politicians were so impressed by the international successes of GDR top-level athletes that they intensified their efforts to study and imitate the GDR sports system. The performance of GDR athletes was attributed to the simple fact of massive doping. However, West German physicians had asserted that anabolic steroids alone were in fact not responsible for the achievements of GDR athletes, but mainly the consistent support and application of those steroids by professional doctors and coaches through a perfectly organized system. The consequence of the decision to follow the model of GDR sports was to call for more support from the state. In other words, the traditional concept of free and private sports was gradually socialized, and the GDR system adopted step by step. Under the conditions of capitalism or so-called social capitalism (*soziale Marktwirtschaft*), as the legendary economics minister and then chancellor of the Federal Republic, Ludwig Erhard, had called this "third way" between state socialism and capitalism, the concept indeed implied a state and tax-financed system of top-level sports on the one hand, but on the other hand, more state control as well. However, the latter did not yet work with respect to doping controls. Accusations of doping were converted into requests for more support and money by the state in order to *reduce* doping.

In consequence, West German top-level sports representatives were confronted with a fundamental ideological dilemma. Whereas the sports philosopher Hans Lenk, winner of the gold medal in rowing (eight) in Rome in 1960, praised Olympic ideals and especially that of sporting achievement through individual endeavor (*Eigenleistung*), the reality of top-level sports had indeed changed. Top performance in sport became less the result of personal activities, and more of social networks offering (to put it politely) specialized expertise. The athlete was of course the most important factor, but still just one cog in the machinery of top-level sports. Inside these social networks, doping in West German sports could take place on a grand scale.

Additionally, West German society of the 1960s was faced with left-wing opposition against capitalism in general and, with respect to sport, against the capitalist structures of performance or achievement sport in particular.[138] This criticism, mostly from left-wing students and academics, confronted their teachers and professors with alternative concepts of body culture and sports. Hans Lenk and Ommo Grupe, for instance, responded by reinventing middle-class ideals of sports.[139] An irony of German history is that this fundamental criticism and opposition against West German civil society, including sports, was indeed pushed by East Germany and its secret service, the Stasi.[140]

CONSEQUENCES OF STATE AND SPORTS POLICIES—THE GRUNDSATZERKLÄRUNG FÜR DEN SPITZENSPORT OF 1977

More money from the state (ultimately from taxpayers) raised the issue of what the sports organizations actually did with it. The public and its representatives in the German parliament and the associated administrations expected better results from West German athletes at international sports events and contests, like the Olympic Games, than was originally the case. However, they also expected state money to be spent appropriately, according to the rules and ethos of sport, that is, without cheating and doping.

When public debates in the press and TV about the doping at the Games of Montreal reached the politicians, they started to ask critically how and on what the money had been spent by the sports organizations. This was a new style of sports politics, because until then, the logic between sports and politics in the West German Bundesrepublik was or at least seemed clear. The state spends money on the noble cause of sport, and the sports organizations are obliged to spend it fairly and correctly. This confidence seemed to be disturbed after the incidents at Montreal with the Kolbe injection as well as the air clyster affair. The chairman of the parliamentary Sports Commission, Hans Evers, therefore asked the following at the opening of a parliamentary public hearing in 1977: "Parliament must get an answer on what we are actually supporting with the money from tax payers. Is it in accordance with the general aims of public support of performance sport as discussed and agreed in the parliament? That is what we are asking in our hearing today."[141]

Beyond this hearing, critical questions of parliamentarians concerning doping were asked, especially between 1977 and 1979.[142] The government and its administrations answered these questions in two ways. First, they emphasized the autonomy of sports, but second, they noted at the same time that public expenditure on sports had to be controlled by the responsible organs of the constitution, just like all other state expenditures. In addition, the administration released an edict in 1978 with respect to the public support of sports that all funds are to be spent subject to the condition that the sports organizations respected the national and international rules against doping or other forbidden technical manipulations. From then on, contracts with federal coaches included a doping clause, stating that breaches of the doping rules could constitute grounds for cancellation.[143]

With respect to the massive increase in the public support of top-level sports by the state, the politicians received the chance, or perhaps more the duty, to control these expenses and how they were used by sports organizations. The public support of sports became a potential instrument for politicians to influence sports development in general and especially to implement anti-doping policies. The sports organizations understood this message—at least to some extent.

The DSB demanded of its member organizations not only compliance and consistent practical applications of the directives against doping from 1970, but also established a commission to overcome the significant moral crisis pervading West German top-level sports after the Olympic Games of Montreal. This commission comprised three people: Heinz Fallak, chef de mission of the Olympic team of Montreal and chairman of the BA-L, Graf Landsberg-Velen, vice president of the DSB and president of the Equestrian Federation, and as chairman Ommo Grupe, professor of physical education at the University of Tübingen. Grupe was an outstanding scholar with a high level of expertise in sports, sports ethics, and sports pedagogy, or physical education. The objective of the commission was to formulate proposals on dealing with medical and pharmaceutical manipulations of performance in top-level sports. Beyond this current question, the sports officials expected more than practical solutions. They ultimately wanted a new ethical constitution and legitimation for top-level sports in West Germany for the future.

It should be mentioned that, for the first time, no sports doctor or other representative of sports doctors was asked to participate at a commission dealing with doping problems. This was indeed a consequence of the behavior of sports doctors with respect to doping and their corrupt image. Sports doctors were no longer expected to contribute toward overcoming the moral crisis of sports caused by doping or to implement consistent anti-doping policies in West Germany.[144] This negative image as doping advocates was reinforced after a congress of sports medicine at Freiburg in 1976, when some sports doctors demanded the relaxation of controls on anabolic steroids, arguing in terms of fairness for West German athletes in the face of the blatantly doped competition from the East.[145] The German Sports Doctors Assocation (Deutscher Sportärztebund, DSÄB) formally criticized "that a commission dealing with questions of pharmaceutical manipulation of sporting achievement does not include people with sufficient expertise to discuss the problems." Herbert Reindell, president of the DSÄB, was not amused (as Queen Victoria might have reacted) that no competent sports doctor or scientific representative of German sports had been asked to join the commission.[146]

However, the commission was established. The essential result of the immense work of this commission, including interviews with more than forty experts, was the Declaration of Principles for Top Sport (Grundsatzerklärung für den Spitzensport) passed in 1977 by the DSB and its various boards.

The so-called Dreierkommission (Triple Commission) attempted to include all possible players or actors of top-level sports who could be tempted to get involved in doping practices. Doping was no longer considered as just a problem of medicine, sports doctors, or training sciences, but as a very real social problem. Social scientists, psychological and pedagogical experts, and politicians and sports officials were requested to discuss the fundamental problems confronting top-level sports in general and doping in particular. However, doping was not to be discussed in isolation from social, cultural, and political contexts.

Even so, the question arose of whether the groundwork of this commission could and should contribute to coming to terms with doping misuse in the past. In fact, the aim of the commission and of the DSB was instead to reconstruct the public image, as well as the moral fundaments, of top-level sports as a whole in German society of the Cold War period. In consequence, the real extent and the details of doping misuse were not researched, but rather trivialized. The claim that only a few sports disciplines were really endangered by doping, and that the detected doping cases were merely exceptions to the rule of clean and fair top-level sports in Germany, was made by the head of the commission, Grupe, at the meeting of the parliamentary Sports Commission in 1977. The majority of athletes were clean and fair, argued Grupe, and they should thus be supported by the state and society.[147] However, at the same hearing of experts, the chairman of the DSÄB, Herbert Reindell, revised Grupe's claim with respect to the estimated number of undetected cases of doping with anabolics. This number was "certainly larger than reported by my friend Grupe."[148]

The Declaration of Principles for Top Sport (Grundsatzerklärung für den Spitzensport) was on the one hand a response to the public and to politicians in the face of a serious crisis of legitimacy of German sports. The spectacular hearing about doping and top-level sports of 1977 in the German Bundestag was a clear sign of this crisis. On the other hand, the declaration was intended to contribute to a new beginning of top-level sports in the Federal Republic. Sports would still be based on the mostly voluntary work of members in clubs and sports associations, but was increasingly dependent on public support, mainly from the state, in order to fulfill the high expectations of the public and political sphere for top performance and success. The declaration was also a moral and structural reaffirmation of the West German sports system in general, which should be both efficient and competitive at the international level, especially compared to East Germany, and morally beyond reproach as well. The declaration would contribute to a humanization of top-level sports. Therefore, the actual title of the declaration was "Der Athlet im Mittelpunkt"—the athlete at the center.[149] Consequently, the concept of the "mature athlete" (*der mündige Athlet*) was propagated as the ideal of an athlete who is able, educated, and competent enough to decide for himself, despite strong constraints and expectations from outside. Humanity in sports and the reference to the moral strength and maturity of the individual athlete could be interpreted not only as a revival of traditional pedagogical ideals of Olympic sports and of German physical education, but also as an alternative to the model of sports and athletics in the socialist part of Germany. "Over there," in the GDR, not the athlete as an individual was the center of sport, but the state. GDR athletes were supposed to be not free and mature, but part of a system. They were compelled to comply with this system and the totalitarian state. If they were not willing to do so, they would be eliminated one way or another.

The Declaration of Principles for Top Sport decisively advocated human and humanized top-level sports without doping or any other unfair manipulation. Anabolic steroids were definitively rejected as unhealthy doping, which indeed contradicted the statements of sports doctors. For the first time in German doping and anti-doping history, the process was no longer considered exclusively as deviant individual behavior, but as a structural problem pervading sports. Various reasons for doping were given, as well as proposals for reducing it. First, there was the expectation of outstanding performance and success. Therefore, the declaration included demands toward the public, media, and politics "to measure the performance and achievement of our athletes not only in medals and records, but also to respect their individual achievements and international rankings."[150] Second, there was the lack of support and social security. Accordingly, the declaration demanded improvements in the assistance of and care for athletes by social workers, psychologists, doctors, and, not least, coaches with generally high levels of expertise, preferably scientific as well. Additionally, athletes should be advised with respect to their broader educational as well as professional careers. Both were regarded as relevant with respect to a humanized sport, optimal conditions for training and competition, and school education and preparation for a professional and social life after the sporting career was over. Compared to athletes of the GDR, the lack of such assistance and care was considered one of the major disadvantages confronting West German athletes.[151] With respect to the prevention of doping, the message of the declaration was that doping could be reduced, at least in the West, if athletes received better assistance and care. Furthermore, this aid had to be paid for by the public and the state—in other words, through social sponsoring for athletes and political sponsoring by the state. For the first time, the Stiftung Deutsche Sporthilfe (Foundation for Aiding German Sports), established in 1967, should be empowered in this context, and the budget for sports had to be increased.

In conclusion, West German athletes and sports organizations were not sanctioned negatively for their morally questionable behavior in Montreal 1976, but in fact rewarded with more money and support from both public and state. The general hope was that doping could be reduced by improving and reforming the Western system of sports. Yet a critical look to the East could easily have revealed that the system with the best-supported athletes by the state was, (regrettably) at the same time, the most doping-contaminated sports system in the world.

However, a consequence of the declaration, as well as of the Montreal Games, with regard to the perspective of international sports, was the fact that anabolic steroids were added to the national doping list of the DSB. In addition, out-of-competition controls were established, but not yet implemented in practice.[152] The practical, political, and logistical conditions were not yet ready for such controls to be put in place. Manfred Donike, as Germany's best-known anti-doping expert, had stated that controlling doping during training would be the most relevant improvement to doping controls and crucial for the fight against doping in the future.[153] Ommo Grupe remained skeptical, fearing for the autonomy of the athlete and the mutual trust among sports, politics, and public. Athletes who are constantly controlled and monitored are no longer free, and the process contravenes the fundamental spirit of free and fair sport.[154]

DOPING ENHANCEMENT IN WEST GERMAN SPORTS

The Declaration of Principles for Top Sport already included some remarks on the structural conditions that are supposed to foster doping. One was the contradiction between the generally excessive public, social, and political expectations for top-level athletes and the demands for an ascetic life without drugs and doping.

In fact, this dilemma could not be resolved. Three main aspects can be identified as anchoring its structure. First, there were criteria for nominating German athletes to participate in the Olympic Games and world championships; second, the criteria for determining the salary of federal coaches; and third, the practice of *Sportförderung* (sports sponsorship) by the state for sports associations via the Bundesausschuss Leistungssport (BA-L, Federal Committee for Achievement Sport).

1. Nomination Criteria

The main relevant criterion for the participation of West German athletes in the Olympic Games is the *Endkampfchance*, which refers to a realistic chance of reaching the final of a competition. This criterion was first practiced before the Olympic Games of Munich in 1972. The BA-L had stated in

1970 that the nomination of national teams for various sports "should not be carried out only with respect to the number of authorized athletes for Olympic Games, world and European championships, but norms of achievement should be referred to as well."[155] This was the initial basis for the discussion of such norms, which were then converted into a specific chance of reaching or even winning a final.

This criterion may sound logical, but it was and always is problematic with respect to doping, because it seemed completely clear that at least in some sports and disciplines, participation in a final was possible only *with* doping. The most striking example of the controversy over this criterion was the nomination or non-nomination of West German female shot-putters for the Munich Games. These athletes, including Brigitte Berendonk, were not nominated by the German Athletics Federation and the National Olympic Committee because they were regarded as unable to reach a final. Their coach, Hansjörg Kofink, argued that these athletes had no chance against the competitors from the East, who almost certainly had doped with anabolic steroids. "You would be punishing athletes who compete according to the rules, by comparing them with the achievements of athletes who have doped (and thus breached the rules), as you very well know," was the accusation of Kofink,[156] who then quit his job as women's athletics coach. Later, Kofink, Berendonk, and other members of this Heidelberg athletics network became the most active and consistent anti-doping campaigners of the Federal Republic of Germany up to the present.

The *Endkampfchance* criterion was again questioned after the Montreal Games of 1976. Herbert Reindell argued during the above-mentioned hearing of the parliamentary Sports Commission in 1977: "This was schizophrenia. If the officials had demanded the limits of physical achievement, they could know that an athlete is able to shot a put maybe 10 meters but not 22. This performance has nothing to do with physiological adaptation by training. Despite this knowledge, these unrealistic norms of achievement were specified. The questioning is therefore justified."[157]

Joseph Neckermann, the founder and first chairman of the Stiftung Deutsche Sporthilfe, and winner of gold medals in 1964 and 1968 in team dressage, therefore requested the removal of this criterion. "I think we should cancel these criteria and participate at international competitions as well as Olympic Games whenever possible."[158]

This *Endkampfchance* criterion has been criticized and questioned again and again, including after German reunification by the so-called Reiter Commission in 1991. However, these norms are still relevant, with the consequence that athletes either have to dope like everyone else at the top, or not be nominated. This unhappy dilemma is in fact an indirect pressure to dope, and that is indeed unfair.

2. Salaries for Federal Coaches

Federal coaches of the Federal Republic of Germany are paid by the state but employed by the German Sports Federation or specific federations. Legally, they are responsible to the sports organization. Their salaries were set by the *Bundestrainervergütungsordnung* (Regulations for the Payment of Federal Coaches) of 1970, which included specific bonuses dependent on the achievements and results of the athletes they are coaching. The reason for these bonuses was to motivate coaches to do a good job and to promote greater achievement. This principle was reformulated in 1979, when the coaches were classified according to different levels of payment. The classification within specific levels was "exclusively dependent on the achievements and results of the athletes for which the federal coach is personally responsible. Raises purely through length of service are no longer possible."[159]

A comparison of the rules of payment for federal coaches over time reveals that the salary increases at the higher levels were far greater than at the lower ones. For example, a federal coach at the highest level earned DM 6,784 in 1984, which was about that of a professor at that time, whereas in 1977, the same coach earned only DM 3,772 a month. This contrasts sharply with federal coaches at the lowest level, who earned DM 3,194 per month in 1984 and DM 2,994 in 1977. In other words, achievement-oriented salaries for top coaches were enforced far more than at the lower levels. In addition, since 1980, special bonuses for truly outstanding success were introduced. A further barrier to higher achievement for (less successful) coaches was the fact that the contracts were not for life. They could easily be terminated by the federation if the athletes were not successful.

Similar to the nomination criteria, these achievement-oriented salaries of coaches in fact encouraged doping. In some sports and disciplines, good or extraordinary results were possible only through doping or other unfair means. If salaries are dependent on results alone, the coach is more or less forced to encourage or at least turn a blind eye to the doping of his athletes. Of course, this still has to be kept secret, because, rather ironically, the contract also includes an anti-doping clause.

3) *Sportförderung*: State Money for Top-Level Sports

As mentioned above, West German sport is autonomous in principle. However, especially top-level sports are supported by the public and the state so that they can fulfill their expected functions or obligations, such as high achievement and success, as well as fair sports and games in representing Germany abroad.

In practice, the system works as follows. Starting in the 1960s, the German Sports Federation (DSB) and the various sports federations filed applications for their needs for the following year. This model was changed at the end of the 1960s in anticipation of the Munich Olympic Games. The funds were now to be allocated according to the level of achievement and success of the federations and their athletes. Planning for the future of the discipline in question would also be taken into account.[160] In 1970, the board of the DSB decided "to privilege sports and disciplines with better chances of success with respect to the allocation of public as well as private funding."[161] Public money was mainly from the budget of the Ministry of the Interior (BMI), and private funds were collected by the Stiftung Deutsche Sporthilfe.

The federal government also mentioned this concept in its program for supporting achievement sports. The concept was officially presented during a debate on sports in parliament and then discussed between the government and the DSB.[162]

This concept of achievement and the success-orientated distribution of funds for different sports federations was developed and refined over time. In 1977, following the above-mentioned declaration of intention in favor of top-level sports, the DSB adopted a "concept of supporting top-level sport." This concept included three levels of development: first, "supporting achievement for the perception of international obligations"—in other words, to enable competition at an international level; second, "further support for top-level sport at the international level"; and third, "optimal support to ensure consistent success."[163] During the 1980s, the previously increasing public means were terminated. Therefore, the concept of achievement was elaborated. The sports organizations were required to develop profiles and set priorities in order to determine which disciplines should be supported first and most urgently.[164] In effect, competition between the sports federations was intensified, and the pressure to achieve and deliver success became stronger. The financial situation of individual federations often depended of the success of just one or a few top-level athletes.

The effects of this concept are well demonstrated by relatively small amateur federations with low levels of economic wealth but a high affinity to doping, such as the Federal Association of German Weightlifters (Bundesverband Deutscher Gewichtheber, BVDG). The chairman of the organization, Otto Schumann, reported in 1971 that he had finally succeeded in convincing the DSB to support the weightlifters before the Olympic Games at home in Munich, although the chances of reaching a final were low. However, the concept of stricter planning and leadership of the federation was successful.[165] Between the Games of 1972 and 1976, the BVDG reformed its concept of training in order to compete successfully according to the criteria of the DSB. A twenty-six-page internal paper of intent provided a concept "of establishing conditions of training similar to those in Eastern Europe in order to achieve the high norms set by the NOK (that is, finishing 8th in the finals)."[166]

Although there is no evidence to support this, it is reasonable to assume that "conditions similar to those in Eastern Europe" include doping with anabolic steroids. According to the Special Principles of Economic Support for Sport, passed by the federal government in 1978, public money could only be spent subject to the condition that the federation accepted and followed the anti-doping rules of the DSB and the international federations. However, in West Germany, there is no evidence that an application for public funding has ever been declined because of a violation of these rules.

Two examples are useful in explaining this typical behavior. The cyclists and the weightlifters have two sports organizations with apparently major doping problems, the former mainly with stimulants and the latter with anabolics. Both reported detected doping cases too late and therefore violated the anti-doping rules. In 1982, a deputy of the Bundestag asked formally in parliament whether the federal government knew about these violations, which meant the government had to terminate financial support for the weightlifting federation. As a result, the administration was indeed ordered to stop the payment and to prove the allegations, after which a detailed investigation including interviews started. The board members of the weightlifting federation were duly interrogated. Finally, the undersecretary of state drew the conclusion "that the federation did not violate its obligations."[167]

The board members themselves felt about these investigations as Henry IV did on his way to Canossa, as they reported.[168] They were very much aware of the consequences of the doping problem for their organization. The images of the federation and of heavy athletics in general were seriously endangered. Without public support, the federation would in fact be financially ruined, and the risk that weightlifting could be banned from the Olympics was also not unrealistic. However, as the minutes of the board meeting stated, "our friends in the German Sport Association and in the Ministry of the Interior did not abandon us."[169]

This example shows that the government and the sports organizations were well aware of the possibility of cutting the sports budget because of violations of the anti-doping rules. However, they did not use this instrument until the end of the 1990s. The structures encouraging doping were apparently stronger than the instruments aimed at achieving the converse.

DOPING AND ANTI-DOPING POLICIES BETWEEN 1977 AND 1989

Anabolic steroids remained the most commonly used and problematic doping substances in top-level sports in the 1980s. Although scientific methods for detecting anabolics were developed, not least by the German biochemical scientist and anti-doping expert Manfred Donike, the strategies for actually testing and controlling were complicated and expensive. National and international sports organizations were unable to introduce consistent out-of-competition controls, although the responsible officials were aware that the fight against anabolics in top-level sports was hopelessly lost without them.

The Medical Commission of the IOC was informed by reports from various sports and doctors about new doping practices, for example with testosterone, cortisone, and adrenocorticotrophin. These are essentially anti-inflammatory drugs, which are used to alleviate pain in the course of or after intensive training, including the inevitable more or less minor injuries. The IOC considered putting these pharmaceuticals on the doping list. The British doping analyst Arthur Beckett informed the IOC Medical Commission about further hormonal drugs like choriongonadotrophin (hCG) and the growth hormone hGH in 1983. In 1988, the Medical Commission acquired information about the use of erythropoietin (EPO), which became the main doping drug of the 1990s, at least in endurance sports.[170] Typical of all these new doping substances and practices was that they aimed at improving performance intensity and are therefore taken on a more or less ongoing basis during training processes and between competitions. Testing and proof of use at competitions is difficult or even impossible if use is stopped sufficiently early before competitions and expected tests. Also relevant is the fact that the optimal timing and mixture of drugs, training, nutrition, and other performance-enhancing means demand high expertise that can no longer be achieved by athletes alone. In addition, the analysis of these new hormone-based drugs is complicated insofar as the difference between such hormones that are produced "naturally" by the body and those that are taken or injected from outside the body and therefore "artificial" is not always evident, given that the biochemical substances are in principle the same. Testosterone and EPO are the best-known examples of this problem. Both are "natural" hormones in that every body produces them, but they can also be taken artificially and additionally to improve either the growth of muscles or of red blood cells, which are necessary for the transport of oxygen in the blood.

In 1977, after the IAAF World Cup in Düsseldorf, Manfred Donike wrote a letter to August Kirsch, president of the German Athletics Federation and director of the Federal Institute of Sports Science, indicating that he "strongly suspected that the athletes competing in Duesseldorf had stopped taking anabolic steroids before the competition, in time to avoid detection. According to my test results, the evidence is there of urine metabolites of testosterone in high concentration, so that it seems very likely that these athletes had substituted anabolic steroids with testosterone."[171]

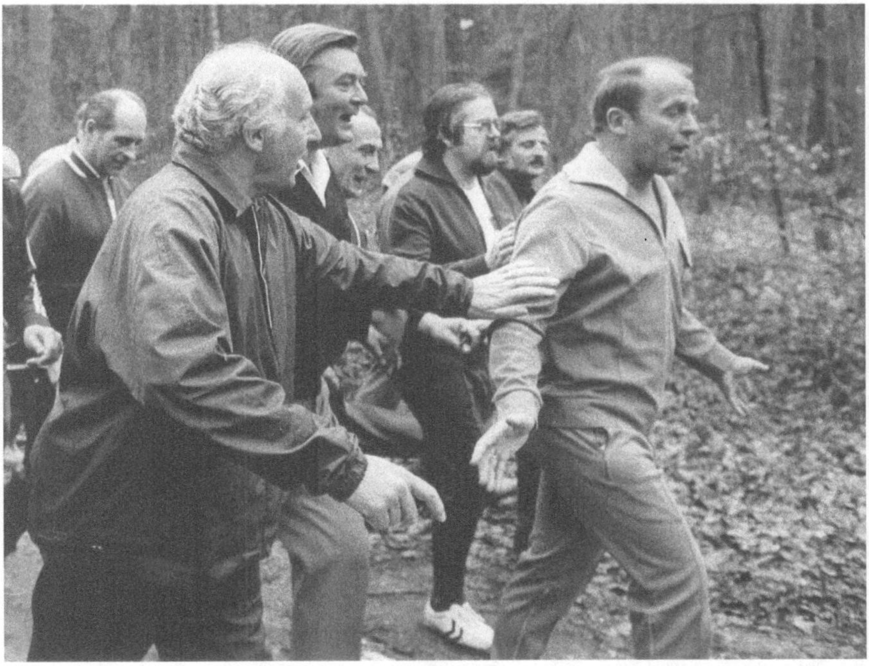

Figure 2.5. August Kirsch (1925–1993), director of the Bundesinstitut für Sportwissenschaft (BISp), the federal institution for the support of sports science in West Germany, at the head of a common jogging event in 1975 with Willi Weyer (1917–1987), at that time president of the German Sports Federation (DSB), and (left) Walter Scheel (b. 1919), then president of the FRG. Kirsch served professionally as director of the BISp and voluntarily as president of the German Athletics Federation (DLV). ***Source: Carl-und-Liselott-Diem Archiv (CuLDA)***

This letter reveals two major steps in the development of doping in top-level sports, namely the application of hormones and the practice of concealing this violation of the regulations by an early termination of use.

In Germany, as well as internationally, sports doctors and scientists (biochemists) were, as usual, working on both sides of the doping front. That is, they were simultaneously enhancing the performance of athletes and, like Manfred Donike, preventing doping and testing (doped) athletes. Two of the former were the German sports doctors Heinz Liesen and Georg Huber.

Liesen was a professor of sports medicine at the University of Paderborn and, among other functions, medical assistant of the German soccer team at the 1986 World Cup in Mexico City. He provided the team with various pharmaceuticals, especially vitamin injections. Liesen argued in favor of improving the pharmaceutical support of top-level athletes and even the "substitution" of testosterone for athletes. The stated reason was the same as for the substitution of vitamins: top-level athletes burn up more testosterone than normal people because of their intense and exhausting training. Therefore, this testosterone—as well as vitamins or minerals or nutrition—needed to be administered in order to help athletes maintain their metabolic balance. Liesen was not alone in this opinion, which was shared by many medical experts and sports officials.

Huber had been the responsible assistant doctor for medical support of the German Cycling Federation (Bund Deutscher Radfahrer, BDR) since the 1980s. The Commission of Experts for Doping Investigations at the University of Freiburg's Institute of Sports Medicine has officially stated that Huber definitely provided cyclists with testosterone, at least in 1987 and 1988.[172]

Both Liesen and Huber are prominent examples of a general tendency in the community of sports doctors involved in top-level sports to provide athletes with numerous pharmaceutical products. The standard argument was that these substances were literally necessary for athletes whose bodies were unable to produce them in sufficient dosages by themselves.

THE CASE OF BIRGIT DRESSEL

A spectacular victim of this thinking among sports doctors was the female heptathlete Birgit Dressel,[173] whose story was reported extensively in the German press.[174] Dressel had finished fourth at the European championship in Stuttgart in 1986 after a rapid escalation of her track-and-field achievements during 1984–1985. In spring 1987, she was admitted to the university hospital in Mainz, where she had trained at the university track-and-field achievement center. She was suffering from severe pain throughout her body. The specialists at the university hospital were unable to control her pain effectively, and could only administer painkillers. Birgit Dressel died after three days of agony, because of a "toxic-allergic shock," as the official diagnosis stated. Up to twenty-four doctors had tried to save her. About two hundred types of drugs could be detected in her body after the autopsy, including the anabolic steroids Stromba and Megrasevit, according to the forensic report of July 23, 1987.[175] Dressel had been medicated by the Armin Klümper of Freiburg, as had the majority of German top athletes from various sports. His clients respected and some even admired him. He became popular because of his so-called Klümper cocktails, injections containing a mixture of anabolic steroids and anti-inflammatory drugs, as well as analgesics of apparently high efficiency, according to the myths about these injections circulating in the community of top-level sports. Klümper even medicated some sports officials, and no one really asked what was in these allegedly miraculous injections.

However, after the death of Birgit Dressel, which was officially denoted as "tragic," the myth of Klümper and his cocktails was soon shattered. A scandal arose and Klümper was accused publicly. Klümper denied everything and shifted the blame to the doctors at the university hospital in Mainz. Dressel had, after all, been medicated by several doctors at the same time, but nobody had been informed about the full details of her treatment and medication. Klümper stated that he had not administered any doping substances to Dressel and that his relationship to her had been very open. The parents of Birgit Dressel stated categorically that they could not imagine their daughter having doped, and the vice president of the Athletics Federation, Inge Bechthold, also declared her conviction that Birgit Dressel had taken nothing forbidden. Medical experts from different sides of the scandal commentated on the deadly scenario. Some sports doctors, like the official doctor of the Athletics Federation, Hartmut Krahl, stated (categorically again) that Dressel died as a consequence not of doping, but of an allergic shock. Her death was a tragic accident but no more. The intensive medication and medical assistance of top-level athletes was necessary and even indispensable. Liesen backed this opinion and stated at a hearing of the parliamentary Sports Commission that Dressel's death was not a problem of sports medicine specifical-

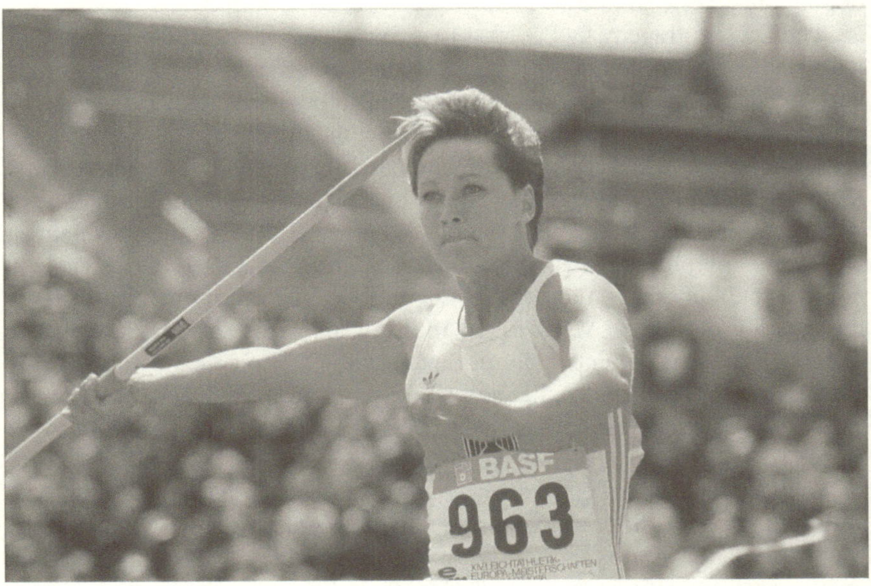

Figure 2.6. Birgit Dressel (1960–1987), West German heptathlete. She died in 1987 after a toxic shock due to the hundreds of drugs that she had received over time. ***Source: Picture Alliance***

ly, but a general clinical one relating to pain relief. Others, like Willi Wülbeck, world champion in the 800 meters, did talk about doping in the context of Dressel's death. There were athletes, he claimed, who were more like "walking pharmacies (or drugstores)" than normal athletes. And Heidi Schüller, former top athlete at the Munich Games, where she had spoken the Olympic oath of the athletes during the opening ceremony, and then a professional mainstream doctor, was disgusted at the fact that the sports doctors had attempted publicly to shift the responsibility and indeed guilt for the death of Birgit Dressel to the doctors at the university hospital in Mainz.[176]

The case of Birgit Dressel was unique in that the doping strategy of some German athletes and sports doctors ended fatally. However, Dressel was by no means unique in her handling of drugs and doctors in order to enhance her performance. With respect to international athletics, Ben Johnson was the most famous representative of these practices in the sprint disciplines. However, anabolic steroids and other alleged miracle drugs were much more common in heavy athletics, even or just in West Germany. As Brigitte Berendonk had already reported in her initial anti-doping book *Doping Documents*, the West German community or social subculture of heavy athletes, including their coaches and networks, was apparently keen on using anabolics consistently. Discus and javelin throwers and shot-putters, both male and female, and both in East and West, did not ultimately seem to differ in their doping practices.[177]

The Dressel tragedy had at least two consequences. First, German athletics and the sports community as a whole were shocked and increasingly convinced that the fight against doping had to be intensified. However, the split between those demanding significant action and others who were trivializing the tragedy as usual became apparent in the question of whether Armin Klümper should be dismissed as doctor of the German Olympic athletes, or whether he should retain his position. Whereas Willi Daume, president of DSB, the umbrella organization of German sports, and also NOC president, declared publicly that Klümper was not guilty of the death of Birgit Dressel, the chairman of the DLV, Eberhard Munzert, managed to force Klümper to resign. In the end, Klümper did not attend the Olympic Games of Seoul in 1988. However, Munzert rather surprisingly retired from his chair in August 1988. With these personal consequences, the Dressel case seemed to be closed.

Second, there were consequences with respect to structural changes in anti-doping policy. Similar to the situation ten years earlier, in 1976, after the Montreal Games, the scandal over the death of Birgit Dressel triggered an increasing interest from the state in doping and anti-doping. The parliamentary Sports Commission of the Bundestag organized a hearing on doping and anti-doping in 1987 against the background of the Dressel case.[178] This hearing was another compelling demonstration of the fact that doping had now become both public and political beyond the borders of the sports community. The responsible politicians and sports officials, as well as the doctors, were aware that new strategies had to be found to reduce doping effectively. Two months after the death of Birgit Dressel, a working group on doping, installed by the Federal Institute of Sports Science, discussed the possibility of introducing out-of-competition controls. Incidentally, this occurred parallel to similar discussions in the IOC and in international sports federations more generally. The experts were still split between those who urgently demanded such controls and others who instead proposed better medical support for top-level athletes. The experts of the sports doctors' lobby argued that the first step should be the establishment of professional doctors for the medical care of top-level athletes, and then the employment of other experts for doping controls. They repeated the familiar argument that damage to health from anabolic steroids had not been proven. Accordingly, they recommended only optional out-of-competition controls and no obligatory out-of-competition tests or spot checks.[179] However, more effective, coordinated, and professional medical care for top-level athletes was a general demand of sports doctors after the Dressel case. After all, better control and central medical coordination could have prevented the chaotic situation that the doctors involved were not informed at all about the anamnesis or the medication that the patient had been receiving. Sports doctors from both the East and West claimed that in the GDR such an accident could not happen because of the professional and centralized system of medical care for athletes.

By contrast, Manfred Donike, head of the Doping-Control Laboratory in Cologne, argued vehemently for out-of-competition controls as soon as possible.

PREVENTIVE CONTROLS

Out-of-competition controls were again a double-edged sword. One is the regular control by official controllers of the anti-doping laboratories, ultimately legitimized by the Medical Commission of the IOC. The other (the exact converse) is control of athletes by experts and sports doctors during training in order to prevent the detection of anabolic misuse at regular competition controls. This principle had been perfected in the GDR, where the Doping-Control Laboratory in Kreischa, officially accredited and even recommended for best practices by the IOC, was in fact used to examine athletes before they left the country for international competitions. This practice can indeed be called "anti-anti-doping." Therefore, no East German athletes had tested positive for anabolics, except for the previously mentioned case of Ilona Slupianek, but never again after this awkward accident.

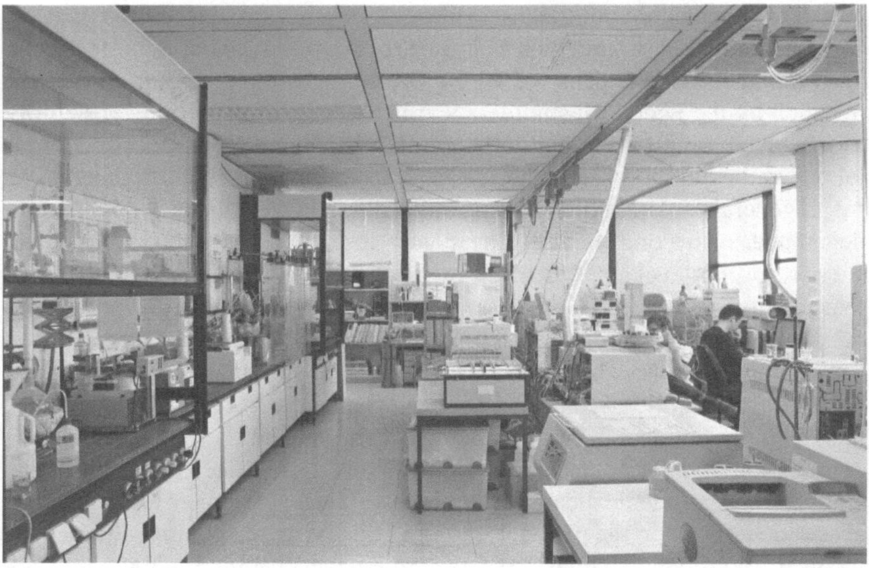

Figure 2.7. The Doping-Control Laboratory in Cologne, one of the world's oldest and best, acknowledged by the IOC since its foundation in 1977 and currently accredited by the WADA. ***Source: DSHS Köln***

However, this practice was not limited to the GDR. There is evidence that Western nations also followed this example cheating the anti-doping system. According to Thomas Hunt, such internal tests were held by the Olympic Committee of the United States before the Los Angeles Games of 1984.[180] The IOC was in fact informed about or at least strongly suspected such unfair practices.[181]

However, it has not been proved that such practices were used systematically in West Germany. There is just one case, that of the cyclist Gerhard Strittmatter before the Los Angeles Games of 1984, that can be interpreted in this manner. Strittmatter received Primobolan from his doctor, Armin Klümper, (purely) for "therapeutical reasons," as Klümper argued. At the German championship, which also served as the qualifications for Los Angeles, Strittmatter tested positive for anabolics, as expected. Strittmatter was then tested several times in Cologne, coordinated with Manfred Donike, to make sure that the depot effect of this substance, measured by metabolites of anabolic steroids, could no longer be verified. The experts were not quite sure about the results, and therefore Strittmatter was not sent to Los Angeles. Afterward, the tests were legitimized, in that the athlete could not be sanctioned because of mistakes made by his doctor, Klümper. The latter was certainly not allowed to administer such medications, but Strittmatter should get a chance to compete in Los Angeles without being detected at a doping control. Joseph Keul additionally criticized his colleague Klümper on the grounds that there had never been any medical reason for the medication with testosterone.[182]

ANTI-DOPING: SOME FACTS AND PROBLEMS

However, the 1970s and 1980s were decades not only of doping, but of anti-doping as well. The number of regular and consistent tests at competitions increased year by year after the Montreal Olympics. First, more federations participated in these controls or at least agreed that their athletes would be tested. Second, the absolute number of controls in West Germany almost doubled in only one year from 465 in 1977 to 853 in 1978, and then climbed to 1,703 controls in 1988. Since 1989/90, consistent out-of-competition controls have been introduced, but the rise of controls in different sports was uneven.[183]

With respect to these statistics, it should be borne in mind that about a third of the controls was for cycling only (31.76 percent), followed by equestrian sports (13.19 percent), athletics (10.76 percent), swimming (8.02 percent), and weightlifting (4.27 percent), as these are the sports federations with an established affinity to doping. Roughly 32 percent of all controls were for all other sports.

As mentioned, all these controls were out of competition. Therefore, the essential problem of doping control at that time was that anabolic-steroid and hormone doping could in fact *not* be controlled, because they were applied during training. This problem was certainly not limited to Germany, but constituted an international phenomenon. In 1978, the European Council asked the Medical Commission of the IOC to determine whether the member states or member federations within the IOC had in fact implemented the recommendations of the European Council declaration of 1967. This revealed that very few organizations had implemented any measures with respect to training controls.[184] The logistics, as well as the organizational and financial barriers, seemed to be too high for effective out-of-competition tests, although there is some doubt as to whether the political willingness of the sports, as well as mainstream policy, was in fact sufficient to overcome these obstacles. However, the situation changed after the Dressel case with respect to Germany, and after the Ben Johnson doping scandal at the Seoul Olympics of 1988 for international Olympic sports "governed" by the IOC.

The introduction of out-of-competition controls raised the question of who could in fact implement these controls effectively and who was able and willing to bear the cost. For Germany, the cost for various activities in the context of doping analysis increased significantly after the end of the 1970s. Manfred Donike identified four reasons. First, the increasing number of tests in general; second, the extension of doping lists and the constant addition of new substances; third, the increasing number of methods of testing, which were becoming more complicated; and fourth, the increasing international communication, cooperation, conferences, mutual visits, and so on, which all required more personal input, time, and money than before. Donike estimated the increase in analytical anti-doping activities during the last ten years at about "a factor of ten or twenty." Therefore, he demanded better equipment and modern facilities,[185] with the consequence that the budget for supporting sports doctors was split after 1979 into specific types of costs for "doping analysis." This type of costs increased disproportionally in the following years, whereas the sum for the usual sports medical research stagnated or even decreased. Therefore, the community of sports medical researchers was split into two sections, doctors and doping analysts. Both fought for the larger piece of the cake, in terms of greater financial support from the state. This conflict effectively demonstrated the emerging self-understanding and reorientation of sports doctors or sports medical research in Germany in the light of doping and anti-doping.

Manfred Donike was a highly respected member of the Medical Commission of the IOC. He had developed the test for externally applied testosterone and attempted to upgrade his Doping-Control Laboratory in Cologne. In order to do so, he also tried to gain financial support from the state. Sports doctors like Joseph Keul of Freiburg or Wildor Hollmann of Cologne feared for their standing within the community of sports medical sciences, with respect to governmental funds, if major parts of the funds were given to doping analysts. This competition was also an important reason why Keul opposed the request of Donike to add testosterone and caffeine to the doping list of the IOC. Keul had always argued that adequate and valid tests for testosterone were lacking and that the performance-enhancing effects of caffeine had not been proved.[186]

Keul then used another strategy to improve the position of sports doctors compared to those doing doping analysis. He argued that a reduction in doping was not possible through the development of doping analysis alone, but needed more and better medical assistance of athletes from sports doctors. "If the government wants to reduce doping effectively," he wrote in a paper in 1982, "not only doping analysis has to be developed, including expensive facilities and substantial investment, but also other initiatives, especially medical assistance for athletes from highly specialized sports doctors."[187]

The Keul paper also influenced the revised Grundsatzerklärung für den Spitzensport (Declaration of Principles for Top Sport) of 1983, which was in fact an update of his 1977 paper. At that time, the traditional group of sports doctors had apparently lost much of their influence on sports policy. The head of the Triple Commission, Ommo Grupe, explained in his introduction to the paper that "Prof. Keul had mentioned in an elaborate paper the difference between doping controls, their immense cost, including high technical and logistic investments on the one hand and therefore, on the other hand, the declining responsibility of coaches and athletes in this context. He also criticized the lack of education and enlightenment of athletes and coaches, as well as the spin-offs from the doping-control system."[188]

In fact, the German Sports Federation followed Keul's advice in several respects. First, the conditions for the medical and physiological assistance of athletes during training were improved, and second, the German sports organizations argued increasingly critically with respect to more controls: "The sports organizations in Germany are convinced that controls are necessary to maintain the rules of fair sport. However, complete and comprehensive control is neither possible nor desirable. Instead, the fundaments of fair sport and sporting rules are the ethics of sports, as well as the ethically based responsibility of all involved athletes, coaches, doctors, assistants and officials. These ethical elements have to be strengthened."[189] Skepticism toward overall controls, and the danger that top-level sports could change radically from a free game and leisure activity to a totalitarian system of controlled work (as in the communist GDR), was an argument that not only Ommo Grupe but numerous other officials and politicians had always used. They worried about the loss of ethics and morality in sport, which in fact revolved around liberty and the free will of mature athletes.

A DOUBTFUL RESEARCH PROJECT: THE STUDY OF REJUVENATION/REGENERATION BY MEANS OF TESTOSTERONE

The debates about out-of-competition controls, the increasing cost of doping analysis, and, not least, the quarrelling inside the community of sports doctors and doping analysts about the effects and proof of anabolic-steroid and testosterone use all formed the background of various questionable research projects surrounding sports doctors in the 1980s, and in particular the so-called *Regenerationsstudie*. This was an allegedly scientific study about the link between testosterone application and the ability of athletes to rejuvenate after intensive training and competition stress. The study was financed by the Federal Institute of Sports Science in Cologne in 1985.[190] Critics asserted that this study, financed by the state, provided proof of systematic doping research in West Germany.[191] They argued that this study did in fact support the use of testosterone in sport, because during the investigation, athletes were even obliged to take testosterone.

In fact, the most relevant background was the differing opinions among sports doctors and sports scientists about the proved effects of testosterone. The male hormone testosterone became increasingly popular among athletes when the application of synthetic anabolic steroids could easily be detected. Testosterone was difficult for biochemists to detect. It then became apparent that testosterone was being used not only in sports like weightlifting or disciplines involving high levels of strength, but also in endurance sports like long-distance running, cycling, and rowing. The relevant and well-known sports doctor Heinz Liesen had asserted at a congress of sports doctors in 1981 that injections of testosterone were also useful for marathon runners in order to shorten periods of rejuvenation or regeneration. Because studies by American sports scientists had shown the level of testosterone to decrease significantly after long-term, intensive sporting achievements, a responsible sports doctor was then obliged to substitute these hormones that had been used up through physical exertion.

Though Liesen's colleague Joseph Keul from Freiburg had also been sympathetic to this theory of substitution some years ago at the doping hearing of the German Bundestag in 1977, in the 1980s Keul now disagreed with Liesen. He asked for clear proof of this hypothesis and for valid scientific studies that could verify the assertion that testosterone could shorten regeneration times for athletes. In fact, the thesis that externally applied testosterone could enhance the ability of athletes to regenerate was not verified at all.

In consequence, the leading sports medicine centers in Germany, namely Freiburg, Saarbrücken, and Cologne, and their leading sports doctors, Joseph Keul, Wilfried Kindermann, and Wildor Hollmann, and indeed Liesen, requested funding for a major project to settle this issue once for all. The BISp agreed and awarded a grant of DM 300,000 for three years to research "whether the application of testosterone or anabolic steroids can really improve the regeneration ability of athletes after intensive long-term achievement."[192]

Finally, the research was organized and supervised by Keul in Freiburg, Kindermann in Saarbrücken, and Liesen in Paderborn, where the latter had obtained a professorship after his service at the Sports University of Cologne. Athletes from different sports and endurance disciplines, from long-distance running and rowing to triathlon, cycling, and winter skating, were tested after the application of testosterone. There were also control groups to adjust for placebo effects. The Ethics Commission of the University of Freiburg stated that there were no ethical doubts about the research, subject to the condition that the testosterone doses were at a "normal" level.

The result of the research project was documented in the final report as follows: The tests had demonstrated clearly "that substitution by testosterone, as well as anabolic steroids, had no positive effects on the regeneration of athletes or on the status of their immune system." The asserted recuperation-enhancing effects for athletes could thus not be proved.[193]

Interestingly, the final report of the regeneration project coincided with the process of German reunification. The history of sports and doping was an issue of general interest within this process. Therefore, in the united German parliament, questions were also asked about this study on testosterone funded by the government. The question was whether this project was in fact a pro-doping research project of the government. In other words, the federal government may have spent money on unethical doping research. The response of the government can be summed up as follows: "The only task of the project was to get answers to the question of whether testosterone could really be used as a means of substitution and regeneration. As mentioned, 'pro-doping research' was not intended at all and the aim was not performance enhancement, but regeneration."[194]

However, the difference between regeneration and performance enhancement was not at all clear. Better regeneration abilities certainly have immediate performance-enhancing effects, because the intensity of training can be raised. Yet in the longer run, the vulnerability of athletes is much higher because of more intensive training. Even so, the research project was indeed not comparable to the secret doping research of the GDR. The process of planning, operating, and evaluating was transparent and publicly discussed. There can also be no doubt that research about such open questions on the effects of certain pharmaceuticals is legitimate. But it was evident that powerful lobbyists of West German sports doctors used the project to entrench their status, demand public funding for a project of questionable merit and value, and ultimately misuse the Federal Institute of Sports Science (BISp) for economic and egoistic motives.

Some responsible administrators of the BISp may have noticed the true motives behind this research. They sharply criticized the short seven-page final report, which had cost German taxpayers more than DM 300,000. The criticism of the medical department of the BISp was unusually strong. The biased presentation was criticized, as was the short report, for being deficient in both form and content, using unsound methodological approaches and analysis, and lacking the reports of the three research groups pursuing the project.

Accordingly, the project and its report can also be interpreted as an example of the arrogance of leading West German sports doctors, their lack of ethics, and their low level of scientific competence compared to the international community.

The research project was in fact doping research only in that doping was researched. However, the allegation that the federal government had agreed to and sponsored doping is certainly unfair. At least two more critical aspects are worthy of mention. First, there was the fact that the tested athletes had really been doped with testosterone or anabolic steroids. Their participation in the project was a clear violation of the existing anti-doping rules at that time. Second, a researcher from the working group of Heinz Liesen in Paderborn was the ex-GDR sports doctor and doping expert Hartmut Riedel.[195] He fled the GDR in 1987 and was immediately employed by Liesen in Paderborn. There, he worked on the testosterone project team. It is clear that doctors like Liesen and others were very interested in the highly confidential GDR doping system. The sports doctor Georg Huber, who was later charged in relation to doping in cycling, was a member of the working group of Joseph Keul in Freiburg. He may have been interested in the testosterone project for his later career as a doping doctor for the German cycling team Telekom.

INTRODUCTION OF OUT-OF-COMPETITION CONTROLS

The possibility of out-of-competition controls had been discussed continuously in international sporting contexts since the 1980s. In 1982, Jacques Rogge, later president of the IOC from 2001 to 2013, but then a member of the working group of the European NOCs, reported on "problems of science and health" that out-of-competition controls had caused in Finland, Sweden, Norway, and Belgium.[196] In England, a pilot project for examining such tests started in 1985.

German sports officials remained hesitant, with only Manfred Donike pushing for the introduction of training controls. Several letters to the Federal Institute of Sports Science, as well as to the German Sports Federation, confirm his initiatives. The only exception among German sports organizations was the German Swimming Federation, which had tested voluntarily during training since 1984 as a consequence of two young female swimmers who had tested positive for anabolics.[197]

The DSB had commissioned a legal opinion in 1983 about the possibility of training controls, with the result that such controls were considered possible in principle, but subject to the condition that contracts between athletes and the controlling authorities had to be signed. However, leading sports officials like August Kirsch and Joseph Keul remained skeptical. Some of the usual arguments were mentioned in a letter from Keul to Kirsch: "Sport controls during training are very problematic, entailing numerous logistical issues and cannot be justified legally in my view. In addition, it seems to me highly problematic to determine how such controls should be organized, because often, the training locations are not even known, and numerous athletes do their training abroad. Another point is that it is not clear who should pay for these expensive controls."[198]

As mentioned above, it is fair to assume that the motives of Keul and of other sports doctors had less to do with solving the doping problem and more to do with the status of sports doctors and sports doctors as essential supporters of German top athletes. The latter should be internationally competitive, and sports doctors, in their social role as medical supporters of top-level athletes, had to be supported, just as the new medical branch of doping analysis was.

The federal government refused to assume responsibility, as usual in West Germany, and passed the buck to the sports organizations: "Based on the principle of autonomy, the sport organizations have to take a stand on these controls [. . .]. The federal government does not intend to influence this decision-making process."[199]

The Ministry of the Interior adopted the traditional principle of the relationship between sport and state in the Federal Republic of Germany. The ministry was in fact authorized to deal with general questions of top-level sports, which were regarded as significant for the image of West Germany abroad. However, with respect to this question of doping controls in the context of international communication, the German attitude became an obstacle for West German politics in general. A principle of West German foreign affairs since the foundation of the Republic in 1949 has always been to conform closely to the nation-states of the Western alliance. However, this position became problematic, as the Western neighbors and their sports organizations had gradually introduced out-of-competition controls. Manfred Donike had mentioned several times since the 1980s that, one by one, more Western sports nations had introduced training controls, even the USSR and the GDR in 1986. The IOC reported in 1987 that 23.6 percent of all anti-doping controls in official, accredited laboratories were out of competition.[200]

When the European Council held a conference on this issue of training controls in 1988 and voted on a recommendation for all member states to introduce training controls, only the Netherlands and the Federal Republic of Germany did not agree. Both countries refused because of their lack of communication and coordination with their unique sports organizations. In fact, this vote was a diplomatic disaster. Therefore, immediately after the assembly of the European Council, the German minister of the interior wrote a circular to all relevant individuals, officials, departments, and sports organizations concerning accepting the recommendation of the European Council, conveying that "with respect to these facts, a rejection of the recommendation of the EC could create the wrong impression about the German attitude towards the doping problem. Therefore, I propose an acceptance of that recommendation, despite several open questions in the Federal Republic."[201]

A few days later, the responsible departments, administrations, and sports organizations, including DSB and NOK, agreed and accepted the recommendation of the European Council as well as the German minister of the interior, who ultimately allocated money to top-level sports in Germany. The simple fact was crystal clear to everybody in sports administration that German sports had to follow these political directives of the minister.

The political pressure on German sports and sports policy increased when, in the same year of 1988, the Conference of European Ministers Responsible for Sport, the European Council, and, not least, the First Permanent World Conference on Anti-Doping in Sport in Ottawa voted for the introduction of training controls. The European Council had wanted a general convention against doping in order to achieve greater international commitment in the fight against doping. The European Council followed an initiative of the British sports ministers and intended to force them to a more effective commitment with regards to options against doping.[202]

However, German representatives were again critical and skeptical of this plan, according to reports of the informal meeting of European Sport Ministers: "The State Secretary of the Federal Republic of Germany stated that his government attached great importance to the notion of long-term prevention, education and protection. It offered support to its sports organizations in the conduct of their controls (laboratory, financial help), but would find it difficult to approve a policy of binding or compulsory out-of-competition controls, which would raise practical and legal problems. It would, however, be able to accept the draft recommendation and would invite sportsmen to submit to such controls, in accordance with the ethical and moral principles of the 1984 Charter."[203]

The German Ministry of the Interior stated that compulsory regulations were in fact a "serious intervention in the autonomy of sport" in Germany. Therefore, the German attitude was still skeptical, although the minister would urgently recommend ignoring these concerns in the light of the increasing commitment of international sports organizations, as well as parliaments and governments, to finding common and consistent instruments for reducing doping, including out-of-competition controls.[204]

In the nick of time, the West German sports organizations agreed to the convention against doping and the introduction of training controls. In addition, the criteria for the nomination of the Olympic team would be reformed so that only athletes who were also willing to be tested outside of competitions could be nominated. At first, a pilot project was to be organized in 1989/90.[205] Four federations participated in this project, namely ice skaters, weightlifters, rowers, and track-and-field athletes. As usual in Germany, the federal Ministry of the Interior paid the bill for this project. After the competition, the project was to be evaluated and extended to all top-level Olympic sports.[206]

Manfred Donike sharply criticized the fact that in Germany, the ministry and the sports organizations were responsible for the pilot project and the training controls.[207] He demanded independent controllers, according to the international discussions on doping controls. In Germany, such independent instruments to control doping could not be implemented before 1992. By then, the process of German reunification had overcome its first and greatest obstacles. New political conditions cleared the way for a more effective, independent doping-control system. In 1992, the (in principle) independent Anti-Doping-Kommission (ADK, Anti-Doping Commission) was founded. The question of how high the costs for doping controls would be and who would pay was and still is critical up to the present. However, the politicians and sports officials agreed that the independence of doping controls had to be guaranteed.[208] The establishment of an independent commission or institution that was responsible for the planning, organization, and evaluation of doping controls was in fact a new step in the process of reducing doping through truly effective controls. This was possible for two reasons. First, the numerous European and international initiatives against doping from sports organizations as well as supernational organizations since the 1980s had produced so much political pressure that the German sports organizations and sports politicians could no longer remain aloof. Germany had to follow the international mainstream of anti-doping policies toward more and better competition as well as out-of-competition controls. Second, intensified anti-doping policies coincided with the end of the Cold War. However, the demise of the Cold War did not imply the end of doping, but did create new opportunities for international and national initiatives against doping. The approval of German sports officials and sports politicians of stricter out-of-competition controls was also the result of concerns about the spread of doping throughout Germany after the collapse of the GDR. Unified Germany wanted to inherit the results and supremacy of GDR sports, but without doping—or at least with less doping. What the process of German reunification implied for doping and anti-doping policies will be revealed in chapter 3.

INTERIM RESULTS—CHANGES TO DOPING AND ANTI-DOPING POLICIES IN THE 1970S AND 1980S

The 1970s and especially the Montreal Olympics of 1976 changed the world of sports and the parallel one of doping. The Cold War was in full swing even on the track, and both sides, East and West, did everything to win. Athletes, sports officials, and sports doctors on both sides were remarkably creative and innovative in finding new ways to enhance performance without violating anti-doping regulations. Most of these practices were common and of course allowed by the rules, such as intensifying training processes and improving training methods. Training became more professional, scientifically based, systematically planned, and controlled by experts. However, when these practices in accordance with the spirit of sports did not provide the expected results and sporting victories, new medical or technical innovations were attempted, like the Kolbe injection and the air clyster technique in 1976. Both demonstrate creativity in finding means to enhance performance without violating anti-doping rules. The most sustainable was by far the use of anabolic steroids, which had been developed by sports scientists, produced by the pharmaceutical industry, and consistently applied by sports doctors, at first in the GDR, but then internationally. Such hormone doping could not be tested and proved for a long time, and was therefore not listed. Sports doctors, sports scientists, biochemists, and pharmacists quarreled about the effects and side effects of these new substances based on "natural" hormones.

These efforts at inventing new substances to enhance performance can also be regarded as a consequence of defining doping in the form of a concrete doping list. This provoked new inventions that were not forbidden but were effective in enhancing performance. However, doping lists also included the need for controls and, in consequence, sanctions, which opened the race between dopers and doping controllers.

Sports organizations throughout the world, including West Germany, hesitated to control doping consistently. Sports were still regarded mainly as "just a game" for amateurs, and the sports federations were thus unable to organize and finance effective and consistent doping controls. Until the Montreal Games, the majority of sports officials could not really accept the reality of the spread of doping in Olympic sports. They considered doping as simply a form of foul play that could be regulated by rules and referees. However, the Games of Montreal may well have opened the eyes of at least some sports officials and politicians.

The "totalization" of sport included on the one hand higher standards of sport, more and more effective training, better organizations, qualified coaches and experts, scientists, and doctors, but also, on the other hand, professional controllers to stop cheating and doping. Sports organizations themselves were not able to organize or to pay for this process of sports professionalization. Because commercialization processes in sports were in their infancy, the state had to play the major role in supporting sports. Sports under communism were the most successful model of top-level sports supported by the state.

West German sports officials and politicians took a long time to overcome their traditional ideology of the autonomy of true amateur sports. GDR sports structures were transferred to the West and adapted to the conditions of the Western Federal Republic. Finally, sports officials and sports politicians accepted that top-level sports without massive support by the state and the taxpayers would not be internationally competitive, at least not with the most modern sporting nation, the GDR, those Germans in the other, socialist part of Germany. It again took a long time to accept that the state had also to assume more responsibility with respect to doping controls and that those who pay the bill usually demand the power to decide what exactly has to be done with the money.

In Germany, these processes were associated with extensive debates on sports generally, top-level sports, and doping in the media as well in public, in sports organizations, and even in parliament after the Games of Montreal and then in further steps in 1980. One major result was the Grundsatzerklärung für den Spitzensport of 1977, the Declaration of Principles for Top Sport, which included a new ethical understanding of top-level sports and its ethos with the German sports movement. It was revised and adapted to changing conditions in sports and society in 1983 and 1988.

The case of Birgit Dressel in 1986 increased the awareness in German sports and politics of the urgent problems confronting top-level athletes and the need for better support as well as better control. This case can be regarded as a German prelude to the internationally notorious Ben Johnson doping scandal of the Seoul Games in 1988. It again challenged the role of sports doctors and scientists in the world of top-level sports. In Germany, a deep rift arose between sports doctors on the one hand, and doping analysts and biochemists on the other. One result was the spectacular study of regeneration, where both sides could "meet." However, this scientific study was and remains highly controversial, for both ethical and scientific reasons. It revealed the dubious quality of West German sports science and medicine at that time.

Finally, international anti-doping initiatives in the 1980s, as well as the fall of the Berlin Wall, opened the door to new ways of reducing doping in Germany, as well as internationally.

NOTES

1. Stalin's decision to take part in the Olympic Games and to abolish the International Red Sport movement occurred in 1937, according to Nikolaus Katzer, "Körperkult und Bewegungszwang: Zur gesellschaftlichen Dynamik des frühen sowjetischen Sportsystems," in *Der deutsche Sport auf dem Weg in die Moderne: Carl Diem und seine Zeit*, ed. Michael Krüger, Studien zur Geschichte des Sports 9 (Berlin and Münster: Lit, 2009), 257–84, esp. 275. See also Nikolaus Katzer, "Am Rande der Vollkommenheit: Aspekte einer Geschichte sowjetischer Körperoptimierung," in *Hormone und Hochleistung: Doping in Ost und West*, ed. Klaus Latzel and Lutz Niethammer (Cologne: Böhlau, 2008), 205–30. The course for a scientifically based sports and doping system in the USSR was set early in the 1930s.

2. The minutes of the IOC Executive Committee after World War II show the efforts made to integrate the athletes of the Soviet Union into the Olympic movement. For example IOC Archives, minutes of the "session du Comité international olympique, Lausanne, 3–6 Septembre 1946," p. 8f. The IOC policies against doping are analyzed by Marcel Reinold, "Arguing against Doping: A Discourse Analytical Study on Olympic Anti-Doping between the 1960s and the Late 1980s: Final Research Report of the IOC Postgraduate Reserach Grant Programme 2011," in *Final Research Report of the IOC Postgraduate Research Grant Programm 2011*, ed. International Olympic Committee.

3. Thomas M. Hunt, *Drug Games: The International Olympic Committee and the Politics of Doping, 1960–2008*, Terry and Jan Todd Series on Physical Culture and Sports (Austin:

University of Texas Press, 2011), 39, supposes that sporting contests were a kind of substitute for war during the Cold War.

4. Mike Dennis and Jonathan Grix, *Sport under Communism: Behind the East German "Miracle,"* Global Culture and Sport (Basingstoke, Hampshire: Palgrave Macmillan, 2012), have emphasized that many Western and democratic nations admired the East German sports "miracle" and attempted to imitate its sports system, even after the breakdown of the Berlin Wall.

5. Kay Schiller and Christopher Young, *The 1972 Munich Olympics and the Making of Modern Germany,* Weimar and Now 42 (Berkeley: University of California Press, 2010).

6. The following chapter refers essentially to Michael F. Krüger, Stefan Nielsen, and Christian Becker, "The Munich Olympics 1972: Its Impact on the Relationship between State, Sports and Anti-Doping Policy in West Germany," *Sport in History* 32, no. 4 (2012): 526–49, doi:10.1080/17460263.2012.756424.

7. Paul Dimeo, *A History of Drug Use in Sport, 1876–1976: Beyond Good and Evil* (New York and London: Routledge, 2007); Hunt, *Drug Games.*

8. *New York Times,* 14 July 1973.

9. Kalevi Heinilä, "Citius—altius—fortius: The Olympic 'Contribution' to the Professionalization of Sport?" in *Sport in the Modern World—Chances and Problems: Papers, Results, Materials; Scientific Congress, Munich, August 21 to 25, 1972,* ed. Ommo Grupe (Berlin: Springer, 1973), 351–55.

10. C. Brissonneau and F. Depiesse, "Doping and Doping Control in French Sport," in *Doping and Doping Control in Europe: Performance Enhancing Drugs, Elite Sports and Leisure Time Sport in Denmark, Great Britain, East and West Germany, Poland, France, Italy,* ed. Giselher Spitzer, Edition Sport & Freizeit 15 (Aachen: Meyer & Meyer, 2006), 145–67.

11. S. Donati, "Doping and Anti-Doping Fight in Italian Sport," in *Doping and Doping Control in Europe: Performance Enhancing Drugs, Elite Sports and Leisure Time Sport in Denmark, Great Britain, East and West Germany, Poland, France, Italy,* ed. Giselher Spitzer, Edition Sport & Freizeit 15 (Aachen: Meyer & Meyer, 2006), 17–56; Robert O. Voy and Kirk D. Deeter, *Drugs, Sport, and Politics* (Champaign, Ill.: Leisure Press, 1991), 103ff.

12. Voy and Deeter, *Drugs, Sport, and Politics,* 174.

13. Schiller and Young, *The 1972 Munich Olympics.*

14. Karlheinz Gieseler, ed., *Der Sport in der Bundesrepublik Deutschland,* Ämter und Organisationen der Bundesrepublik Deutschland 35 (Bonn: Boldt, 1972), 118ff.

15. Uta Andrea Balbier, *Kalter Krieg auf der Aschenbahn: Der deutsch-deutsche Sport, 1950–1972. Eine politische Geschichte,* Sammlung Schöningh zur Geschichte und Gegenwart (Paderborn: F. Schöningh, 2007), 131, 253.

16. The constitution of the 1. Sonderausschuss für Sport und Olympische Spiele took place on 13 November 1969. Its designated role was the parliamentary supervision of the 1972 Olympics and the FIFA World Championship in 1974. Doping and anti-doping were not mentioned as main topics. The first success of this parliamentary board was that the government had to provide a report every four years (once during each election period) on the development of sports. Deutscher Bundestag, ed., *40 Jahre Sportausschuss* (Berlin, 2009); Peter Danckert, *Kraftmaschine Parlament: Der Sportausschuss und die Sportpolitik des Bundes,* Hauptsache Sport (Aachen: Meyer & Meyer, 2009).

17. Anne Martin, ed., *Wir gegen uns: Sport im geteilten Deutschland* (Darmstadt: Primus-Verl, 2009).

18. The competition was introduced in 1969. A contemporary description of change in the elite sports system in West Germany is provided by Arnd Krüger, *Sport und Politik: Von Turnvater Jahn z. Staatsamateur* (Hannover: Fackelträger-Verlag, 1975), 143ff.; also Michael Krüger, "60 Jahre Sport in Deutschland," *Sportwissenschaft* 39, no. 3 (2009): 237–50.

19. Krüger, "60 Jahre Sport in Deutschland," 243.

20. During this conference, the young sports physician Joseph Keul of Freiburg presented a paper about his research on anabolic doping, sponsored by the Bundesinstitut für Sportwissenschaft (BISp). The title itself was a euphemism: "Fundamental Metabolic Problems in Sport," in *Sport in unserer Welt,* ed. Ommo Grupe, 525–28.

21. Ommo Grupe, "33 Jahrgänge 'Sportwissenschaft,'" *Sportwissenschaft*, no. 35 (2005): 336–38.
22. Gieseler, *Der Sport in der Bundesrepublik Deutschland*, 135.
23. The name *Zentralkomitee* in Germany has usually been used for important boards of the Catholic Church or of the Communist Party in the GDR.
24. Supplement 4 to Prot. Nr. 5 of the Sports Commission of 11 May 1973, in Parlamentsarchiv Berlin.
25. Report of a meeting of the BA-L, 28 April 1970, in B 106/49957, Bundesarchiv Koblenz.
26. Bundesarchiv Koblenz, B 106/49958.
27. Andreas Singler and Gerhard Treutlein, "Doping in der Bundesrepublik Deutschland: Historische und soziologische Aspekte abweichenden Verhaltens im Spitzensport," in *Hormone und Hochleistung: Doping in Ost und West*, ed. Klaus Latzel and Lutz Niethammer (Cologne: Böhlau, 2008), 41–65.
28. N. Allen, "Heat May Affect Performances," *Times*, 7 July 1967; *Times (London)*, 10 September 1968.
29. Charles L. Dubin, ed., *Commission of Inquiry into the Use of Drugs and Banned Practices Intended to Increase Athletic Performance* (Ottawa: Canadian Government Publication Centre, 1990), 553.
30. Hunt, *Drug Games*, 32ff.
31. *Extracts of the Minutes of the 65th Session of the International Olympic Committee*, 95. Also *Olympic Review* 5 (February 1968): 71; *Olympic Review* 10 (July 1968): 264.
32. Hunt, *Drug Games*, 27–29, 32–36.
33. *Minutes of the IOC Executive Board*, Lausanne, 2–5 February 1973.
34. Brundage to de Merode, 22 April 1971, Avery Brundage Collection, Box 99, Folder Medical Commission, 1970, 73, cited in Hunt, *Drug Games*, 40.
35. See *Minutes of the IOC Executive Board*, Lausanne, 2–5 February 1973.
36. Dimeo, *A History of Drug Use in Sport*, 116.
37. IOC Brochure, *Doping* (1972).
38. *Olympic Review* 43 (April 1971): 202ff.
39. Dimeo, *A History of Drug Use in Sport*, 116.
40. Ibid.
41. See the analysis of West German newspapers about doping by H. E. Meier, M. Reinold, and A. Rose, "Dopingskandale in der alten Bundesrepublik: Öffentlicher Diskurs und sportpolitische Reaktionen," *Deutschland Archiv: Zeitschrift für das vereinigte Deutschland* 45, no. 2 (2012): 209–39.
42. DSB to BMI, 11 July 1968, in DOSB Archive.
43. Bundestagsdrucksache, 5.WP, 196. Sitzung, 15 November 1968, 10556. Juristic reflections about a specific law against doping in sports were at that time repeated at various opportunities by Federal Public Prosecutor Max Kohlhaas. See, for example, M. Kohlhaas, "Doping aus rechtlicher Sicht," in *Rekorde aus der Retorte: Leistungssteigerung im modernen Hochleistungssport*, ed. H. Acker (Stuttgart, 1972), 53–57; M. Kohlhaas, "Gesetzliche Grundlagen für ein Verbot von 'Doping,'" *Sportarzt und Sportmedizin* 17, no. 2 (1966): 64–81.
44. Brigitte Berendonk, "Züchten wir Monstren," *Die Zeit*, no. 49, 5 December 1969.
45. Bundestagsdrucksache, VI/1480, B 185/1997, Bundesarchiv Koblenz.
46. Bundesarchiv Koblenz, B 185/1997.
47. For the whole case see: Bundesarchiv Koblenz, B 322/9.
48. Statement of Donike during a hearing of experts in the Sixth Meeting of the Sports Committee on Wednesday, 28 September 1977, in Bonn.
49. Anabolics were first tested during the Montreal Games in 1976. Experts like Donike or Keul knew very well that these tests were mostly useless, because evidence of anabolic use could be covered by simply stopping their use in time. Therefore, Donike requested controls to be implemented in the training stage. Manfred Donike, "Zum Problem des Nachweises der anabolen Steroide: Gas-chromatographische und massenspezifische Möglichkeiten," *Sportarzt und Sportmedizin*, no. 1 (1975): 1–6.
50. Hunt, *Drug Games*, 43.

51. Protocol of the Meeting of the Board, 2 March 1972, in B 106/113210, Bundesarchiv Koblenz. However, for the IOC, Schlickenrieder became a persona non grata, and de Merode explicitly forbade an engagement of Schlickenrieder in the context of the doping controls in Munich. Comment on Doping Controls at the Olympic Games of 31 May 1972, in B 185/1999, Bundesarchiv Koblenz.

52. The full names of these persons are not used because of data privacy protection.

53. *Times (London)*, 9 August 1971.

54. Letter from Hansjörg Kofink to the NOK for Germany, 5 August 1972, http://www.cycling4fans.de/uploads/media/Offener_Brief_an_NOK_5.8.72.pdf, accessed 20 July 2013.

55. Bundesarchiv Koblenz, B 322/9.

56. Bundesarchiv Koblenz, B 185/1996.

57. The nickname of Donike was "Kanüle" (syringe needle) because of his experiences with doping as a cyclist. See the unpublished thesis of S. Thyssen, *Manfred Donike und das Institut für Biochemie der Deutschen Sporthochschule Köln: Geschichte und Leistung im Kampf gegen Doping* (2010).

58. Protocol of the meeting of 12 June 1970, in B 185/1999, Bundesarchiv Koblenz.

59. Comment in Department I v. 5.5.1970, in B 185/1996, Bundesarchiv Koblenz.

60. Bundesarchiv Koblenz, B 106/30678.

61. For a list of the *Probeläufe* (trial runs), see B 185/1999, Bundesarchiv Koblenz.

62. D. Clasing and A. Klümper, "Dopingkontrollen bei den Spielen der XX. Olympiade München 1972," *Leistungssport*, no. 2 (1972): 130–34.

63. Ibid., 131.

64. Ibid., 134.

65. Les Woodland, *Dope: The Use of Drugs in Sport* (Newton Abbot, UK: David & Charles, 1980), 57, 193.

66. D. Clasing et al., "Dopingkontrollen bei den Spielen der XX. Olympiade München 1972 (III)," *Leistungssport*, no. 4 (1975): 306.

67. The East German laboratory in Kreischa was evaluated positively and with strong recommendations from the IOC all the time. Even so, everybody knew that Kreischa was being misused by the GDR politicians and physicians for pretests of athletes before international events. See also the unpublished final research report of M. Reinold, "Arguing against Doping," 48, sponsored by the IOC. Kreischa obtained the highest ranking for "good performance" in the report of the IOC Medical Commission, Reaccreditation Procedure 1989, Annex 1 of the Minutes of the Subcommission Doping and Biochemistry, 5 February 1989, file Procès-verbal Commission Medicale 1989.

68. K. Jung, "Normen, Ziele, Prioritäten der Sportpolitik," *Tutzinger Studien*, no. 1 (1974): 49.

69. Ibid., 56.

70. Quoted in Helmut Acker, ed., *Rekorde aus der Retorte: Leistungssteigerung im modernen Hochleistungssport,* Ein X-Buch (Stuttgart: Dt. Verl.-Anst, 1972), 52.

71. Dimeo, *A History of Drug Use in Sport, 1876–1976*, 103.

72. Klaus Latzel, *Staatsdoping: Der VEB Jenapharm im Sportsystem der DDR* (Cologne and Vienna: Böhlau, 2009). The archives of several sports federations and responsible persons confirm this fact. See, for example, the estate of the former president of the DLV (German Athletics Federation) August Kirsch, archived in the Carl and Liselott Diem Archive in Cologne (folders 85 and 111), and the reports and minutes of the Medical Commission of the IOC (IOC Archives). See also Reinold, "Arguing against Doping."

73. *Leichtathletik* 43 (1970), 1568.

74. This discussion can be seen in the DLV journal *Leichtathletik* of the 1970s and according to the competition rules of the DLV, here 1972, rule 16.

75. *Athletik* 5 (1972), 20.

76. Ibid., 13.

77. Ludwig Prokop, "Zur Geschichte des Dopings und seiner Bekämpfung," *Sportarzt und Sportmedizin* 21, no. 6 (1970): 130.

78. Minutes of the 72nd session of the IOC, p. 28, IOC Archives.

79. Special edition of the conference of the British Association of Sports Medicine, published by the *British Journal of Sports Medicine* 9 (1975): 110.

80. This ethical and philosophical question about what is "natural" and "artificial" in sports, training, and doping is discussed extensively by Claudia Pawlenka, *Ethik, Natur und Doping,* Ethica 19 (Paderborn: Mentis, 2010).

81. Patrick Laure, *Le dopage: Pratiques corporelles* (Paris: Presses Universitaires de France, 1995), 138; C. Brissonneau and F. Depiesse, "Doping and Doping Control in French Sport," 145–67.

82. Giselher Spitzer, *Doping in der DDR: Ein historischer Überblick zu einer konspirativen Praxis; Genese—Verantwortung—Gefahren*, Wissenschaftliche Berichte und Materialien des Bundesinstituts für Sportwissenschaft 1998, 3 (Cologne: Sport und Buch Strauß, 1998), 221; Brigitte Berendonk, *Doping: Von der Forschung zum Betrug*, 2nd expanded ed., rororo Sport 8677 (Heidelberg: Rowohlt, 1992), 91, 168.

83. Andreas Singler and Gerhard Treutlein, *Doping im Spitzensport: Sportwissenschaftliche Analysen zur nationalen und internationalen Leistungsentwicklung (Teil 1)*, 6th ed., Sportentwicklungen in Deutschland 12 (Aachen: Meyer & Meyer, 2012); Martin Lames, "Leistungsentwicklung in der Leichtathletik: Ist Doping als leistungsfördernder Effekt identifizierbar?" *dvs-informationen* 17, no. 4 (2002): 15–22.

84. *Sports International* 6 and 7 (1987).

85. Correspondence in various archives of federations evidently prove the unsystematic practice in different sports. See, for example, the documents in the Bundesarchiv Koblenz (B 322/9), in the CuLDA (esp. estate of August Kirsch), and the archive of the BISp.

86. C. Schrange, "'Kompliment, Herr Hangstein . . . Das war präsidentisch!' Verhandlung gegen Dieter Leitner," *Radsport*, no. 34 (1971): 7–8.

87. *Leichtathletik* 40 (1970): 1409.

88. For more detail, see Marcel Reinold, "Arguing against Doping," 19ff., 22ff.; Bund Deutscher Radfahrer (BDR), Sportordnungen, 1970 and 1975, paragraph 138: Doping; Deutscher Sportbund (DSB), Rahmen-Richtlinien zur Bekämpfung des Dopings, Beschlossen am 26. September 1970 durch den Hauptausschuss des DSB in Mannheim, 1970, § 4; Deutscher Leichtathletik-Verband, Amtliche Leichtathletik-Bestimmungen, 1971, rule 16/1.

89. Deutscher Leichtathletik-Verband (DLV) Archiv, Folder 1, decision of the FLVW advocate against Klehr, 4 December 1972.

90. Carl und Liselott Diem-Archiv (CuLDA), Nachlass Kirsch, Folder 111, DLV 4 (Council of the Federation), minutes of the meeting of the chair, 10 August 1978, p. 3ff.

91. Ibid.

92. H. Nolte, "Presserklärung des Sportausschusses Niedersachsen," *Radsport*, no. 26 (1973): 10.

93. Manfred Donike, "Dopinganalytik bei Olympischen Spielen," in *Rekorde aus der Retorte: Leistungssteigerung im modernen Hochleistungssport*, ed. Helmut Acker, Ein X-Buch (Stuttgart: Dt. Verl.-Anst, 1972), 46–52, esp. 49.

94. International Olympic Committee, *Le Mouvement olympique de lavenir: Thème 3. XIe Congrès olympique à Baden-Baden 1981* (Lausanne: CIO, 1982).

95. For more detail, see Henk E. Meier and Marcel Reinold, "Performance Enhancement and Politicisation of High-Performance Sport: The West German 'Air Clyster' Affair of 1976," *International Journal of the History of Sport* 30, no. 12 (2013): 1351–73, doi:10.1080/09523367.2013.784273.

96. Giselher Spitzer, *Siegen um jeden Preis: Doping in Deutschland: Geschichte, Recht, Ethik, 1972–1990* (Göttingen: Verlag Die Werkstatt, 2013); Henk E. Meier and Marcel Reinold, "Dopingskandale in der alten Bundesrepublik: Öffentlicher Diskurs und sportpolitische Reaktionen," *Deutschland Archiv: Zeitschrift für das vereinigte Deutschland* 45, no. 2 (2012): 209–39.

97. Archiv Willi Daume in der Deutschen Olympischen Akademie, 105.14, report of Alois Mader on the effects of Berolase (Cocarboxylase) and Thioctacid (Alpha Liponsäure) for sporting performance in short and middle distance running, including a letter from Mader to Nöcker, 3 September 1976, p. 7.

98. Archiv Willi Daume in der Deutschen Olympischen Akademie, 105.14, letter from Mader to Nöcker, 3 September 1976; Bundesinstitut für Sportwissenschaft (BISp), Doping E-Z, letter of Reindell to Grupe, 14 December 1976; letter of Reindell to Kirsch, 2 November 1978.

99. The BA-L was founded in 1968/69 for allocating financial support from the federal state to the various sport organizations. This commission became a very powerful "state within the state" of German sports. Meier and Reinold, "Performance Enhancement and Politicisation of High-Performance Sport," 1359.

100. According to the report of Meyer in the journal *Der Schwimmsport* 21 (1977): 418.

101. These activities are well documented by the Sports Commission of the German parliament, held in the Parlamentsarchiv (PA), see especially the letter from the Swimming Federation to the Ministry of the Interior, 16 June 1976.

102. Parlamentsarchiv (PA), letter of the BMI to the DSV, 21 June 1976.

103. *Der Schwimmsport* 21 (1977): 418; G. Heydn, "'Luftduschen' nutzen nichts," *Der Deutsche Schwimmsport*, no. 6 (1977): 140.

104. See chapter 3 on the role of the Stasi and the West German Bundesnachrichtendienst (BND). The Cold War on the track is well described and researched by Balbier, *Kalter Krieg auf der Aschenbahn*, for Germany. See also Mike Dennis, "Securing the Sports 'Miracle': The Stasi and East German Elite Sport," *International Journal of the History of Sport* 29, no. 18 (2012): 2551–74, doi:10.1080/09523367.2012.719881; Dennis and Grix, *Sport under Communism*.

105. According to the memories of the East German president of the DTSB, Manfred Ewald and Reinhold Andert, *Manfred Ewald—Ich war der Sport: Wahrheiten und Legenden aus dem Wunderland der Sieger,* EP 526 (Berlin: Elefanten Press, 1994), 182.

106. *Der Spiegel* 34 (1977): 179. The West German journal *Der Schwimmsport* reported extensively about the successes of the GDR swimmers, here 24 (1976): 441.

107. Public meeting during the thirty-seventh session of the German Bundestag Committee on the Status of Sports Science and Sports Medicine in the Federal Republic of Germany, 17 March 1976, 75ff.

108. Giselher Spitzer, "Gab es in der DDR Spionage des Bundesnachrichtendienstes?" (Was there any spying by the BND in the GDR about sport?) *Sozial- und Zeitgeschichte des Sports* 13, no. 3 (1999): 28–40; Hans J. Teichler, "Die Ausspähung des westdeutschen Sports durch das Ministerium für Staatssicherheit der DDR" (Spying of the West German sport by the Stasi), in *Der geteilte deutsche Sport: Tagung der DVS-Sektion Sportgeschichte vom 24.–26. März 1995 in Potsdam*, ed. Giselher Spitzer and Harald Braun, Berichte und Materialien des Bundesinstituts für Sportwissenschaft 97/3 (Cologne: Sport und Buch Strauss, 1997), 65–98.

109. The DSB organized so-called *Akademiegespräche* (academy talks), where athletes of the GDR were openly asked about their experiences in GDR sport. Gunter Holzweissig, *Sport und Politik in der DDR* (Berlin: Holzapfel, 1988), 55ff.; the case of Renate Neufeld was reported comprehensively in *Der Spiegel* 12 (1979). See also http://en.wikipedia.org/wiki/Doping_in_East_Germany, accessed 18 May 2014; Neufeld also published a book including her experiences as a GDR top athlete. Renate Neufeld-Spassov, Dimitrov Pentschon, and Johannes Hampel, *Politik und Sport* (Munich: Olzog, 1980).

110. Jutta Braun, "'Republikflucht' und 'Fluchthelfer': Ein verdrängtes Kapitel deutsch-deutscher Sportbeziehungen," in *Vergessen, verdrängt, abgelehnt—Zur Geschichte der Ausgrenzung im Sport: Tagungsbericht der 10. Hoyaer Tagung zur Sportgeschichte vom 10. bis 12. Oktober 2008*, ed. Arnd Krüger, Schriftenreihe des Niedersächsischen Instituts für Sportgeschichte Hoya e.V. Reihe 1, Wissenschaftliche Reihe 21 (Berlin: Lit-Verl, 2009), 106–16, esp. 109ff.

111. Der Bundesbeauftragte für die Unterlagen des Staatssicherheitsdienstes der ehemaligen Deutschen Demokratischen Republik (BStU), MfS, AGM, Nr. 476, p. 169.

112. For more detail, see Jutta Braun, René Wiese, and Claudia de La Garza, *ZOV Sportverräter: Spitzenathleten auf der Flucht; Begleitbuch zur Ausstellung; Eine Ausstellung des Zentrums Deutsche Sportgeschichte Berlin-Brandenburg e.V. (ZdS) in Zusammenarbeit mit der Künstlerin Laura Soria und der Ausstellungsagentur Exhibeo*, with the assistance of Gloria Fochs, (Berlin: Zentrum Deutsche Sportgeschichte Berlin-Brandenburg, 2011); Jutta Braun and

Laura Soria, *ZOV Sportverräter—Spitzenathleten auf der Flucht: Eine Ausstellung des Zentrums Deutsche Sportgeschichte Berlin-Brandenburg e.V. (ZdS) in Zusammenarbeit mit der Künstlerin Laura Soria und der Ausstellungsagentur exhibeo; Begleitbuch zur Ausstellung; 22. Juli–28. August 2011, Willi-Brandt-Haus, Berlin* (Berlin: Zentrum deutsche Sportgeschichte, 2011).

113. Der Bundesbeauftragte für die Unterlagen des Staatssicherheitsdienstes der ehemaligen Deutschen Demokratischen Republik (BStU), MfS, A 637/79, vol. 2, p. 45.

114. Michael Krüger, "Vorbild DDR? Neuorientierung im westdeutschen Sport," in *Wir gegen uns: Sport im geteilten Deutschland*, ed. Anne Martin (Darmstadt: Primus-Verl, 2009), 98–107.

115. Der Bundesbeauftragte für die Unterlagen des Staatssicherheitsdienstes der ehemaligen Deutschen Demokratischen Republik (BStU), MfS, A-637/79, vol. 2, p. 55ff.

116. Ibid., vol. 2, p. 210ff.

117. Ibid., vol. 2, pp. 279, 281, 225. With respect to the Stasi documents it ought to be mentioned critically that the reports of the Stasi were neither true nor objective. The spies or "Informelle Mitarbeiter" had an interest in telling their supervising officers about successful missions.

118. Ibid., vol. 2, pp. 285–86.

119. Ibid., vol. 1, p. 296ff.

120. Arnulf Baring and Manfred Görtemaker, *Machtwechsel: Die Ära Brandt-Scheel* (Stuttgart: Deutsche Verlags-Anstalt, 1982).

121. Doping tests at the Olympic Games in 1976, by Alexandre de Merode, http://library.la84.org/OlympicInformationCenter/OlympicReview/1979/ore135/ore135i.pdf, accessed 20 May 2014.

122. Robert Hartmann, "Das Trauma Anabolika," *Leichtathletik* 47: 1660–61.

123. Berendonk, *Doping*, 242, 277, 279. However, the quantity of doping applications cannot be determined.

124. With respect to the international process of medicalization, see Ivan Waddington and Andy Smith, *An Introduction to Drugs in Sport: Addicted to Winning?* (London: Routledge, 2009), esp. 65–68.

125. Bernard Asbell, *Die Pille und wie sie die Welt veränderte,* Fischer 13662 (Frankfurt am Main: Fischer-Taschenbuch-Verlag, 1998).

126. Bundesministerium des Inneren (BMI), *Sportberichte der Bundesregierung* (Bonn, Berlin, 1973–2010), 1970, p. 22; 1976, p. 36; 1978, p. 34.

127. Bund Deutscher Radfahrer (BDR), Sportordnungen, minutes of the meeting of 1972, p. 22, and 1974, p. 37.

128. Bund Deutscher Radfahrer (BDR), Sportordnungen, minutes of the main assembly in 1971.

129. Carl und Liselott Diem-Archiv, folder 85, trials on doping, letters from Schuch to Kirsch, 23 April 1975, and Pfeifer to Kirsch, 28 April 1975. Deutscher Leichtathletik-Verband, Amtliche Leichtathletik-Bestimmungen, trial Klehr, folder I, Bavarian Track and Field Association, note on Kirsch trial, Bechtold, Klehr, 28 March 1978.

130. Gehrmann had delivered hormone doping systematically to female athletes. Berendonk, *Doping*, 270ff.; Parlamentsarchiv (PA), minutes of the hearing of the sixth meeting of the Sports Commission, 28 September 1977, 119; Deutscher Leichtathletik-Verband, Amtliche Leichtathletik-Bestimmungen, trial Klehr, folder I, statement by Manfred Steffny, 11 October 1976.

131. The CV of Kofink and his fight against doping are extensively documented under http://www.cycling4fans.de/index.php?id=4523, accessed 22 May 2014, including documents on his communication with leading officials in the 1970s.

132. Parlamentsarchiv (PA), minutes of the Sports Commission, 1977, 56.

133. Interview with Willi Weyer in the newspaper *Tagesspiegel*, 11 May 1977, cited by Andreas Singler and Gerhard Treutlein, *Doping im Spitzensport,* Sportentwicklungen in Deutschland 12 (Aachen: Meyer & Meyer, 2000), 213.

134. Deutscher Sportbund, ed., *Berichte des Präsidiums,* 3 vols. (1982), 238.

135. For more detail, refer to Balbier, *Kalter Krieg auf der Aschenbahn*, 133.

136. Peter Danckert, *Kraftmaschine Parlament: Der Sportausschuss und die Sportpolitik des Bundes,* Hauptsache Sport (Aachen: Meyer & Meyer, 2009).

137. Bundesministerium des Inneren (BMI), *Sportberichte der Bundesregierung* (Bonn, Berlin, 1973–2010), Sportförderung des Bundes, 1970, pp. 15, 21; Sportberichte, 1973, pp. 9, 25; 1976, p. 36; Günter Pelshenke, "Stiftung Deutsche Sporthilfe" (Univ, 1999); in general, Krüger, "60 Jahre Sport in Deutschland"; Krüger, "Vorbild DDR? Neuorientierung im westdeutschen Sport," 98–107.

138. Bero Rigauer, *Sport and Work,* European Perspectives (New York: Columbia University Press, 1981), first published in German in 1969, was the work in which the Marxist concept and criticism of capitalist sports had been initiated.

139. Hans Lenk, *Leistungssport: Ideologie oder Mythos? Zur Leistungskritik und Sportphilosophie,* Urban-Taschenbücher 826 (Stuttgart: Kohlhammer, 1972); Ommo Grupe, *Bewegung, Spiel und Leistung im Sport: Grundthemen der Sportanthropologie,* Reihe Sportwissenschaft 18 (Schorndorf: K. Hofmann, 1982); Michael Krüger, "Ruhmsucht und Rekordfimmel: Zur Geschichte der Leistung im Sport," in *Für einen besseren Sport: Themen, Entwicklungen und Perspektiven aus Sport und Sportwissenschaft*, ed. Hartmut Gabler and Ulrich Göhner (Tübingen: Institut für Sportwissenschaft der Universität Tübingen, 1990), 343–62.

140. Hubertus Knabe, *Honeckers Erben: Die Wahrheit über die Linke* (Berlin: Propyläen, 2009), argues in this manner.

141. Parlamentsarchiv (PA), Sports Commission, 1977, p. 9.

142. These discussions are well documented in Parlamentsarchiv (PA), Sports Commission, eighth election period, 1977, various meetings, esp. eighteenth and twenty-fifth meetings.

143. Printings of the Bundestag 8/2850, here on p. 9.

144. Ommo Grupe, "Der Athlet im Mittelpunkt: Einführung in die Grundsatzerklärung," in *Grundsatzerklärung für den Spitzensport: 17. Sitzung des Hauptausschusses des Deutschen Sportbundes am 11. Juni in Baden-Baden*, ed. Deutscher Sportbund (1977), 5.

145. Singler and Treutlein, *Doping im Spitzensport.*

146. Bundesinstitut für Sportwissenschaft (BISp) Archive, B 322/444, letter of Reindell to Gruppe, 14 December 1976.

147. Parlamentsarchiv (PA), minutes of the hearing of the Sports Commission of the Bundestag, 28 September 1977, 15.

148. Ibid., 37.

149. Ommo Grupe, "Der Athlet im Mittelpunkt: Einführung in die Grundsatzerklärung."

150. Ibid., 12.

151. Karlheinz Gieseler, "Soziale Hilfen für den Spitzensport," in Deutscher Sportbund, *Berichte des Präsidiums* (see note 80), 144.

152. Deutscher Sportbund, ed., *Grundsatzerklärung für den Spitzensport: 17. Sitzung des Hauptausschusses des Deutschen Sportbundes am 11. Juni in Baden-Baden* (1977), §1.

153. Parlamentsarchiv (PA), statement of Donike at the meeting of the parliamentary Sports Commission, 1977, 43.

154. Ommo Grupe, "Der Athlet im Mittelpunkt: Einführung in die Grundsatzerklärung," 8ff.

155. Bundesarchiv Koblenz, B 106/49957, report of the meeting of the BA-L, 28 April 1970.

156. The whole story can be read online at http://www.cycling4fans.de/index.php?id=4604, here letter of Kofink to the NOK, 11 August 1972, accessed 2 July 2014.

157. Parlamentsarchiv (PA), hearing of the Sports Commission, 28 September 1977, 66.

158. Josef Neckermann, "Die Abkehr von Normen," *Der Deutsche Schwimmsport*, no. 1 (1977): 6.

159. Bundesministerium des Inneren (BMI), *Sportförderung des Bundes* (1970ff.), 1982, p. 32.

160. Balbier, *Kalter Krieg auf der Aschenbahn*, 178ff.

161. Bundesarchiv Koblenz, B 106/49958.

162. Bundesministerium des Inneren (BMI), *Sportberichte der Bundesregierung* (Bonn, Berlin, 1973–2010), 1976, p. 53.

163. Deutscher Sportbund, *Berichte des Präsidiums*, 1978, pp. 249–53.

164. Bundesministerium des Inneren (BMI), *Sportförderung des Bundes* (1970ff.), 1982, p. 16; 1986, p. 30.

165. Bundesverband Deutscher Gewichtheber (BVDG), minutes of the board meeting, 13 November 1971, 1.
166. Ibid., 1 November 1975, 1.
167. Parlamentsarchiv (PA), Bundestagsdrucksache (BT) 9/1292, p. 8, response of Undersecretary of State von Schoeler, 14 January 1982.
168. When Henry IV walked to the pope at Canossa in 1076, he both paid penitence for his sins and tried to be absolved from the ban by the pope and the church in order to gain better opportunities to act as he wished.
169. Bundesverband Deutscher Gewichtheber (BVDG), folder minutes of the meetings, 12 June 1982, 3.
170. For more detail, see the report of Marcel Reinold, "Arguing against Doping."
171. Carl und Liselott Diem-Archiv (CuLDA), heritage Kirsch, folder 91, Doping 1971–1977, letter Donike to Kirsch, 21 October 1977.
172. Evaluierungskommission Freiburger Sportmedizin unpublished manuscript (accessed 29 May 2014); "Abschlussbericht der Expertenkommission zur Aufklärung von Dopingvorwürfen gegenüber Ärzten der Abteilung Sportmedizin des Universitätsklinikums Freiburg" (23 May 2009; 12 May 2009) unpublished manuscript, p. 35 (accessed 29 May 2014).
173. Meier and Reinold, "Dopingskandale in der alten Bundesrepublik," esp. 228–37.
174. See the cover story of the journal *Der Spiegel*, 7 September 1987.
175. Documented in Berendonk, *Doping*, appendix, 4B.
176. On the hearing of the Sports Commission, see Deutscher Bundestag, "Humanität im Spitzensport: Öffentliche Anhörung des Sportausschusses des Deutschen Bundestags am 14. Oktober 1987 in Bonn," (1988), unpublished manuscript, 109.
177. Brigitte Berendonk, *Doping Dokumente: Von der Forschung zum Betrug* (Berlin and New York: Springer-Verlag, 1991), 233–70.
178. Ibid.
179. Joseph Keul, "Freiwillige Dopingkontrolle während des Trainings empfohlen," *NOK-Report*, no. 3 (1987): 16.
180. Thomas M. Hunt, *Drug Games*, 68–70.
181. Marcel Reinold, "Arguing against Doping," 44.
182. Carl und Liselott Diem-Archiv (CuLDA), heritage Kirsch, folder 101, Doping 1, betr. Gerhard Strittmatter, summarized analysis by Gerhard Huber.
183. These numbers are from the reports of the Bundesinstitut für Sportwissenschaft (BIS) from 1975 to 1990.
184. Laure, *Le dopage*, p 193.
185. Carl und Liselott Diem-Archiv (CuLDA), heritage Kirsch, folder Doping 86, letter of Donike to Kirsch, 27 January 1982.
186. Discussions on these issues are broadly reported in the documents on the legacy of August Kirsch in ibid.
187. Carl und Liselott Diem-Archiv (CuLDA), heritage Kirsch, folder Doping 86, position paper of Joseph Keul, 29 June 1982.
188. Carl und Liselott Diem-Archiv (CuLDA), heritage Kirsch, folder Doping 86, introduction of Ommo Grupe to the Grundsatzerklärung für den Spitzensport, 3 December 1983.
189. Carl und Liselott Diem-Archiv (CuLDA), heritage Kirsch, folder Doping 86, decision of the main committee of the German Sports Federation, in accordance with the National Olympic Committee, with respect to the Grundsatzerklärung für den Spitzensport, 5 November 1983.
190. Bundesinstitut für Sportwissenschaft (BISp) Archive, 0408/1 Forschungsauftrag "Regeneration" W 1.1 1986–1990; the following according to these documents.
191. Giselher Spitzer, ed., *Doping in Deutschland: Geschichte, Recht, Ethik: 1950–1972*.
192. Carl und Liselott Diem-Archiv (CuLDA), heritage Kirsch, folder 87, Doping 3, 1985–1986, Top 2 of the minutes of the working group on doping, 31 January 1986.
193. Bundesinstitut für Sportwissenschaft (BISp) Archive, 0408/01 Forschungsauftrag "Regeneration" W 1.1 1986–1990, final report of Keul/Jacob, December 1992.
194. Parlamentsarchiv (PA), printing 12/1781, p. 7.
195. Berendonk, *Doping*, 401–7.

196. Carl und Liselott Diem-Archiv (CuLDA), heritage Kirsch, folder Doping 86, report of the meeting of the working group on problems of science and health of the European NOCs, 13 January 1982 in Brussels, p. 2.

197. These cases, as well as the initiatives of Donike, are documented in the legacy of August Kirsch in the Carl und Liselott Diem-Archiv (CuLDA), the Bundesinstitut für Sportwissenschaft (BISp) Archive, and the archive of the Deutscher Schwimm-Verband (DSV).

198. Carl und Liselott Diem-Archiv (CuLDA), heritage Kirsch, folder 87, Doping 3, 1985–1986, letter of Keul to Kirsch, 25 November 1985.

199. Parlamentsarchiv (PA), printing 11/404, response of the federal government to the "short questionnaire" on "humanity in top level sport," 3 June 1987.

200. Carl und Liselott Diem-Archiv (CuLDA), heritage Kirsch, folder 89 on doping, several letters of Donike to Kirsch. Similar letters are collected in the archive of the Deutscher Olympischer Sportbund (DOSB), 1322/B6.5/4B 12.

201. Carl und Liselott Diem-Archiv (CuLDA), heritage Kirsch, folder 88, Doping 5, circular letter, 15 March 1988.

202. Ibid.; Council of Europe, Recommendation No. R (88) 12 of the Committee of Ministers to Member States on the Institution of Doping Controls Without Warning, adopted 21 June 1988 by Committee of Ministers; IOC Archives, Final Declaration of the First Permanent World Conference on Anti-Doping in Sport from 26.–29.6.1988. Annex I of the minutes of the 94. IOC Session, 13.–16.9.1988, p. 104.

203. Ibid.; Report of the Thirteenth Informal Meeting of European Ministers Responsible for Sport, Athens, 1–2 June 1988.

204. Carl und Liselott Diem-Archiv (CuLDA), heritage Kirsch, folder 88, Doping 5, circular letter, 26 August 1988.

205. Deutscher Olympischer Sportbund (DOSB) Archive, folder 4026/B 6.5/KII1=B, collection of important decisions of the NOC to reduce doping.

206. Carl und Liselott Diem-Archiv (CuLDA), heritage Kirsch, folder 89, Doping 6, letter of DSB, 30 March 1989.

207. Carl und Liselott Diem-Archiv (CuLDA), heritage Kirsch, folder 89, Doping 6, Donike to Keul, 30 March1989; Donike to Hansen, 12 April 1989.

208. Deutscher Olympischer Sportbund (DOSB) Archive, folder Anti-Doping Commission, minutes of the opening meeting of the Anti-Doping-Commission, 27 February 1992.

Chapter Three

Doping and Anti-Doping in the Process of German Reunification

In order to achieve a better understanding of the development of top-level sports in general after the breakdown of the Eastern bloc in the late 1980s, and especially the history of doping and anti-doping in Germany through the German reunification, it should be borne in mind that during the period of the Cold War, both Germanies, East and West, were leading sporting nations. West Germany, the Federal Republic of Germany (FRG), developed its sporting system according to the western world, guided by the Anglo-American model of free sport, and based on its traditions of sporting and gymnastics clubs before the Nazi dictatorship. East Germany, the German Democratic Republic (GDR), looked on sports as a means of developing socialism in this "other" (or "second") Germany, under the control and support of the socialist state and its single political party, the Sozialistische Einheitspartei Deutschlands (SED). Both countries were members of the Olympic family, and both were keen to demonstrate their superiority in all spheres of life, namely political, social, economic, and cultural, including sports.[1] At the Munich Olympics of 1972, they were the most successful teams after the superpowers, the USSR and the United States. The GDR gained twenty gold medals, seven more than the West German athletes. As Willi Daume, the chief organizer of the Olympics, commented: "The GDR gets most of the medals, and we are the hosts and proudly present these wonderful, fair, and cheerful Games to the world. That is why both sides can be pleased."[2]

The GDR became the most successful nation after the USSR at the 1976 Olympics in Montreal, measured by the medal count. At the Winter Olympics of 1980 in Lake Placid, the GDR athletes gained more medals than any other team, even more than their socialist "brother," the USSR. The GDR sports politicians and sports organizers expected to become number one in world top-level sports in 1984.[3]

However, everybody in sports, and the public, knew—or rather could have known—that the enormous increase in achievement in top-level sports and the advance over athletes from other countries in specific sports were possible only through "sustaining means." This was the official term for doping substances that had been invented in the sports medicine laboratories of the GDR, as well as throughout the world of top-level sports. No doubt, the GDR system (in some selected sports and disciplines) was the most successful—at any rate in this dubious context. Otherwise, it would be impossible to explain why a small state with fewer than twenty million inhabitants could become number one at the Olympics. But it was well known and indeed obvious that on the "bright" (or should that be the "right" side) of the Iron Curtain—outside the "empire of the devil," as Ronald Reagan used to call the USSR and its satellites—doping and manipulation were practiced as well, and particularly vigorously. Finally, the Montreal Olympics of 1976 presented the writing on the wall for many problems, constituting a crisis of modern top-level sports, beginning with the anachronism of amateurism and culminating in the huge but not then really evident doping problem.

When the Berlin Wall came down or was "torn down" in 1989/90, as President Reagan had challenged the most powerful person in the USSR, Mikhail Gorbachev, to do in his famous Berlin speech of 1987, clean sports and anti-doping seemed to be getting a new chance to do things right. Regrettably, this opportunity was not converted into reality. The situation in German sports after the collapse of the GDR was ambivalent. On the one hand, sports politicians and lobbyists of top-level sports from both former Germanies believed that all-German Olympic teams could be unbeatable in the future if the political process of unification succeeded in sustaining the successful structures of the East, combined with the individual and commercial motivation of athletes from the West. Evidence of this opinion is provided by the fact that the continued existence of basic institutions that led to the "miracle" of GDR sports were guaranteed by the official treaty of German unification (*Vertrag zur Deutschen Einheit*). This had been negotiated and drafted mainly by Wolfgang Schäuble, then a minister of the West German chancellor Helmut Kohl and former minister of the interior, which includes sports. The Forschungsinstitut für Körperkultur und Sport (FKS, Research Institute for Body Culture and Sport), a scientific institute closely associated with and located near the German University for Body Culture and Sport in Leipzig (Deutsche Hochschule für Körperkultur und Sport, DHfK), the Doping-Control Laboratory in Kreischa, and the scientific institute for developing and researching sports utilities and equipment in Berlin, was to be transferred to the unified Germany in order to "save" the scientific heart of the GDR sports system, on the one hand.[4] On the other hand, as all insiders of sports in East and West Germany were well aware, these institutions were also responsible for, or at least involved in, the comprehensive doping system of the GDR. In fact, the laboratory at Kreischa, which was accredited by the IOC and praised for its high scientific quality, was misused to protect GDR athletes from detection prior to international competitions.[5]

This was the initial position of sports, doping, and anti-doping in the context of German unification. Two weeks after the fall of the Berlin Wall, the government responded to a *Große Anfrage* (literally "major request") from the parliament concerning doping and anti-doping in German sports: "The federal government started early combating doping in German sport. German sport has even declared to the public and to the federal government that the clubs and sport federation have the doping problem under control. [. . .] The government believes that the use or misuse of doping substances is very different in various sports. Doping should make no sense in most sports, because these methods would not contribute to better achievement and performance."[6]

It is obvious that this response was completely incorrect. The problem was not at all under control, neither by the government nor by the sports organizations. It should be added that the international sports organizations, led by the IOC, were helpless and impotent in the face of this problem, as were the governments and sports organizations of many other countries. In Germany, revelations about the *Staatsdoping*[7] in the GDR showed that such activities were far more widespread than politicians and even sports experts and organizers could possibly imagine. The revelations in the GDR ultimately had the consequence that doping in West Germany came into the focus of a critical and sensitized public. The West German public had already been shocked three years previously by the case of Birgit Dressel, the West German heptathlete who died in 1987 in Mainz after an allergic reaction from essentially poisoning herself by the misuse of various medications over an extended period, including hormones, anabolics, and analgesics.[8]

In addition, new doping scandals in the unified Germany brought the full nature of the practices to light. At the beginning of the 1990s, the case of Katrin Krabbe, a top-level female track-and-field athlete, dominated the headlines of German and international papers (and the media generally). Krabbe was very much a "product" of the GDR sports system. She ran first in the 100 and 200 meters at the 1990 world championship in athletics in Tokyo, where she beat Gwen Torrence and Merlene Ottey, and became the top female athlete in the world in 1991. At the first European championship after the Cold War, in 1990 in Split, Croatia, she won three gold medals as part of a unified all-German athletic team. She was praised by the media and became the "glamour girl" of unified German athletics. For the Germans, she embodied the hope of reunified German sports, coming from East Germany, educated by coaches, pushed by doctors and advisers of the vanished or vanishing GDR, and achieving success, glory, and wealth in the new commercialized and mediatized sports system of the West. In 1992, she and Thomas Springstein, her coach since her youth at the SC Neubrandenburg, were accused of hormone doping with clenbuterol (a substance used in cattle breeding) and banned from competition for two years by the International Association of Athletics Federations (IAAF). Her comeback in 1995 failed, as she was unable to perform even close to her old level.

The Katrin Krabbe scandal is worth mentioning for two main reasons. First, the case has not been researched scientifically until now, and second, Krabbe was the first athlete who succeeded in obtaining a substantial compensation payment (DM 1.2 million) as a result of her ban. The German courts in Munich agreed to her claim against the IAAF that the ban contravened the fundamental right of freedom to choose and perform a job. After this judgment, the sports organizations became and remained very cautious about banning or sanctioning athletes. The Krabbe case is therefore significant for the process of "juridification" (*Verrechtlichung*) of modern society and sports in general, and specifically of the controlling and sanctioning of doping rules.

These spectacular doping cases and their enormous public resonance provoked intervention by politicians and sports organizers. With the Cold War over, and "won" by the West, the politicians felt free to demonstrate their policies in favor of fair and clean sports, meaning doping-free. Rudolf Seiters, minister of the interior in the government of Helmut Kohl, the chancellor of German unification, even questioned the traditional partnership between sport and the federal German state. If sports organizations were not willing and able to develop and implement "concrete plans against doping," he warned the president of the German Sports Federation, Hans Hansen, the sponsoring of top-level sports by the federal state could be withdrawn.[9]

This letter is a sign of the changing relationship between the state and sports organizations in unified Germany, caused directly by doping issues. The federal government, especially the minister of the interior, became more critical toward the tax-financed support of top-level sports as a (routine) matter of course. The aim of the following chapter is to clarify the changing relationship between sport and state in Germany in the process of and after the German reunification. First, the relationship between state and sport in Germany will be described and explained. It seems necessary to recapitulate some of the above-mentioned general effects of this relationship in order to understand how and why the political situation of sport was somewhat complicated in Germany after 1989/90. In unified Germany, the West German sports system was maintained in general, but unified Germany also retained elements of the East German system, which were adapted to the conditions of West German society. Second, the role of the media is considered, because the changing nature of sports policies cannot be explained without dealing

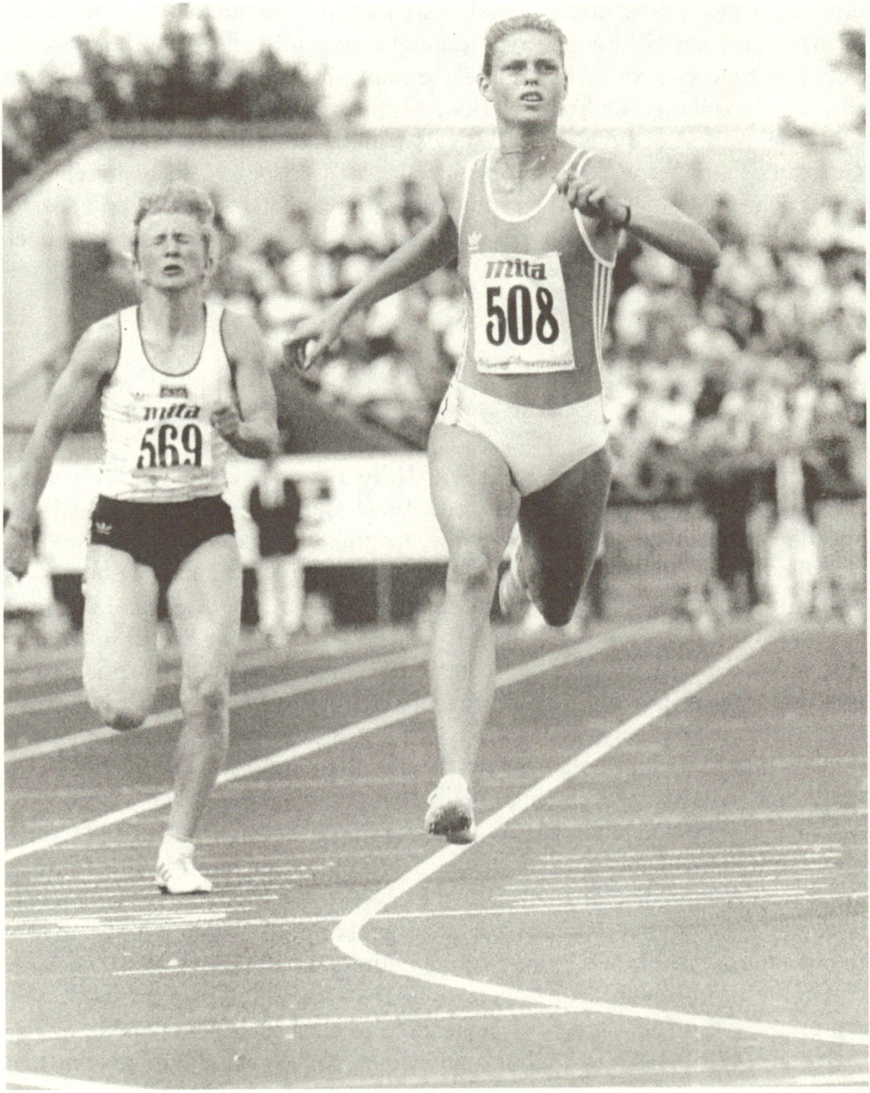

Figure 3.1. This official photo from the East German press agency ADN shows Katrin Krabbe during her victory at the European Athletics Cup in Gateshead, Great Britain (1988). She ran the first 100 meters in 11.14 seconds and was one of the East German *Fräuleinwunder* of GDR athletics. She also competed in reunified Germany. In 1992, she was charged with doping. *Source: Bundesarchiv/ Bild 183-1989-0805-024/ Peter Koard*

with the pressure put on politicians by journalists. Third, the efforts of sports and politics to combat doping reliably are placed in an international context.

The question of how and why doping issues influenced the relationship between state and sport in unified Germany has not been researched and discussed explicitly. Only the work of Andreas Singler[10] and Gerhard Treutlein,[11] as well as of Jutta Braun,[12] deals with doping issues during the era of German reunification from the perspective of the social and historical sciences. They also touch on the problematic fundamental relationship between the state and sport. However, the period of the 1990s has definitely not been researched systematically in that context of the historical or political sciences.

STATE AND SPORT, DOPING AND ANTI-DOPING IN WEST GERMANY BEFORE 1990

As mentioned above, after World War II, two completely different systems of sports were developed in East and West Germany by the political and sporting authorities. In East Germany, originally occupied by the Soviets, and then by the GDR government, organs of the state and the state party SED, including its "mass organizations" Freie Deutsche Jugend (FDJ, Free German Youth) and Freier Deutscher Gewerkschaftsbund (FDGB, Free German Trade Union) attempted to control the sporting activities of the people and to integrate sports into their broader sphere of influence and administration. In West Germany, under the control of the US and British authorities (and in the German southwest by the French), sport was regarded as an individual activity for free people pursuing enjoyment and as a leisure-time activity. The responsible officers of the US and British armies even looked upon free and independent sports as a means of reeducating the German youth.[13] The influence of any political party or even state administration was rejected. This was not only a political demand of the Western Allies, but also the common will of the German sports authorities after the disaster of Nazi dictatorship, in which sports were politically exploited and misused. The representatives of the former civilian and workers' sports movement in Germany, as well as of the Catholic and Protestant sports clubs, agreed that politics and ideology should not have any influence in future sporting affairs. But they also agreed that sports should not be divided into social, political, or cultural sectors, as in the Weimar Republic years of the 1920s and early 1930s. This fragmentation of free sports clubs and associations was considered one reason why the Nazi Party succeeded so easily and quickly in securing the control of sports. In December 1950, when the Deutsche Sportbund (DSB, German Sports Federation) was founded by the free will of all its members and without any state influence or party politics, the charter established the political, religious (confessional), and racial neutrality of this new umbrella organization of the German sports and gymnastics movement.[14] The DSB was intended to become an alternative model of free sports compared to the East German model of state sports, as well as to the obsolete model of totalitarian Nazi sports, although many of its new (but in fact old or previous) leaders had worked *in* and some of them very much *for* Nazi organizations and Nazi sports. The basis of the relationship with the state and with the public administration was the ideology of autonomy and self-organization of sports clubs, associations, and federations in the Federal Republic of Germany. This autonomy included a sound and fair partnership with political and state administrations. This implied the will of and need for the state and politics to support the efforts of autonomous sports clubs and federations in all issues concerning the interests of civil society in Germany and its representation of the German nation—for example, international sporting events and the Olympic Games. In contrast to the GDR, where "body culture and sports" were part of the constitution, in West Germany, sport was not a responsibility of the state and its administration. Rather, sport is part of the *gesetzesfreie Verwaltung*, administration without recourse to law. Of course, this did not imply that there were no rules or laws in sports. This was certainly not the case, but in sports, the rules of sports counted first, and only then the laws of the state. Sports were looked on as an *Eigenwelt*—a world of their own, an element of civil society and not a duty of the state to be financed by taxpayers.

This ideology of sports autonomy was very strong and compelling in the early days of the Federal Republic of Germany, but never prevailed in reality. In fact, high-level sports were always supported by the sponsoring state, since West German athletes participated at international competitions and especially the Olympic Games. This occurred first in Helsinki in 1952. Since then, the financial backing of sports increased year by year during the Cold War, peaking at Munich in 1972. Of course, this largest and most important sporting event of the old Federal Republic of Germany could not have been realized without enormous financial support from the federal state, as well as from the state of Bavaria and the city of Munich.[15] In spite of the ideology supporting the autonomy and liberty of sport, various German governments during the Cold War era did not hesitate to use sports as a means of foreign policy—for example, in the Hallstein Doctrine. This implied that the West German government would cut diplomatic relations with any state or government acknowledging the status of the GDR as an autonomous nation-state according to international law.[16]

Doping and anti-doping did not play a major role in the relationship between sport and state until the 1970s. Until that point, a common consensus and moral assessment of doping did not exist, either in the world of sports or in politics.[17] Doping was not regarded as a risk or danger for amateur sports and their moral integrity, but as an inevitable reality of commercialized professional sports. Furthermore, "professional sport is not sport," Carl Diem, the grand old man of German sports and "Mister Olympics 1936," had claimed in his influential work *Wesen und Lehre des Sports und der Leibeserziehung*, first published in 1949 and in various subsequent editions.[18] That is also one reason why the state authorities saw no need to communicate with sports authorities about the doping issue.

The situation changed gradually after the mid-1960s, when the Council of Europe discussed a resolution against doping and, given spectacular doping cases like that of Knud Enemark Jensen at the 1960 Olympic Games in Rome, where this talented cyclist died from amphetamine misuse. Jensen was an amateur athlete, whereas Tom Simpson, who died at Mont Ventoux during the 1967 Tour de France, and Jupp Elze, who died after a boxing fight in Hamburg, were professionals.

The doping or doping-related cases in the West German team after the Montreal Games of 1976 were alarming signs that even amateur sports were not "clean." In the late 1970s, various debates on doping took place in parliament and the relevant parliamentary commission. Sporting politicians, officials, and managers were required to report on, explain, and respond to these doping cases and to suggest ways of dealing with this "cancer" of modern sport, which risked not only the health of athletes, but the morality and fairness of sport itself. As a result, the Deutsche Sportbund (DSB) concluded a Declaration of Principles for Top Sports in 1977. The sports organizations in Germany confirmed their solidarity with top-level athletes and the principle of free, autonomous sport. They demanded financial support from the state, because of the importance of top-level sports for the nation, but doping was rejected completely. The DSB also promised to formulate specific plans to develop anti-doping. One main aspect was to improve coaching, with special respect to psychological and medical counseling for the athletes. This was an important argument for obtaining more money from the state, because it was maintained that better conditions for top athletes were the best means of preventing them from doping and cheating.

In 1987, as noted above, the tragic death of Birgit Dressel shocked the West German sporting community. Despite medical, forensic, and legal investigations, and after public hearings in parliament, the politicians and federal administration neither intervened nor changed their fundamental opinion that solving the doping problem was the responsibility of the sports organizations and not of the state. The state, they thought, should limit its engagement in sports to the principle of subsidiarity. Concerning anti-doping, this seemed (to them) to be fulfilled by financing the Doping-Control Laboratory under Manfred Donike in Cologne from 1974 and by supporting scientific research on anti-doping.[19] Until German reunification, this position did not change fundamentally, although in fact the expenses of the state for supporting top-level sports were increasing annually. They were also used for the support of anti-doping.

REVELATIONS OF DOPING BY THE GERMAN MEDIA AFTER UNIFICATION

In spite of there being little concrete evidence, it was well known on both sides of the wall that doping took place in sports. The details, however, remained unclear. Doping practices in the GDR were reported in the FRG by athletes, coaches, scientists, doctors, and other experts who were fleeing to the West during international competitions, tournaments, or congresses. The medical expert Alois Mader and the athlete Renate Neufeld were the most useful sources for the West. There is also some evidence that the West German secret service was interested in and had knowledge of the East German sports and doping system.[20]

Brigitte Berendonk's 1969 article in the *Die Zeit*, a weekly newspaper read mainly by well-educated people and intellectuals, called "Züchten wir Monstren?" (Are We Breeding Monsters?), and her 1977 interview with the German doctor Joseph Keul in the popular sporting show "Das aktuelle Sportstudio," were important turning points. Thereafter, the West German public was informed about doping in the West through numerous articles and revelations in the press.[21] After the death of Birgit Dressel, each case was followed by parliamentary hearings, resolutions, and declarations, as well as a large number of publications in the press. However, the interest of the media and politics in doping and anti-doping was not really sustainable and faded over time.

This situation changed in 1990, after the fall of the Berlin Wall. From then on, an extensive general debate began in the press and media about doping in Germany. In *Der Spiegel*, the German "little brother" of the American *Time* magazine, a series of critical articles about doping was published throughout 1990. The subtitle of the series was: "So wird in der Bundesrepublik von Medizinern, Trainern und Athleten manipuliert"—How doctors, athletes, and coaches in the Federal Republic manipulate. The names of well-known West German athletes who had doped consistently were cited. The scandal swept across the German border to Switzerland when the Swiss champion in shot put, Werner Günthör, was included in public accusations with respect to anabolic doping.[22]

The general sentiment was that doping was still practiced in East and West Germany, that sports managers, doctors, and politicians were neither able nor willing to solve the doping problem, and that unification in sport would be a "disastrous alliance of doping experts from East and West."[23]

Stern, another critical and popular magazine with a broad circulation, published an article in November 1990 titled "Doping—The evidence: How the GDR produced champions."[24] The article was based on documents from Manfred Höppner, deputy head of the GDR sports medical service and chief administrator of the Doping Program 14.25 of the GDR government. Ten years later, Höppner received an eighteen-month suspended sentence for aiding and abetting a criminal assault in doping crimes of the GDR. The documents of Höppner, various Stasi papers, and testimonies in court contributed to the public being informed in considerable detail about doping practices in the GDR, including athletes who were still active at that time.

Some days later, *Der Spiegel* reacted and published its own investigative article about the so-called *Hammer Modell*. The name relates to the sports club in Hamm (Westfalia), where athletes, coaches, doctors, and managers worked together in a *Trainingsgruppe*. Our research about doping in West Germany revealed that these doping networks were typical or symptomatic of West German doping practices. They can be regarded as the free Western equivalent of the state-run doping model behind the Iron Curtain.

The conclusion drawn by *Der Spiegel* was that doping was not regarded as cheating and foul play within these networks and athletes, and neither athletes nor managers and officials openly conceded any doping. There was no "public confession" of doping, as *Der Spiegel* explained. The West German sports system was ruled by a "gang of four," the journal added: "ambitious athletes, coaches who are addicted to prestige and success, ruthless doctors, and officials who were fond of travelling."[25] Politicians, managers, and officials would probably maintain the wall of silence on doping and there would be no revelations on doping for many years. *Stern* agreed and published an article about "The scandal after the scandal" and summarized: "The revelation of forbidden practices in sports was without consequences. Athletes and coaches who are caught, keep on doing their sport and doping as if nothing had happened."[26]

Brigitte Berendonk's book *Doping-Dokumente: Von der Forschung zum Betrug* (From research to cheating) was published in September 1991.[27] The effects of this book cannot be overestimated. It was not only read intensively by a specific German audience, but even abroad and by a wider public. The author and her husband, Dr. Werner Franke, collected and saved secret documents of the doping system in the GDR from the Stasi and various other archives. Without their initiatives, many important documents would probably have been destroyed forever. The book can also be regarded as an impulse and source for John Hoberman's work *Mortal Engines*, first published in 1992.[28] Berendonk documented doping practices in detail not only in the GDR, but in West Germany as well. Her message was that German top-level sports were completely contaminated by doping, both in East and West Germany. The sports organizations and their officials would not be able (and some were not willing, either) to cure sports of this grave societal disease. The new, unified German state and its responsible administrations and politicians were looking passively at (or perhaps away from) the disastrous processes in top sports. Consequently, German sports unification would be a unification of dopers, cheaters, liars, and former Stasi agents. This summary can be seen as the message of the anti-doping media campaign in Germany in the early 1990s, which took place during the process of unifying both German sporting systems.

RESPONSES FROM SPORTS AND POLITICS

A first, but rather late response to the revelations and the media campaign was provided by the Reiter Commission, named after its chairman, Heinrich Reiter, president of a high German court, the Bundessozialgericht. As he claimed in the preliminary remarks of his report in 1991, the commission had been installed because of the danger to the reputation of German top-level sports posed by media reports about doping in sports in the East and West. The DSB and the NOK motivated the introduction of this commission, but the minister of the interior financed it. This was the classic model in West German sports policy—the sports organizations act, and the state pays. No sports officials belonged to the commissions, nor did physical educators or ethicists; rather, it was dominated by lawyers, doctors, and scientists with natural-science expertise. This constellation implies that doping was looked on as a medical, legal, and scientific problem, rather than as an ethical or pedagogical one. The political aim was clearly to demonstrate to the critical public that both sport and state were willing and able to examine and reveal what was going on and enforce the appropriate consequences. The commission met ten times and published a report half a year later.[29] The order to the commission was to develop proposals on what to do and how to prevent and combat doping in the future. The basis for these proposals was to be the "experiences of the past." The commission asserted "that the responsible officials in West German sports knew or could make an educated guess of the misuse of anabolic steroids in high level sports, at least since 1976. [. . .] They limited themselves to a series of resolutions, declarations, and other activities which can really be considered as mere after-the-fact actions and/or justifications." Concerning the GDR, the commission asserted that "doping methods were ordered and controlled centrally by the government, scientifically researched and implemented, specifically used in different sports, and therefore systematically and extensively applied to promote high achievements in sports."[30] The commission did not name specific people as responsible or guilty of these criminal offenses.

As a consequence, the commission expressly rejected the proposal to introduce a specific law against doping. The commission repeated the traditional opinion about the relationship between sport and state: "Sports have to be free of regulation by state and politics. The state fulfills its duties through its own distinct responsibility and self-government."[31]

As an effective means of anti-doping, the commission recommended extending out-of-competition controls and improving analytical methods. The system of the payment for coaches was to be evaluated and improved. The background to this recommendation was the fact that the salaries of coaches were and still are dependent on the success of their athletes. Finally, the rules for the nomination of athletes for international competitions and events like the Olympic Games would be revised. Many experts had (and still have) the opinion that the desired sporting achievements were possible only with doping.

One recommendation of the commission was particularly controversial. The commission proposed a general pardon for all doping cases and misuses by athletes before January 1, 1991. However, for coaches, managers, doctors, and other members of athlete networks, a general pardon would *not* be given, but provided case by case, if a guarantee of clean and correct behavior in the future could be given. This would take the form of a written statement.

The proposals of the allegedly independent Reiter Commission for a general pardon were advocated by the sports organizations, which were keen on integrating the potential of GDR sports into the new, unified German sports movement. However, this *Schlussstrichmentalität* (line-drawing mentality) was also controversial with the public. The victims of GDR doping felt this recommendation to be insulting and scandalous. They organized themselves into a club—the Doping-Opfer-Hilfe-Verein—and fought with the sports organizations and the government for both acknowledgment and compensation. Eleven years later, in 2002, a law addressing "financial support for victims of doping in the GDR" was passed by the German Bundestag.[32] Finally, and after long legal battles, the acknowledged victims of doping agreed to a compromise settlement with the Deutscher Olympischer Sportbund (DOSB) and a one-time compensation. Since then, all claims of former victims of doping in the GDR have been legally resolved.

In political matters, the recommendations of the Reiter Commission moved along familiar, conservative lines. The autonomy of sport was backed, and the commission trusted in the capability of the free sports organizations to resolve the doping problem. The responsibility of the state and governmental administrations was neglected, and the question of a unique German anti-doping-law was not discussed. The mistakes or failure of anti-doping policies by sports and governmental administrations or policies was not regarded as a structural failure of the West German model of sporting autonomy, but as deviant individual behavior.

In this context, it is interesting to note that another commission, the Richthofen Commission, was convened by the German Sports Federation (DSB) and the NOK für Deutschland. Its members were all officials of the sports federations. The chairman was Manfred von Richthofen, vice president of the DSB.[33] The function of this commission was "to evaluate the current doping cases, and to advise the main sports federations on how to act and resolve the problems."[34] The Richthofen Commission had no means of obtaining further or confidential information, or of sanctioning anyone. Its work had a mere advisory character. Therefore, its information and knowledge was not and could not be more detailed than that of the Reiter Commission or even of the investigative journalists of *Der Spiegel* and *Stern*. In the DSB archive, we found handwritten protocols in which names in magazine articles had been highlighted, indicating people who were subsequently invited to the commission. The information provided by the commission concerning people with a past tainted by doping activities was often ignored by the federations. In fact, they even gave formal apologies to these people, including those who had held high positions in sports in the former GDR.

The federal government regarded the work of these commissions as satisfactory, such that the problems of doping in German sports were considered "acceptably cleared." The federal government had no intention of "instituting a further investigation"—this was the response of the undersecretary of state, Eduard Lintner, to the demands of Bundestag representative Wilhelm Schmidt from January 21, 1992.[35]

In reality, at that time, there was an exodus to the West of hundreds of competent, highly educated athletes, coaches, and other experts who became unemployed after the collapse of the GDR. The West in fact meant not only West Germany. The knowledge and skills of GDR coaches were much sought after by former rivals in many countries. Some found jobs in Austria or in other German-speaking countries, where the language barrier did not apply. The rise of China as a sporting world power can also be associated with the work of former experts from the GDR. In general, "sport under communism" was looked on as a model for and reflection of the effective organization of postcommunist top-level sports, as Mike Dennis and Jonathan Grix maintain.[36] East German top-level sporting expertise—sports "Made in Germany"—became an *Exportschlager* (export hit) on the one hand, and on the other hand, the unified German sports federations and their officials feared a kind of "brain drain" in sports, sports sciences, and sports medicine. East German sporting expertise always included knowledge of the technical and tactical issues of sports, as well as of medical and even doping issues.

THE PARLIAMENT VETO: BUDGET CUT IN 1991/92

The parliamentary Sports Commission (Sportausschuss des Deutschen Bundestages) was not satisfied with the anti-doping policies of the DSB and NOK after the publication of the findings of the Reiter and Richthofen Commissions. This constituted a clear break from the statements of the government and the Ministry of the Interior. The chairman of the Sportausschuss, Representative Ferdinand Tillmann (CDU), required Heinrich Reiter and other members of the commission to conduct a private (nonpublic) hearing, which was reminiscent of the great doping hearings of the 1970s and 1980s. "In all these meetings and hearings [in 1977 and 1987], we were always assured by the sports organizations that there was no doping problem, that German sports were clean. But now, Mr. Reiter, your commission found that this was not true. I put it to you that we representatives were not informed correctly or in sufficient detail, to put it mildly. Or, we were misinformed intentionally and deliberately, to put it bluntly and clearly."[37]

This criticism was a new and unfamiliar situation for the sports officials in West Germany. In the past, the Sportausschuss had always been their faithful partner in attempts to get money from the government, but now the wind was changing. Members of parliament articulated tough criticism of the German sports officials. Anti-doping policies were not sufficient; anti-doping rules were not integrated consistently into the rules of the federations; doping misuse was not controlled and sanctioned enough; doping allegations against athletes, coaches, and doctors were trivialized. All in all, the representatives were angry that the sports officials in the federations "had drawn a picture of a doping-free sports life in Germany, despite knowing better."[38] Further investigations were required to shed more light on the realities of doping and cheating in sports.

After extensive discussions, the Bundestag decided for the first time to cut the budget for the sports organizations by about 10 percent for 1992, subject to the condition that the sports federations would present a future strategy on the following issues: planning and organizing doping controls (including out-of-competition controls); changing rules and charters to integrate sanctions for doping; and integrating doping sanctions into contracts of employment. Doping was to be sanctioned through job loss. The representatives on the commission argued that "clear and unmistakable signs of serious anti-doping measures" should be communicated to the sports and the public through these actions.[39] Two days later, the sports federations were informed formally by the Ministry of the Interior and requested to communicate their anti-doping strategies as soon as possible.[40]

The recommendation of a budget cut for sports was new. Peter Danckert, later chairman of the parliamentary commission, interpreted it as a "*Warnschuss*"—a shot across the bows of the German sports organizations. However, it was also a sign of distrust from the parliamentary representatives of the responsible Ministry of the Interior.[41] The representatives and the public were no longer convinced that the sports organizations themselves were willing and able to fight doping, and even less so able to win. A budget cut for sports expenses had never been possible during the Cold War period. Now, with the Iron Curtain raised, parliament seized the opportunity to investigate, in a new and critical way, the support of top-level sports, financed by the taxpayer. This implied changing the traditional relationship among sports, government, and parliament in Germany.

In the following weeks and months, several meetings took place, dealing with further questions and investigations. The parliamentary commission led by Representative Schmidt (SPD) considered installing a formal board of inquiry through the Bundestag. Some representatives, like Helmut Sauer (CDU), drew attention to the danger of nominating athletes and coaches of the former GDR with a possible doping past for the Olympics in Albertville and Barcelona in 1992. The critical German media would surely use this to discredit German sports.[42]

The impending Olympics were fundamental for the officials of the sports federations. Harm Beyer, chairman of the German Swimming Federation (DSV), made a clear statement to the representatives: "Swimming was the best of GDR sports if you look at the results. Yet, according to the investigations of the Reiter and Richthofen Commissions, swimming and other sports were pervaded by a detailed program of doping. On the one hand, the Swimming Federation wants to maintain the high level of achievement, even after the unification of East and West, but on the other hand, almost every coach, athlete and official was involved in these doping practices."[43]

Beyer remarked on the fundamental dilemma after German unification. The high potential of GDR sports offered the chance to become number one in world top-level sports. "Should we abandon this chance," he asked the representatives, merely "because some journalists and a critical public want to squabble about the past?"[44]

After a long and heated debate, the parliamentary commission distanced itself from the proposal of a budget cut and favored a single evaluation and investigation of every federation.[45] The budget commission of the German parliament, however, decided to freeze the budget at about DM 5 million. The minister of the interior, Rudolf Seiters (CDU), assured the president of the DSB "that we will succeed in getting the financial support as planned by spring 1992," in time for the Barcelona Olympics. He also promised "to continue the good partnership between sport and state in Germany and maintain the close cooperation between the Ministry of the Interior and DSB." Top-level sports would also be sponsored by the federal government in the future. The autonomy of sport in Germany would not be jeopardized, and the request from the ministry to present a strategy for anti-doping by the DSB and the sports federations should not be interpreted as doing so.[46] That is, the ministry claimed that sports autonomy would not be threatened. However, the reality was different. Despite the claim of the government, the autonomy of free sport in West Germany was indeed limited. The budget cut was dropped, and financial support for the German sports organizations was assured, just before the Olympic Games in Barcelona.

The budgetary conflict over the financial support of top-level sports after German unification made two things clear. First, the politicians and representatives in the German parliament had become more sensitive to criticism from the sports organizations concerning their willingness and ability to implement anti-doping actions effectively. The opinion of the representatives with respect to sports also changed, because of the critical public mood against cheating and doping. Second, the sports organizations were still sufficiently strong and influential to stop the pending budget cut. Politicians in parliament and government remained supporters or sponsors of sports rather than financial controllers.

EUROPEAN AND INTERNATIONAL PERSPECTIVES

The change in policy toward anti-doping in Germany took place in both European and international contexts. What the case of Birgit Dressel implied for German sport, that of Ben Johnson in Seoul 1988 did for the international Olympic sports scene. These scandals revealed that throughout the world, top-level sports were penetrated by a serious doping malaise or "cancer," as many officials like the German Willi Daume appropriately described the severe and chronic problem. Various investigations demonstrated that the international sports organizations alone, with the IOC at the top, were neither willing nor able to get on with the job of countermeasures. The Dubin Commission, installed by the Canadian government after the Seoul Games of 1988, uncovered many international doping networks, also including those between Canadian and German athletes and coaches.[47]

The late 1980s and 1990s were characterized by growing international cooperation in anti-doping measures and a growing involvement of state-related, governmental interests in anti-doping. Barrie Houlihan speaks of an international, political anti-doping regime taking place during the course of and after the end of the Cold War.[48]

An important milestone on this long road was the Convention against Doping of the European Council in November 1989.[49] According to legal experts, it is looked upon as the "first international and binding law against doping."[50] The convention provided an essential impulse to activities against doping by individual states and through national laws.[51] In contrast to previous European initiatives, this convention listed specific actions for implementation by national parliaments and governments. The overarching aim was to win the fight against doping. A precondition was seen in international cooperation by states and governments, as well as between governmental and free sporting institutions. The contracting partners reassured each other that they would coordinate anti-doping policies and introduce laws, declarations, and administrative actions against doping, in order to restrict the availability and use of forbidden doping measures and doping substances. The support of sports federations and athletes was to be ensured by their adherence to anti-doping rules. The control of and sanctions against doping should be maintained by the various national states. Such controls and transparent sanctions could be implemented effectively by states and sports organizations, and the contracting parties would take part in these controls. Each contracting party promised to establish an anti-doping laboratory and install educational programs to prevent doping. The introduction and organization of out-of-competition controls was also a consequence of this convention. The World Anti-Doping Agency (WADA) and the National Anti-Doping Agencies (NADA), which were institutionalized step by step after 1999/2000, continue to deal with this difficult and (financially) expensive problem of out-of-competition controls, as part of the ongoing fight against doping.

Germany took part in advising this convention, but it took until May 1992 for the minister of the interior to sign the contract and another two years before the Bundestag ratified it. The main reason for this delay may have been the serious concerns of German sports policy makers about intervention by states and governments in the autonomy of sport. Another reason was that the proposed anti-doping actions led to high expenditures, which ultimately had to be paid by taxpayers.

In Germany, article 4 of the convention was the subject of controversy. The requirement was that states would promulgate "laws" against doping. The undersecretary of state, Eduard Lintner, declared to members of the Sports Commission in the Bundestag that the European convention did not in fact imply a separate anti-doping law in Germany, as many politicians were requesting.[52] The amendment of existing laws like the *Arzneimittelgesetz* (pharmaceutical law) would be sufficient, at least according to the convention.

In line with its Anti-Doping-Bericht (Anti-Doping Report) in May 1994, the federal government still preferred and praised the "self-cleansing power of the autonomous sports organizations." The European convention on anti-doping would still be respected fully within the German anti-doping system. Nonetheless, the main responsibility for anti-doping would remain firmly in the hands of the free and autonomous sports organizations. The government did not see the need for a specific anti-doping law in Germany.

THE CASE OF DIETER BAUMANN—A BLOW TO THE FIGHT AGAINST DOPING

The difficult times after the German reunification seemed to be over when, in 1999, the famous German runner Dieter Baumann tested positive for the anabolic steroid nandrolone. This result was a shock for both the sports community and the German public. Baumann was one of the most successful West German athletes, winner of the silver medal at the 1988 Olympics in Seoul and the gold medal in Barcelona in 1992, both for 5,000 meters, his favorite distance. He was one of the athletes who had experienced Germany and German sports before and after the German reunification, during the Cold War and afterward in the unified Germany. Both athletes, the above-mentioned Katrin Krabbe of the GDR and Baumann of the Federal Republic, represent the two types produced by the East and the West, and also the somewhat typical fates of East *and* West German athletes after the fall of the wall. Whereas Katrin Krabbe had been a product of the East German sports system, Baumann was from the West. Krabbe was always dependent on her "collective," that is, people close to her like her coach Thomas Springstein. What she had in common with Baumann is failing as a proven doper. Krabbe was in fact also a victim of her East German sports education and the networks responsible for her triumphs in the GDR, ultimately culminating in her deep decline after the reunification.

Baumann, on the other hand, wrote a book entitled *Ich laufe keinem hinterher*, which translates as "I run behind no one." This sentiment reflects the self-conscious, individualistic attitude of athletes in the "free" West. He and the public also cultivated this image of the "mature" athlete, which was in fact a kind of antimodel of the athlete's education in the East. Baumann was one of the few top athletes of the West who was able to compete successfully with the East German sports "comrades" and even with the outstanding runners of Africa. When Baumann rather surprisingly won the final 5,000-meter race at Barcelona, the first time that a unified German team competed at the Olympics, the former superiority of East Germany already seemed forgotten and a thing of the past. The indirect message of the victory of Dieter Baumann in Barcelona was that the West had both better athletes and ones who had not doped like Katrin Krabbe. In a broader context, this was the real message of German reunification. The West had won, and the East had both doped and cheated; the West were the honest winners, and the East the losers who had lost deservedly.

In addition, Dieter Baumann not only was an excellent athlete, but also had the courage to argue vehemently against doping in public. He was a front man of the athletes' fight against doping in Germany before and after German reunification.[53] Therefore, it was all the more shocking for him as well as for the whole German public when it was revealed that his urine tested

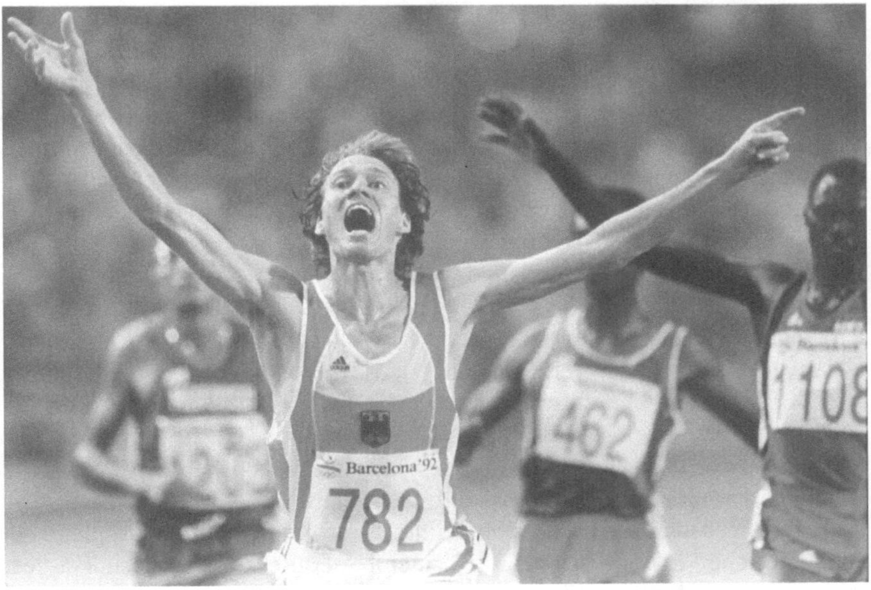

Figure 3.2. Dieter Baumann (b. 1965), at his "gold" race of 5,000 meters at the Barcelona Olympics. As one of the best-known athletes in Germany, he was active against doping in the 1990s. However, in 1999, he was involved in one of the most mysterious doping cases and banned from international competitions from 2000 to 2002. *Source: Picture Alliance, dpa-Fotoreport/ Franck Kleefeldt*

positive for the anabolic steroid nandrolone in 1999. The substance was proven to be ten times as high as the normal level.

Baumann at once stated adamantly that he had never taken any doping substances, but could not explain how this substance had found its way into his body. Baumann was banned by the German Athletics Federation (DLV) and the IAAF. He was also not allowed to participate at the Sydney Olympics in 2000. Interestingly, he had not been pronounced as guilty by the legal committee of the German Athletics Federation. Intensive investigations were undertaken after Baumann legally contested the allegations against him. The prosecutor and police investigated in every possible direction, among others that nandrolone was consumed together with dietary supplements, or in the form of eye drops, given that Baumann wore contact lenses. There was another strong suspicion that the doping substance had been placed by a third party in Baumann's toothpaste, which he had used during a common training camp of the German athletics team. In fact, rather surprisingly, nandrolone could be found in various toothpastes used by Baumann, but it was not possible to explain how the substance got there and who could possibly have put it there. Finally, after long months of investigation, the responsible prosecutor closed the case in 2000 without any conclusive result. Baumann remained banned from international athletics competitions until 2002, but had a comeback at the European championship in 2002, when he finished second.

The case is both compelling and cryptic in several respects. The first is the basic dilemma of whether an athlete can validly be considered as doped, given the principle of "strict liability." This principle was included in the doping rules of the Medical Commission of the IOC and was later adopted by the WADA in its Anti-Doping Code. The principle means that only the athletes themselves are responsible for their bodily integrity. The only relevant fact is whether anything forbidden is found in the body and not any explanations or excuses as to how and why the substance came to be there. However, the case of Dieter Baumann raised the general question of whether it is fair to ban an athlete who swears under oath that he has not taken the substances that have been found in his blood or urine. Given that nobody in fact knows the truth, the strict-liability principle would be deeply unfair if Baumann had not doped, at least not intentionally. If he had doped unintentionally, because of a criminal contamination of food or dietary supplements (or some other devious means), the principle of strict liability seems at best inappropriate. However, if he had doped intentionally and knowingly, he would have merely been a common liar. If that was indeed the case, Dieter Baumann was just one more link in the long chain of liars and cheaters in doping history—*mundus vult decipi*, the world wants to be cheated, is an old Latin saying.

Second, the case of Baumann sheds some light on the broader situation in German sports after reunification. Following the suspicion of Baumann himself and other experts that his toothpaste had really been "spiked," it seems plausible that former East German competitors or networks could well have been the perpetrators of this truly disgraceful action. Werner Franke, one of the most enthusiastic anti-doping campaigners in Germany and worldwide, argued in an interview with the weekly magazine *Der Spiegel* that he was convinced that Baumann had *not* doped and that former Stasi agents had put nandrolone into his toothpase: "I am sure that it was a form of assault. Bauman has always been so committed to anti-doping. His toothpaste was contaminated, which is a well-known Stasi trick. Baumann was abused by these people."[54]

If this suspicion, which could never be proved, was in fact justified, Baumann was a victim of the long shadow of German history and politics.

INTERIM RESULTS: REUNIFICATION, REHABILITATION, AND NEW BEGINNINGS

In the years after the fall of the Berlin Wall, German sports officials and politicians faced pressure to justify their policies and to react to the various doping scandals and revelations. Their first response was to set up boards of inquiry. One fundamental question was whether the federal government was still justified in investing in a sport system that was (and still is) so obviously contaminated by doping and cheating. This allegation was directed not only toward athletes, coaches, and officials of the former GDR sports system, but to the West as well. The commissions and boards of inquiry were installed not by parliament—as was the case for similar anti-doping commissions in other European countries—but by the sports organizations themselves. This meant that they did not have sufficient democratic legitimation or legal power to obtain really new and detailed information about doping networks in East and West Germany, or even to prosecute guilty coaches, doctors, and athletes.

German politicians and sports officials were faced with a serious moral dilemma. On the one hand, they saw the chance to become number one in world sports after German unification by exploiting the competence of the former GDR sports system. On the other hand, it was obvious, and a public scandal, that the "secrets of GDR sports" were simply about doping. Sports in the unified Germany should not start the new era with this fundamental moral flaw.

This dilemma should also be considered against the background of German society as a whole in the 1990s. How could one deal with the totalitarian past of sixteen million new Germans from the East? Who were and still are the victims, and who were the perpetrators? How was German unification to be financed? Who was really guilty of a crime or misdemeanor, as opposed to merely having been an uncritical follower of the totalitarian system? Was the East German political system and regime actually a tyrannical dictatorship? Such problems continue to occupy public debate in Germany, and sport has been a major forum for these extremely awkward and challenging questions.

The result was a compromise—in both sports and society as a whole. Whenever possible, sports and politics tried to integrate East and West German authority in order to maintain high levels in international sports. The threat of the parliamentary Sports Commission to cut the budget for sports organizations and top-level sports because of inactivity, incompetence, and nontransparency did not materialize. The ideological basis of the autonomy of sports federations was not changed, but politicians were eager to evaluate and control sports more effectively and to be stricter about tax-funded expenditures. State politics was going to play a major role in anti-doping and sports politics. The changing opinions of politicians concerning their responsibility in anti-doping were also motivated by international developments in anti-doping. German sports policies could not be divorced from the recommendations for anti-doping that had been proclaimed by the European Council in 1989.

The financial support of top-level sports by the federal government is the most effective means of improving quality, as well as of fostering achievements and results in international competitions and events. The threat of cutting, freezing, or even reclaiming this money could thus also constitute the strongest possible instrument at the disposal of the sports organizations for promoting anti-doping. The German parliament tried to use this instrument only once, in 1991/92, but never again. The great coalition of sports and politics continued through the crisis in the 1990s, but the controls remained relatively lenient and ineffectual. More than fifteen years later, in the summer of 2007, the so-called Projektgruppe Sonderprüfung Doping (Project Group to Investigate Doping), established by the Ministry of the Interior, maintained: "The Bundesverwaltungsamt (Office for Controlling State Expenditure) has never checked whether the sports federations had really observed their doping paragraphs, which were a precondition for the government to spend money. [. . .] All in all, it must be stated that a systematic and regular controlling of compliance never took place."[55]

In spite of the events and doping crisis of the 1990s in the context of German sports unification, the axioms of the relationship between sport and state in Germany were never really questioned—namely, autonomy, self-government, partnership, and subsidiarity. Doping was then and remains a problem that provokes governmental interest and responsibility in sports, but has resulted in fundamental change to a model of state sports that is surely still far too similar to that of the former GDR. Perhaps, the principle of autonomy changed to one of *limited* sports autonomy, and the solidarity of state politics, with sports moving to a more critical and questioning solidarity. Accordingly, Udo Steiner, former judge at the High Court of the Federal Republic of Germany and chairman of the anti-doping commission of the DSB, argues that Germany needs neither a specific anti-doping law nor a specific paragraph about sports in the charter.[56] In fact, without state sponsorship, top-level sports would not be competitive, nor would effective anti-doping measures be possible. Thus, controlling the funding is *the* key to resolving the persistent and so far perennial doping problem. This situation prevails throughout the world and is by no means unique to Germany.

INTERNATIONAL STRATEGIES OF ANTI-DOPING: GERMANY ON THE PATH TO THE WORLD ANTI-DOPING AGENCY (WADA)

The international world of sports was shocked by the doping case of Canadian sprinter Ben Johnson at the Olympic Games of Seoul in 1988. The dramatic fall of this sportsman occurred just one year after the death of the German heptathlete Birgit Dressel. Whereas the German sports community regarded the death of Dressel as a tragic accident and a signal to improve the medical supervision and support of top-level athletes, the Canadian sports representatives as well as several Olympic sports officials drew different conclusions from the Ben Johnson case. The Canadian government established a commission to investigate this spectacular case, which had shattered the world of Olympic sports and was expected to initiate a radical turn in international anti-doping strategies. The so-called Dubin Commission, named after its chairman, Charles Leonard Dubin, former chief justice of Ontario, painted a chilling and indeed disastrous picture of top-level sports. Not only did a large proportion of top Canadian athletes consistently take anabolic steroids, according to the final report, but doping was declared as a pervasive phenomenon of international sports. Dubin and his colleagues did not hesitate to make serious allegations against the international sports federations, and the IOC at the apex, because of a lack of effective initiatives and practical measures for effectively reducing doping in sport.[57] The work of the Dubin Commission can also be considered as the starting point of the career of the Canadian sportsman, IOC member, and advocate Richard (Dick) Pound as an Olympic campaigner against doping in his role as the first chairman of the World Anti-Doping Agency (WADA), more than ten years after the Ben Johnson affair.[58] It seems remarkable that Pound did not regard the athletes themselves as core of the doping evil, but rather their entourage of doctors, assistants, officials, sponsors, and so on. Pound had even defended Johnson at his trial and declared to the Dubin Commission that Johnson had not even known what anabolics were and especially stanozolol, the substance for which he had tested positive. Instead, his coach Charlie Francis and doctor Jamie Astaphan were the key culprits. However, one way or the other, Ben Johnson had doped and was finally banned from athletics.

As a result of the Dubin Commission report, the conviction arose among the sports communities of numerous countries that the IOC strategies against doping, as well as those of various important international sports federations, had been completely insufficient and ineffective in the past and should be reformed urgently.[59] Sports politicians from several countries started to become more active against doping. Apparently they no longer trusted in the will and ability of the international sports organizations to reduce doping in sport.[60] In fact, the governments of the major Commonwealth countries, namely Great Britain, Canada, and Australia, signed an International Anti-Doping Agreement in 1990. New Zealand, Norway, Sweden, and the Netherlands joined in 1998. The Nordic states had already entered into an agreement in 1996 to harmonize doping controls and doping sanctions. Other European states, except Germany, intended to coordinate anti-doping initiatives at the level of governments and administrations.[61]

These governmental activities to reduce doping seem rather remarkable, given the paradigmatic change in sports policies of the Western states after the Cold War. The Western ideology of the *Eigenwelt* of sports, including the overall responsibility of free organizations for sports in general, or for achievement, top, or competitive sports, had essentially lost its validity. In addition, after the Cold War, there was no reason to retain this superseded ideology to demonstrate a visible contrast to state sports and state amateurs of the now defunct communist East. Finally, top-level sports had become an important part of international and national life affecting business, the media, the public, culture, science, and politics. Politicians and governments apparently believed they could no longer ignore this phenomenon of modern society. The doping problem, which the sports organizations were in fact unable to resolve satisfactorily, was a means of keeping their foot in the door of top-level sports, including its commercial and media potential.

Houlihan argues that these political activities were the first steps toward a political "Anti-Doping Regime."[62] This notion describes the attempt of state organizations, governments, and even parliaments and parliamentary commissions, as well as transnational and international political organizations like the European Council and UNESCO, to reduce doping in sports by means of conventional, international state politics. The days when sports and doping had only been affairs of nongovernmental organizations (NGOs) like the sports associations and federations were really and truly over. It does not seem coincidental that this paradigmatic change coincided with the end of the Cold War on the track, as well as the rise of international sports within the world of big business.

The international anti-doping regime did not stop at the German border, either. In contrast, the German doping and anti-doping activities of sports and politics were part of this process of increasing interdependence between national and international actors of sports and anti-doping policies. The specific German role in this network will be analyzed in the following section. Looking back, the West German government or even parliament was, for the first time in recent history, concerned about sports and doping, when in the 1960s, the European Council initiated a series of papers, resolutions, and declarations on sports, physical education, and even doping. These statements motivated West German politicians to deal with this aspect of society, which was intended to be set apart from state politics according to the post-war ideology of the West. In other words, international networks and international initiatives against doping were a strong reason for West German politicians to become active in anti-doping policies. West German state politics did not wish (again) to pursue a "German *Sonderweg*" (unique German path), but to be in accordance with European and international politics. However, they were confronted with a dilemma between the principle of sports autonomy, which was in fact a relic of the past, and the current need to conform to international sports politics, which were planning to limit the autonomy of sport and increasingly influence international sports.

The doping problem was in fact one of international concern. Doping affected almost every top sport in every country and at every competition, at least potentially. In addition, scientific research on anabolic steroids was on the agenda of sports medical research all over the world, motivated partly by the potential use by top athletes, but also by the will and compelling need to detect misuse in various sports.[63]

THE ESTABLISHMENT OF AN INTERNATIONAL POLITICAL ANTI-DOPING REGIME

Barrie Houlihan refers to the development of an anti-doping policy regime in the context of the theory of political regimes in general, first conceptualized by political scholars Robert Keohane and Stephen Krasner.[64] With regard to this theory of political institutions, regimes are structural occurrences of international cooperation intended to handle international political conflicts. For such political regimes, single states were essentially unable to solve these problems by their own means, but only in systematic cooperation with others. Apparently, this also applies to doping and anti-doping. However, numerous governments not only called for international cooperation concerning anti-doping, but interfered increasingly in sports affairs back home. At a meeting of European sports ministers in 2000 in Bratislava, Slovakia, it was reported that at that time, fourteen European countries had introduced specific anti-doping laws, and thirteen, among them Germany, had discussed and decided on laws against drug dealing, including dealing with doping substances.[65]

Typical of this developing international anti-doping regime, if we follow the logic of Houlihan, was the characteristic that public scandals, or at least key public sport events, led to political actions. The case of Ben Johnson was thus the temporary end of a longer journey beginning in the 1960s with Knud Enemark Jensen's death at the Rome Olympics of 1960 and the Tom Simpson tragedy at Mont Ventoux in 1967. Both of these key doping and anti-doping incidents provoked actions by sports organizations as well as political reactions. The IOC finally established its Medical Commission and started the first doping tests in history at the Mexico Olympics of 1968.[66] In the political arena, the European Council, as a transnational organization of European countries, introduced a new definition of doping in 1963, which can be regarded as the first transnational or international political initiative against doping.[67] Numerous declarations and resolutions followed, with the parliaments of France and Belgium even passing specific anti-doping laws in 1965.[68]

In retrospect, given the Ben Johnson disaster of 1988, all these anti-doping efforts seemed insufficient, incompetent, and quite futile—rather like the anachronistic concept of amateur sports, which had not corresponded to the reality of top sports for many years. National laws against doping failed, first, because of their inherent national limitations, and second, because of the problematic conversion of laws into the practical punishment and sanctioning of dopers. Therefore, the French parliament reformed its anti-doping law in 1975, because of its ineffectiveness in practice. From then on, the sports organizations were obliged in principle to sanction dopers.[69] However, they were in fact not compellingly motivated to do so, as was regrettably the case throughout the world of sports.

The anti-doping initiatives at the levels of intergovernmental and transnational cooperation, like those of the Council of Europe, the meetings of sport ministers, or UNESCO, lacked commitment in the form of international law. As the law historian Judith Schmidt has argued, all these declarations entailed somewhat vague moral commitments.[70] The political, social, and sporting conditions, as well as the attitudes of the numerous states toward doping and anti-doping, were ultimately responsible for the failure of effective anti-doping policies since the 1960s. This unhappy situation could not be overcome, at least in part, until the end of the Cold War.[71]

One of the most important documents in the current history of anti-doping is the International Convention against Doping, which was in fact the first convention reflecting a higher level of legal commitment from the participating nation-states. Schmidt has characterized this document as a "milestone of anti-doping policies of the Council of Europe."[72] However, the practical application and real impact of this document was less than expected. The main reason for the disappointing results was probably its limitation to Europe. However, in Germany, the convention provided an important impulse for changing the current drug law in the 1990s. Dealing with doping substances was now treated as a criminal offense, similar to conventional drug dealing. Although UNESCO had asked its member states to join the European Convention, numerous non-European governments refused to do so. Therefore, UNESCO prepared an anti-doping-convention of its own.[73]

Apparently, the common view spread internationally was that doping constituted a rapidly escalating source of serious problems for both society and politics, similar to organized crime, as John Hoberman argues, and that these problems could ultimately endanger the worldwide system of sports and even pose a threat to governments and states.[74] Only joint international activities against doping could reduce the problem. This understanding was the basis for establishing an international political anti-doping regime. In addition, as Houlihan asserts, at the end of the Cold War, the breakdown of the communist bloc states dispelled at least some serious obstacles for international anti-doping activities by states. In fact, the Eastern bloc had successfully prevented international anti-doping policies in the past.[75] In general, the globalization of sports opened the door to new political solutions for reducing doping. Whereas previously, sports organizations had been rather skeptical of political influence in sports, as well as hesitant in looking for new ways out of the doping trap, the conditions had now changed fundamentally. The political pressure placed by the international community on sports organizations was strong enough to induce a relevant step forward, which would at least contain doping in international sports. The foundation of the World Anti-Doping Agency (WADA) marked the end of this process, for the time being.[76]

In Germany, spectacular public doping cases since the 1990s again motivated a closer cooperation of sports organizations with political actors against doping. Whereas at the beginning of the 1990s work on the heritage of the GDR dictatorship dominated the public debate in Germany, including the debate about sports and doping, doping at the end of the 1990s was dominated by the scandals of the Tour de France, especially that of 1998, which is broadly known as the Festina scandal. At the same time, the first trials of former GDR sports officials, coaches, and scientists on sports and doping started and produced sticking newspaper headlines. The German public became aware of the extraordinary dimensions of GDR doping and its deep moral abyss. The trials were associated with discussions about the victims of GDR doping and the political responsibility for those crimes by the state with regard to possible compensation. In addition, all these cases involved doping victims who had never been exposed by doping controls at international competitions or the Olympics. Therefore, the credibility and efficiency of IOC doping controls were seriously questioned. Finally, the moral credibility of the IOC as a "world government of sports" was challenged.[77]

Doubts were arising as to the credibility of the repeated statements from sports organizations that they could overcome the doping problem alone. These doubts increased substantially when the Festina scandal revealed the doping horrors in professional cycling in 1998. In France, after the Festina scandal, three sports doctors and a masseur associated with cycling teams were charged with doping according to a French law of 1989, which provided for cases of medical treatment with forbidden substances at sports events. The Festina scandal thus challenged the tradition and future of the Tour de France in general by uncovering the prevalence of systematic doping for many years. As a result, the image of this great national French sports event with international significance was destroyed, although everybody knew that doping had characterized the Tour since its beginnings, as it had cycling in general. However, the state and other sponsors of the Tour and various cycling teams hesitated to sponsor the event in the future. Some, like the German phone company Telekom, terminated their sponsorship of their cycling team when systematic EPO doping of some team cyclists was revealed. With respect to the future foundation of the WADA, it was highly relevant that the doping scandal at the Tour de France, as well as forbidden doping practices in cycling in general, could be detected only through state intervention, specifically by the police and public prosecutors. The sports organizations had never been as successful as the state in detecting doping "crimes"—this was at least a crucial message of this doping scandal.[78] However, we should bear in mind the irony that the worst doping crimes were in fact committed by states.

Simultaneously with these occurrences, the credibility and even legitimacy of the IOC, as head of the international sports movement, was challenged because of rumors about corruption concerning the allocation of the 2002 Winter Games to Salt Lake City.[79] The US Olympic Committee (USOC) and the US Department of Justice had ordered investigations and accused IOC members of corruption, including the IOC president Juan Antonio Samaranch.[80] The IOC was criticized worldwide and doubts about its moral integrity were articulated, particularly as to whether the Olympic leaders were ethically capable of organizing the Olympic Games and maintaining the Olympic spirit credibly in the future.[81]

In sum, all these occurrences revealed that the traditional relationship between politics and sports had changed fundamentally, not only internationally, but also and indeed especially in Germany. Whereas before, the attitude of the state and leading politicians toward sports had been rather distanced, with sports being regarded as "the most beautiful pastime in the world" (*die schönste Nebensache der Welt*), they now recognized sports as too important a political field to be left to nongovernmental organizations.

With regard to the other side of sport, it is a fair comment that the sports organizations had succeeded in keeping politics out of the game for a long time. They were able to avoid the intrusion of public law as well as political influence in sporting affairs, even those concerning doping and anti-doping. Doping could be kept "in-house," as D. V. Handstad, A. Smith, and Ivan Waddington have commented.[82] However, after the various sports and doping scandals of the 1990s, politicians throughout the world seemed to be able and willing to influence and care for the integrity of world sports. It was hoped that sports crises could also be mastered by means of state politics and laws from democratically elected parliaments. The sports organizations, headed by the IOC, did not have the same democratic legacy as regular states. The IOC attempted to react appropriately to these new conditions and to the efforts of politicians to assume more power in sports.

FROM LAUSANNE TO THE WADA

The most important benchmark in the process of founding the WADA was the World Conference on Doping held from February 2 to 4, 1999, in Lausanne. The IOC was the organizer and had invited, as usual, relevant representatives of sports organizations, but also, for the first time, representatives of national governments and the United Nations.[83] The IOC mainly intended to improve its image through hosting this conference. In addition, the IOC wished to demonstrate its leadership in international sports and avoid the influence of the state and governments in its sports policy. The administration of the conference was strategically planned so that the present political representatives would praise the new, reestablished power of Olympic sports and the IOC. The strategy was to include political representatives in solving the doping problem while keeping things, as usual, in the hands of the IOC and the international sports federations. The IOC plan proposed a distribution of various obligations to reduce doping by transferring crucial responsibilities to the Olympic movement and further functions to "public authorities."

The essential element of the reform concept was the establishment of a worldwide anti-doping organization named the Olympic Movement Anti-Doping Agency.[84] Although the authority of this new organization against doping was to entail much more than mere doping controls, the IOC was eager to retain its overall responsibility and power. The IOC was to preside over the agency as a member organization of the Olympic movement. Eighteen persons were to compose the board, but just three of them from outside the Olympic movement, as independent members of governments.[85]

The conference in fact took another, somewhat more dramatic course than planned by the IOC. Members of the invited governments did not adopt the IOC concept. Therefore, the conference is considered a turning point in the contemporary relationship between the IOC and the community of constituted states with respect to reducing doping systematically.

The then German minister of the interior, Otto Schily, and the British sports minister Tony Banks played the leading parts in this drama. Incidentally, both ministers were members of recently elected New Labor governments in Europe. Schily was the first political speaker at the conference, due to the fact that Germany presided over the European Council at that time. He fostered his image as a campaigner for a social-democratic understanding of law, order, and justice. In interviews, he had referred to the IOC as something like an anachronistic sporting monarchy. With respect to Samaranch, he had stated that everybody should know when it was time to quit.

Tony Banks was closely connected to the British sports movement, which was traditionally skeptical toward the IOC. Banks criticized the IOC leaders openly for their unhappy legacy, including a fundamental lack of democracy and integrity, which rendered them incapable of representing the international Olympic movement without radical reform. After all, they were unable to win the confidence of the athletes themselves. The German minister Schily followed his British colleague and demanded a complete reorganization of the IOC. Other representatives of state governments supported Banks and Schily. During the subsequent debate at the conference, they insisted on an independent, autonomous, and transparent anti-doping office. That the leadership of this new organization should not be retained by the IOC was a precondition. Although IOC president Samaranch himself tried to resist these demands, the politicians finally succeeded in convincing the conference that their concept was the best possible and most realistic model for an effective international organization to combat doping in top-level sports. A crucial argument of the politicians was the fact that the IOC and other international sports federations lacked the democratic legitimacy to impose worldwide rules against doping that would carry a high level of commitment across the borders of nation-states.[86]

Finally, the Lausanne Declaration on Doping in Sport added a new dimension to the international fight against doping, as well as the beginnings of a reform of the international Olympic sports movement, in an attempt to regain legitimacy and confidence.[87] However, the price for this reform was in some way a loss of power by the IOC in international sports policies. The various states and governments had demonstrated their will and power to participate in solving the international doping problem, but at the same time they requested more power and influence in international sports or the associated nongovernmental organizations. According to Houlihan, the Lausanne conference marked the beginning of an international anti-doping regime.

WADA AS THE NEW CENTER OF THE INTERNATIONAL FIGHT AGAINST DOPING

The WADA was founded officially in November 1999. The essentially new aspects of the WADA as a private-public partnership in sports included, first, the participation of states or governments in the worldwide fight against doping, and second, the worldwide establishment of rules concerning doping controls and sanctions. Every sports organization would be obliged to follow these rules. The first point, the participation of the state, was evident in the organizational structure. Fifty percent of the board is filled by representatives of the Olympic movement, and the other 50 percent by state representatives. The same 50 percent rule applies to the finances. The substantial need for money, experts, and equipment for the new institution can be divided into demands by shareholders, the sports themselves, and politics.[88]

The first and most important product of the new institution was the World Anti-Doping Code (WADC), a book of detailed regulations about doping and anti-doping aimed at harmonizing the worldwide fight against doping in all sports. Sport organizations and states wanted to set up common rules and strategies to counter the use of forbidden performance-enhancing methods and substances. The WADC came into force on January 1, 2004. At that time, thirty-three sports organizations had already signed the Code. Three years later, more than 570 sports organizations, among them all Olympic sports federations as well as all national Olympic and also Paralympic committees, had joined the WADC.[89] Therefore, it seemed likely that the WADA would be highly acknowledged worldwide in both sport and politics.

However, the problem remained that some of the doping activities forbidden by the WADC could be neither controlled nor sanctioned by the WADA itself or by sports organizations, but only by state authorities—for example, like dealing with conventional drug offences.[90] The WADC also included the principle of "strict liability," which means "that each athlete is personally liable for the substances found in his or her body, and that an anti-doping rule violation occurs whenever a prohibited substance (or its metabolites or markers) is found in a bodily specimen, whether or not the athlete intentionally or unintentionally used a prohibited substance or was negligent or otherwise at fault."[91] This principle is remarkable and problematic because, in contrast to a crucial principle of constitutional states, in which the prosecutor has to prove the violation of the law and not the other way around, the accused person has to prove his innocence.

An essential problem during the process of implementing of the WADC in national law was the fact that the constitutions of numerous states did not accept contracts with nongovernmental organizations (NGOs). In order to resolve this problem, UNESCO set out to establish an international convention against doping, allowing such states to adopt the WADC within their specific national laws. The International Convention against Doping in Sport, concluded by the general assembly of UNESCO at the meeting on October 19, 2005, in Paris, was accomplished by numerous consultations at various levels of international sports politics. The second World Conference on Doping of the WADA in Copenhagen in 2003 cleared the way for this process of establishing a political anti-doping regime, according to Houlihan. The UNESCO convention was to be combined with the anti-doping declaration of the European Council and based on the WADC as well as the concept of a common working group of European Council and UNESCO. The UNESCO convention included in annex 1 the WADA's "2005 Prohibited List" and "International Standards," and in annex 2 the WADA's "Standards for Granting Therapeutic Use Exemptions." These exemptions had always been problematic in the past, in terms of how to decide whether an athlete was truly doped or generally needed therapeutic substances. Furthermore, the UNESCO convention, which came into force on February 1, 2007, provided for all 193 member states of the UN to implement these anti-doping rules within their specific national legal system.[92]

The convention against doping was in fact a broad compromise, including a high degree of flexibility for all participating member states. However, all states in the UN entered into binding commitments against doping, specifically against illegal drug dealing, and to support doping controls and tests, as well as activities or programs for the prevention of doping. Athletes, coaches, assistants, or sports organizations that breached the anti-doping rules would not receive any financial support from the states. By 2011, 162 states had signed the convention, among them Germany.[93]

EFFECTS OF THE INTERNATIONAL ANTI-DOPING MOVEMENT ON GERMAN ANTI-DOPING POLICIES: FROM THE ANTI-DOPING COMMISSION OF THE GERMAN SPORTS FEDERATION (DSB) TO THE NATIONAL ANTI-DOPING AGENCY (NADA)

International developments in sports, including anti-doping policies, implied a fundamental change in German sports policies. The traditional concept of the autonomy of sport and the principle of subsidiarity in the relationship with state authorities could not be adopted to the same extent as before. Anti-doping policies in Germany had always been a matter of sports and not of state policy. A specific law against doping, as in France and Belgium, was not even discussed in Germany. The various anti-doping initiatives of the German sports associations and federations were the fundaments of the fight against doping in Germany. Now, at least after the foundation of the WADA, sports and politics in Germany were aware that this era was over.

Of course, the shift from the pure principle of the autonomy of sport to more pragmatic state politics in sport was long-term and complex, as mentioned above. However, since 1992, the Anti-Doping Commission of the German Sports Federation has been in principle responsible for combating doping in Germany (see above). This commission was intended to be independent of the state and sport, at least formally. In fact, it was a commission comprising various sports organizations and formally private. Now, when the WADA had been founded and the process of implementing the WADA principles and the WADC was in progress, the structures of the German anti-doping institutions had to be changed.

Otto Schily, minister of the interior of the FRG, who had been a front man in Lausanne in 1999, when the course for the WADA was set, now asked for more independence for the Anti-Doping Commission (ADK) from German sports organizations. Independence and transparency were two central notions of the international anti-doping movement and were also to be implemented in Germany. Clemens Prokop, president of the German Athletics Federation, argued that German sports had to react to this "pressure to imitate" by conforming to the international levels of anti-doping on German conditions.[94]

After the Lausanne conference, representatives of German sports organizations and the ADK held a meeting with Schily. He argued that the ministry was ready for long-term cooperation with sports organizations only if they were willing to create new structures for the ADK, according to international developments in anti-doping. In other words, Schily required fundamental reforms if his ministry, which was in fact the main sponsor of top-level sports, was to continue to support top-level sports in the future. Central requests were that the ADK had to become more independent of sports, conflicts of interest had to be avoided, and the main practical measures for reducing doping should be centralized. The responsibility for doping controls should be shifted from the sports federations to the ADK as a central office in the national fight against doping. An independent arbitration court would be installed to deal fairly with doping cases. Schily promised the support of the federal state for these reforms, but stressed the crucial responsibility of sports organizations. These reforms could be implemented "cooperatively between state and sport and not against sport," as he commented. But there was no doubt that "the German Sports Federation is the first representative of sporting interests and it is therefore up to the sport to reflect on future developments and to set clear benchmarks for doping and anti-doping."[95]

The federal government retained the autonomy of sport in principle, but requested more political responsibility for national sport. The official turn of phrase for this political strategy could be read in the federal government's ninth report on sports: "The German Sports Federation has a unique responsibility with respect to optimizing the fight against doping in Germany and implementing the anti-doping declaration of the Council of Europe. German sport must especially consider its specific powers and obligations in the fight against doping."[96]

From then on, the process of sports policy making proceeded at various levels. The ADK and its chairman, the lawyer Ulrich Haas, were to propose a concept of the reformed ADK according to these conditions. Various expert reports had to be prepared, the parliamentary Sports Commission discussed these papers including proposals made to the minister of the interior, and the national sport organizations—at the top, the DSB, NOK, and ADK—defined the framework conditions. Finally, all parties in the policy-making process planned the path for an independent National Anti-Doping Agency (NADA), according to the model of the international WADA, in the legal form of a foundation. The main objectives of the office were to be doping controls at and out of competition, as well as education about and prevention of doping. Volunteers were to lead the board, controlled by a commission of representatives of sports and politics on a basis of parity, supplemented by representatives of business and the economy. Sports officials and politicians hoped that the financial basis of the foundation would essentially be secured by sponsors from German business.[97]

Well-known companies were personally asked by the minister to donate more to finance the anti-doping foundation, whereas smaller companies were to be motivated by public relations. Otto Schily, for example, asked the boss of Deutsche Telekom, Ron Sommer, the main sponsor of the German cycling Team Telekom, for financial support to the tune of DM 2 million. However, not only this attempt failed. The German economy and business community was apparently not willing to support the NADA. The foundation fund included mostly public, tax-based money from the federal state (DM 5.1 million) and the regional states or *Länder* (DM 1.02 million). The sports organizations could add only small amounts of about DM 10,000 each, and private companies sponsored less than DM 150,000. The total capital of the fund was DM 6.65 million. For all participating members of the foundation, this was insufficient, disappointing, and considerably below what was needed.[98]

The lack of financial support was certainly the most serious problem at the beginning. Two further problems had to be overcome. One was the question of legal and practical access to both doping-control laboratories in Germany, one in Cologne and the other in Kreischa. It took until 2006 for access to these laboratories to be transferred from the Federal Institute of Sports Science (BISp) to the NADA, after which the objectives of the BISp were to be limited to supporting research on doping and doping analysis.[99]

The issue of establishing an independent arbitration court for doping cases was difficult, insofar as this court also needed to be independent of financial support from the NADA. But who else could and should spend money on this institution? The solution was that the court was attached to the German Institute for Arbitration (Deutsches Institut für Schiedsgerichtswesen) and strictly separated from sports organizations as well as from the NADA. However, this solution could not be achieved until 2008.[100]

Despite these serious problems from the beginning of the new institution, the NADA was officially founded on July 15, 2002, in Bonn, the former capital of the old Federal Republic before reunification. The heaviest burden of the NADA, however, was the lack of funding from the beginning. Otto Schily had clearly declared that the Federal Republic would not be able or willing to spend more than DM 5.1 million for the basic fund. All other needs had to be financed by other institutions, the regional counties, and the German business community,[101] but they all refused to spend enough money. Some argued that top-level sports are the responsibility of institutions by virtue of the constitution, and others that business did not see any need to invest in anti-doping. They wished to see and support winners, not dopers or athletes who neither doped nor won.

GERMAN ANTI-DOPING CRISIS OF 2007

Since the establishment of the German NADA, each annual report lamented the precarious financial situation of the foundation. In 2004, the manager of the NADA, Roland Augustin, revealed that the budget of the NADA constituted just 1 percent of overall support for German top-level sports. At least double this sum would be needed to achieve the objectives of the foundation. Important obligations like doping prevention and education, which are both essential aims of the NADA and an important part of the WADA recommendation, could not even be initiated, let alone conducted on an ongoing basis.[102] In 2007, manager Augustin quit his job. The NADA report in 2009 summed up the first years of the foundation as follows: "The first five or six years since the establishment of the NADA have been characterized by an ongoing imbalance between huge expectations on the one hand, and far too small a budget on the other. This discrepancy culminated in an existential crisis in 2007."[103]

This crisis became public when a research study from Werner Pitsch and others revealed that, according to anonymous interviews, about half of all German top athletes in the upper achievement squads had doped at least once in their careers.[104] These results were not at all compatible with the doping tests of the NADA, according to which only 1 or 2 percent of all athletes had doped. When the NADA manager commented on this scenario in the press, saying that he was indeed not surprised by the results of the research—"I know about this from my international colleagues"—he was forced to resign. The press commented that the NADA was apparently unable to do a good job, and especially not its boss. In addition, specific mistakes in implementing doping controls were reported, and the suspicion was articulated that the NADA would really rather *cover up* doping cases than reveal them. "Step by step, it is becoming apparent," commented the critical German press, "that the NADA is as hopelessly underfunded as it is generally unable to do its job properly. The German NADA is no more than a 'token institution.' For doping sinners with half a brain, the NADA is in fact no danger at all."[105]

A TV feature revealed in 2007 that most of the unannounced out-of-competition controls in Germany could not be implemented as requested by the WADA. The controllers did not even meet the athletes, and the federations had not been informed correctly by the NADA about the timing and the exact procedures of the tests. In fact, the "Missed Test Policy" could not be realized by 2007, as the NADA conceded, although the WADC included this means of anti-doping. The NADA manager Augustin himself spoke of "pure chaos" regarding the test procedures, while the officials of sports and politics had praised the German control system as "most effective."[106]

WADA chairman Richard Pound was surprised, because he had always thought that the German anti-doping system was working well. The test failures should be investigated, and the German NADA reformed. Recently, Pound had kept on criticizing the German NADA. "If the NADA is unable to do its job because of a lack of finances, this is not a good sign [. . .]. What message does this send about German sport? What does this say about the commitment of Germany to fair and clean sport? The German NADA had never been well equipped. If the funding of a poorly financed agency is again cut, this may be a sign that nobody is truly interested in reducing doping."[107]

The crisis of the NADA additionally revealed more doping cases, including confessions by German top athletes of having doped. In the context of doping scandals at the Tour de France, German top cyclists like Jan Ullrich, winner of the Tour de France in 1997 and one of the strongest competitors of the notorious doper Lance Armstrong, as well as Eric Zabel, Andreas Klöden, and others of the German Team Telekom, were detected as dopers. Referring to these scandals, the question was discussed in public of whether tax money had been spent on doping, either directly or indirectly. The German cyclists had been medically supported by doctors of the sports medical center at the University of Freiburg. The scandal about this West German center of sports medicine is still being researched by lawyers and various experts, and two doctors were convicted in court.[108]

Therefore, the minister of the interior, Wolfgang Schäuble, established a task force—Projektgruppe Sonderprüfung Doping (Project Group to Investigate Doping). Its aim was to determine whether any tax money from the Federal Republic had been spent on actually doping athletes or on (pro)doping research, directly or indirectly, or whether money had been given to doctors, athletes, or federations that had doped or were suspected of doping. This task force included nine independent persons from various ministries and administrations, but none from sports organizations. It seems remarkable that for the first time in contemporary German sports history, such an independent investigation of sports organizations took place without the participation of sports officials. All Olympic sports federations and associations were investigated, as well as twenty Olympic Training Centers (OSP) and four Federal Training Centers of Sport (BLZ), to determine "whether the anti-doping conditions of approval letters were in fact met or not." The job of the project group included proving the doping-oriented relationships among sports federations, athletes, and doctors at the sports medical center at the University of Freiburg who were employed and paid by the regional state of Baden-Württemberg.[109]

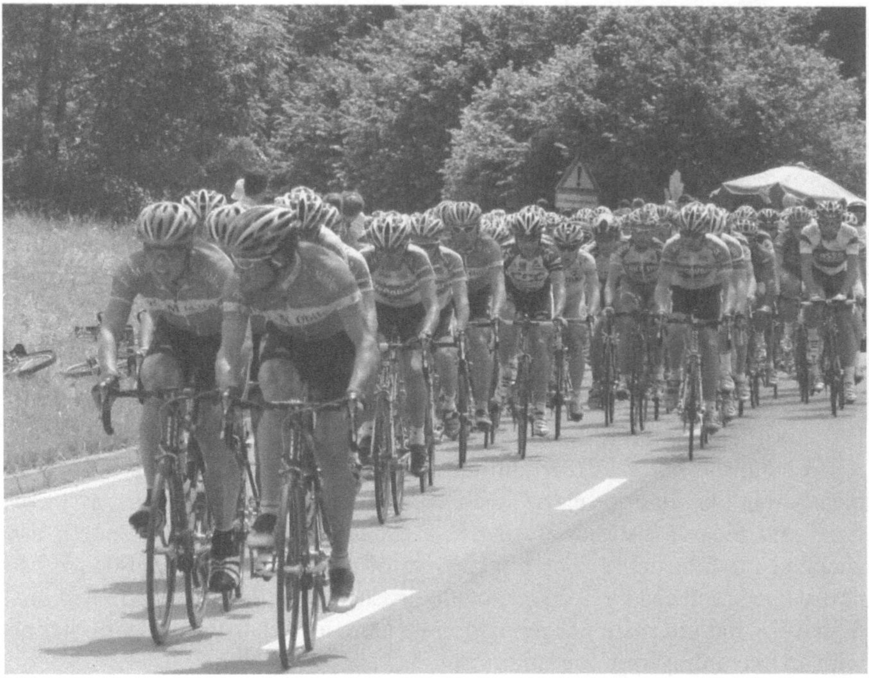

Figure 3.3. The German top cyclist Jan Ullrich in the middle of the peloton during the Tour de France in 2005. Ullrich (b. 1973 in Rostock, GDR) was the most successful cyclist of Germany, educated in the sports system of the GDR, winner of the Tour de France in 1997, and gold medalist at the 2000 Sydney Olympics. His duels with Lance Armstrong are unforgettable. In 2006, he resigned from Team Telekom because of doping allegations. In 2013, he confessed to blood doping; however, he maintains that he never "cheated" anybody.
Source: Picture Alliance

The task force criticized numerous deficits of the German anti-doping system and the NADA, ranging from the control and information system of athletes to the tests. Failures of the sports organizations as well as of political administrations were listed. However, the crucial question of whether tax money had been spent on doping was denied. "Money from the federal state was neither given directly to athletes who doped nor to doctors, coaches or other persons who assisted the doped athletes or assisted in doping them. However, these people profited indirectly from these funds." At the sports medical center of the University of Freiburg, research projects, supported by the federal state, had frequently been operated. By no means all sports federations had conformed to the anti-doping conditions of the approval letters. Some had even clearly violated these conditions. However, the task force argued that currently and due to the legal conditions, it was not possible to reclaim the money from the doped athletes or the federations. The task force also criticized the public administrations and their officials for failing to prove whether the recipients of the tax-financed support had truly met the anti-doping conditions.[110]

The task force recommended various activities to improve anti-doping. Approving and controlling the use of financial support for top-level sports, athletes, sport federations, Olympic Training Centers, and Federal Training Centers should be improved, anti-doping clauses in approval letters had to be truly harmonized and controlled, drugs of any kind (not only forbidden doping substances) should not be financed by public means in general, research projects that can be regarded as doping-related were no longer to be funded, and, finally, cooperation between federal administrations, especially the Ministry of the Interior, on the one hand, and the NADA, on the other, had to be intensified and improved urgently.[111]

In sum, the report of the anti-doping task force of the minister showed clearly that the relationship between state and sport, between sport organizations and federal institutions spending tax money on top-level sports, had changed fundamentally. The atmosphere of mutual trust or confidence had partly been replaced by skepticism and distrust. The federal government also feared for the international reputation of Germany as a fair sporting nation with an exemplary anti-doping system.

The skepticism of German politicians toward sports organizations and their representatives, combined with the public debate on the crisis of the NADA, as well as the report of the Projektgruppe Sonderprüfung Doping, motivated some sports officials and politicians to demand a specific anti-doping law in Germany.

THE DEBATE ON AN ANTI-DOPING LAW

Since the 1960s, the question had arisen frequently in German sports politics of whether a law against doping should be considered by parliament. This notion was rejected just as frequently. The anti-doping initiatives of the European Council in the 1990s again provoked initiatives by some German counties to protect sports as a whole from doping. The sports organizations were regarded as increasingly unable to keep the cultural asset of "sports" clean and fair. This debate was fueled by the fact that the Tour de France doping scandals could only be revealed thanks to the anti-doping law in France. Without this law, the French police would not have been allowed to raid the Tour. The recommendation of the European Council in 1992, the model of anti-doping laws in France and Belgium, and, finally, the crisis of the German NADA, again put this question of an anti-doping law on the agenda of German sports politics.

Until then, the essential arguments for rejecting demands for an anti-doping law were as follows. First, the German Arzneimittelgesetz (AMG, Drug Law) was regarded as sufficient to prevent doping, together with controls and sanctions by the sports organizations. Second, as the federal government had responded to a specific question in parliament with regard to sanctioning an athlete by law because of doping: "In principle, a person should not be punished because he might harm himself, and this includes athletes."[112] Third, the federal government did not see any need for an anti-doping law in Germany deriving from the convention of the Council of Europe, especially with regard to the principle of the autonomy of sports, and given the existing German drug law. Fourth and finally, athletes should not be criminalized, argued the officials of the German sports organizations.

Minister Schily, who had promoted the foundation of the WADA, followed the tradition of his predecessors when he argued that there was indeed no need for a new anti-doping law in Germany. The autonomy of sport in Germany would not be constrained, and therefore, the sports organizations were mainly responsible for reducing doping. The German system of doping control and doping sanctions by the federations and associations of sports was one of the best worldwide. No country in the world operated as many doping controls as Germany, both doping-control laboratories in Cologne and Kreischa were acknowledged worldwide, and the system of sanctioning dopers by the sports organizations would work well. The official tenth report of the federal government on sport in 2002 emphasized the "high level of doping reduction in German sport."[113]

Despite these official statements, within the ministry, as well as in the public and sports arenas, discussions about an anti-doping law continued, and various ideas about how to do it were considered. A proposal of the department chief for sport in the Ministry of the Interior even included a legally binding doping list of forbidden substances and methods.[114]

The German Sports Federation (DSB) proposed the establishment of a commission to prepare a catalogue of legal requirements for a better, more effective, and more consistent fight against doping. The commission was finally installed after a number of meetings of sports politicians from various political parties and sports officials of sports federations. The opinion of representatives of the German sports organizations was always clear. They did not at all approve of a special anti-doping law, because they were keen to avoid a criminalization of athletes, as sports officials were arguing frequently.[115] As expected, the final report of the commission confirmed the opinion of the DSB officials. The fight against doping was up to the sports organizations, and not the police or prosecutors. Actions by the state law could only be "supplementary means." Changes in state laws like that pertaining to conventional drugs were conceivable in order to control doping and drug dealing more effectively. Another option was the establishment of so-called *Schwerpunktstaatsanwaltschaften,* that is, special prosecutors to control and prosecute drug dealing. In addition, a realistic proposal was the establishment of a centralized arbitration court for doping cases. Both national and international sports organizations were increasingly concerned about court cases seeking compensation for athletes who had been banned due to positive doping testing, like Katrin Krabbe (see above).[116]

All these aspects and issues were finally discussed during a public hearing of the Sports Commission of the German Bundestag on September 27, 2006. However, the experts, sports politicians, and sports officials were unable to find a satisfactory solution to the dilemma of German anti-doping policies. The distribution of power, responsibility, and duties in sports in general and especially with respect to doping and anti-doping remained problematic. On the one hand, sports officials constantly repeated the mantra of the autonomy of sports, but complained on the other hand about the lack of support by the organs of the state, both for top-level sports in general and for reducing doping specifically. Some experts like Helmut Digel, a scholar of sports sociology and an official of the Athletics Federation, criticized the German drug law as a "dead duck" with regard to doping prosecution. This law, he claimed, was useless for reducing doping in Germany.[117]

The federal government responded with a Maßnahmenpaket der Bundesregierung gegen Doping im Sport (Package of Federal Government Measures for Reducing Doping in Sport). This referred to participating relevant groups and parties in the fight against doping, which included the sports organizations themselves, federal institutions like ministries and the parliament, and finally the sixteen counties of Germany, which partly financed achievement centers for top-level sports, as well as coaches of youth squads for different sports. The counties were also to share in the costs for the NADA, but refused to provide sufficient financial means—according to the federal government and sports organizations. However, the federal government repeated once again that doped athletes should not be prosecuted by the state, but only by sports organizations. These sanctions, which entailed seriously enforced bans from competitions, were considered as sufficient, both by sports politicians and sports officials. In addition, bans from competition for professional athletes imply temporary bans from their profession, which indeed threaten their professional existence. In consequence, athletes are able to take sports organizations to court with the aim of obtaining compensation.

After all, the federal government was eager to support the international measures against doping from the Council of Europe and UNESCO by ratifying several anti-doping conventions and additional meeting minutes obliging Germany to intensify the fight against doping. Most relevant was the extension of the drug law by including prosecution for dealing in doping drugs. Medicines that could be used for doping were to be labeled as such. Finally, state prosecutors would be authorized to tap the telephones of suspected doping dealers, who could also be athletes. The counties were advised to appoint special prosecutors according to their constitutional powers. All participating parties of anti-doping, namely the federal institutions, sport organizations, and counties, were urgently requested to provide more financial support to the NADA, and to increase its funding.[118]

The responsible Minister of the Interior, Wolfgang Schäuble, summarized the problem in a speech to the German parliament as follows: "During the next few months, we need to discuss better cooperation of autonomous sports organizations with the state, or the legislator and his responsibility for reducing doping. My opinion is that we can deal effectively with the problem if the legislator, prosecutors and sport organizations really cooperate with each other. If the legislator claimed to reduce doping rather than the sport organizations, we would not achieve what we really want."[119]

An extensively discussed aspect of the amendment of the German drug law was the fundamental question of whether an athlete could be prosecuted by the state for merely possessing doping substances. The representatives of the sports organizations were strictly against this alleged criminalization of athletes. Others, like the minister of justice of Bavaria, Beate Merk, favored such regulations. She argued that the state should demonstrate far more power and commitment to reducing doping. Bavaria was, by the way, the first county to install a specific prosecutor against dealing with doping.

Finally, the amended drug law was passed by parliament on July 5, 2007. The relevant undersecretary of state, Christoph Bergner, emphasized solidarity with German sports, and the German Olympic Sports Federation (DOSB) stated its satisfaction with the law. In addition, the board of the DOSB concluded an Anti-Doping Action Plan (Anti-Doping-Aktionsplan) as early as 2006. The obligations of the sports organizations, as well as of the NADA, were concretized and summarized, including improvements in doping controls, doping prevention, sanctions, sports and arbitration courts, and various further details. The plan was praised by the DOSB itself as proof of a "zero-tolerance policy" of German sports against doping. Critics, however, like the former chairman of the parliamentary Sports Commission, Peter Danckert, referred to the plan as a reiteration of the usual "platitudes and routines."[120]

INTERIM RESULTS: DOPING IN THE CONTEXT OF SPORTS, STATE, AND SOCIETY

The foundation of the WADA was indeed a new phase in the development of modern sports. As Houlihan has stated, an international political "anti-doping regime" had been established. The days were over when only nongovernmental organizations like the IOC and other international sports federations exercised power in international sports. With respect to an absolutely crucial problem of modern sports, these sporting NGOs had to share their power with states and governments. The WADA is still a joint project on sports and anti-doping from sports organizations and governments. Both governments and international sports organizations finance the WADA administration, including their responsibility for doping controls according to the internationally valid WADC. Both also define international anti-doping policies, so that the doping problem was also an instrument for states to influence sports in general.

The WADA supported the process of harmonizing the anti-doping rules and procedures for controlling and sanctioning athletes by the WADC. The worldwide awareness that doping in sports is morally wrong and must be forbidden could be strengthened. A consequence of the WADA foundation was that national anti-doping agencies were founded in the same spirit as the WADA. However, it is debatable whether any real success in reducing doping was achieved. Effective actions in the fight against doping, as with organized crime in international networks, were in fact more likely to be achieved by the police and state organs, based on national anti-doping laws as in Italy, France, and Spain.[121]

This paradigmatic shift to parity between sports and states with respect to anti-doping policies was not at all a matter of course. By contrast, the states required power and influence in international sports, as the remarkable Lausanne Conference in 1999 had demonstrated. Whereas the IOC had planned to act as usual and keep international sports completely under control, the representatives of several states demanded a different strategy. From their perspective, the participation of state politics in reducing doping was urgently needed, because doping was regarded by numerous states as a danger to the health of athletes and as an icon of deteriorating societal health.

One can speculate as to why state organs were so interested in resolving such a difficult problem as doping. The expectation of succeeding in solving the problem had always been low, at least for realistic experts on sports and doping. In fact, the odds were similar to those for criminality in general, fraud, or drug use. That is, everybody knows that such behavior cannot be eliminated, and can at best be reduced. In addition, whereas doping in sports is forbidden by anti-doping rules and in some countries even by law, similar performance-enhancing strategies are accepted by other elements of society, like arts and music, and even in everyday life and to some extent at work. Why should athletes be forbidden what is open to everyone else?

And again, why are governments and politicians interested in keeping sports free of doping, and why not arts and music and others? And why do they not leave the problem to the nongovernmental organizations of sport? Why do politicians run a race they can never win? Who can doubt that the sports-political doping game is not a field of honor and success, but rather of defeat and frustration?

Some more answers to these difficult questions may be attempted. Certainly, caring for the health of athletes and the population in general is a crucial motivation for politicians to become involved in the fight against doping. Doping in sports increased parallel to the medicalization of modern societies. Doping-free sports seem to indicate that health and achievement are also possible without drugs. Another argument is the fact that top sports have become a worldwide media, commercial, and professional phenomenon. States cannot afford to leave this important field only to nongovernmental organizations. Rather, they have to be concerned with societal developments and tendencies in order to legitimize their political power.

Following the theory of the process of civilization of Norbert Elias, the participation of governments in reducing doping in sports may be interpreted as part of the process of centralized institutions gaining monopoly power. Sports are part of this process, and doping may be an instrument for securing more control over a phenomenon of modern societies, implying high relevance to the ruling classes both within and beyond politics. This may explain why both sports and politics share their power over and responsibility for international top-level sports and anti-doping.

Whatever the case, the fact is that the WADA became the model for national anti-doping organizations. Founding the NADA was the national reaction to the WADA in Germany. The WADA concept of public-private partnership in reducing doping was even difficult for Germany to accept, because of the tradition of autonomy of sport. In addition, the German experiences with and recent memories of state sport in the former GDR did not lead to a preference for state politics or sports administrations, whereas in fact the state had already become the essential sponsor of top-level sports in Germany. In some way, the strong support of top sports by the state was a heritage of the Cold War, when the idol of the successful state sports system of the GDR was even being imitated. After German reunification, when the high cost of the successes of GDR sports became apparent—in German Marks and Euros as well as in human tragedies and doping victims—skepticism against more state in sport was hardly surprising.

These are some essential reasons why the process of installing a political anti-doping regime in Germany developed rather hesitantly and in a complicated manner. German sports politicians were challenged by several dilemmas. First, there was the traditional skepticism of the fact that the state sponsored top-level sports extensively. Second, there was the need and will to be successful in international sports in contrast to the moral obligation toward the national and international public to reduce doping effectively. Third, the strong ideology of the autonomy of sport contrasted with the international tendency toward state controls and anti-doping laws. The political elite in Germany was clearly motivated by a desire to conform to international political trends. Therefore, the politicians willingly followed all European initiatives, as well as those of international institutions like the European Council and UNESCO. German sport was not to go its own German *Sonderweg*—neither in politics nor sports.

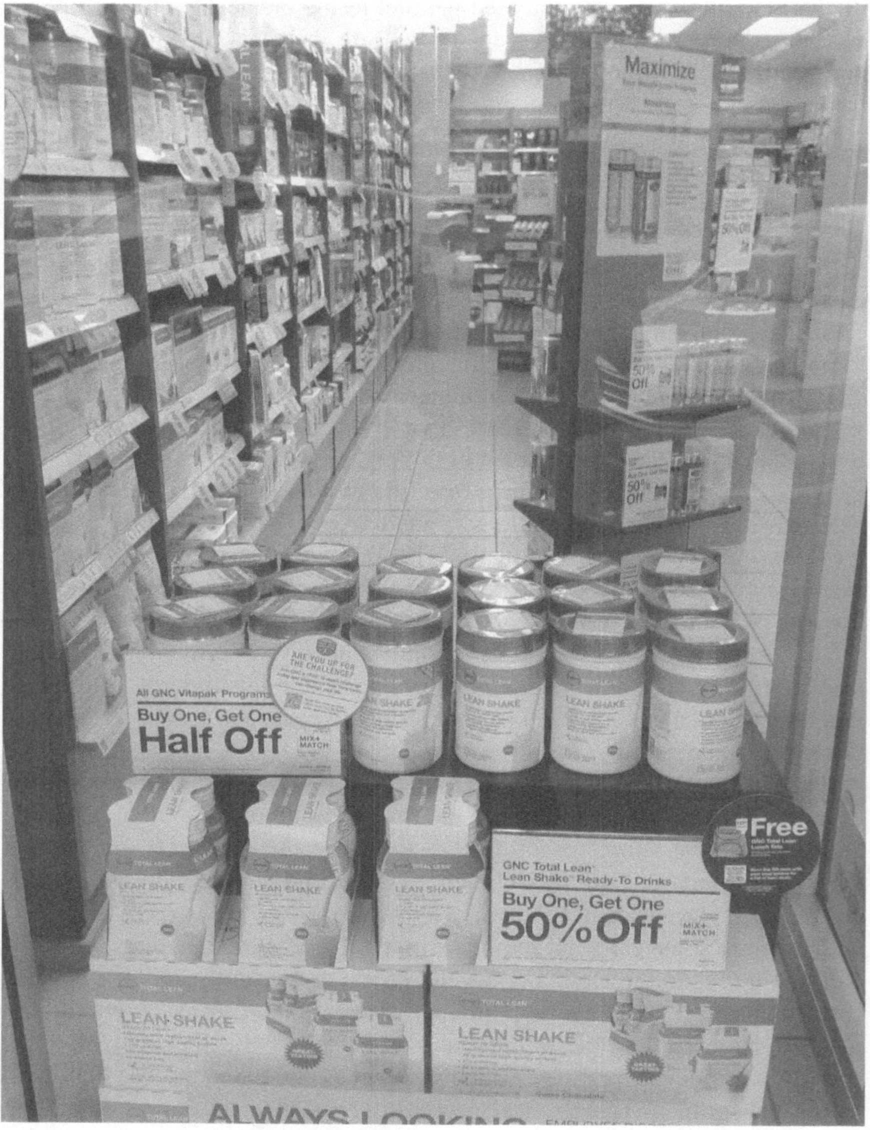

Figure 3.4. Enhancement products, vitamins, and testosterone boosters are freely available in supermarkets and drugstores in many countries, including here in the United States. ***Source: Courtesy of the author***

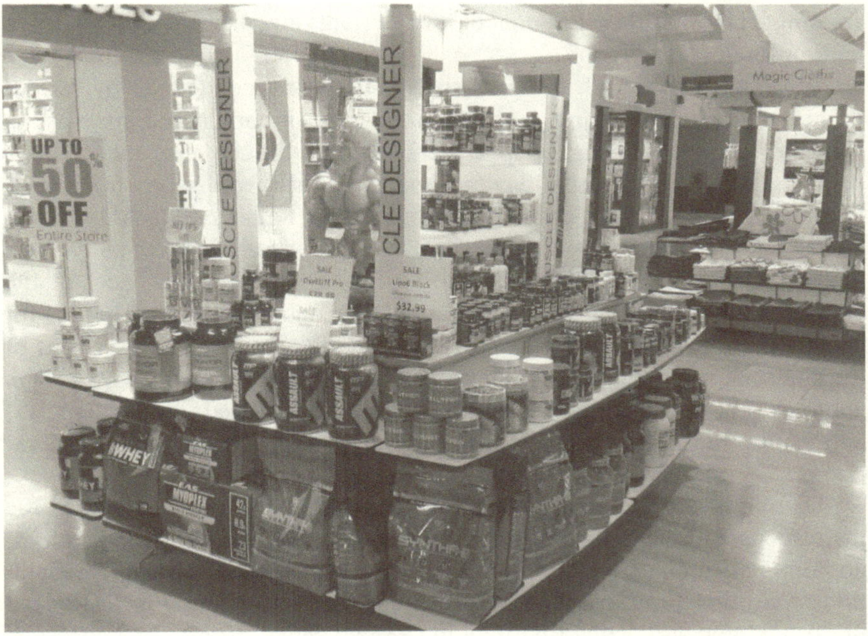

Figure 3.5.

Long, controversial, and sometimes highly complex debates in public and in sports forums, in various boards of the sports organizations, in special commission and committees, partly filled with experts, sports officials and politicians were held accountable, and acceptable compromises had to be found. Numerous reports were written as well. One compromise was that despite the still significant principle of autonomy, partnership, and subsidiarity, the state or, more precisely, various state administrations are obliged to intervene in sports if problems arise that concern society in general. This is indeed the case with doping, because it affects the general health of the population and relates partly to drug dealing as a criminal act.[122]

In addition, organized sport is able to define its own rules; the *Eigenwelt des Sports* does not need to conform absolutely to public law. This occurs, for example, when sports institutions or public-private partnership organizations like the WADA and the NADA are acting according to the principle of "strict liability" to prosecute doped athletes. The application of this principle in the context of constitutional states can be legitimized only by the fact that an athlete accepts, by his own choice, the unique rules or laws of sport, including the principle of "strict liability." Another important factor was the transparency of doping controls, in contrast to principles of the protection of privacy, according to the laws of constitutional states. Modern top athletes are obliged to limit their personal or human rights and privacy if they wish to participate in competitions.

The establishment of the German NADA was accompanied by serious problems from the beginning, of which the most important and long-lasting was the lack of funding. Hopes were quickly dashed that the German counties, which are constitutionally responsible for school sports but not for top-level sports, or the German economy would support the NADA financially. The German sports organizations, except football (soccer) and tennis, were also unable to contribute significant sums to the fund. Most of the German sports organizations are in fact relatively poor amateurs. The fees for sports clubs are traditionally low, and so, therefore, are the contributions of the clubs to the federations. Top-level sports are financed mainly by the state, and only at a low level by private sponsors. As mentioned, football (soccer) and tennis are relevant exceptions to the rule of poor German sports federations.

Therefore, the German government or Ministry of the Interior, as the main sponsor of the top-sports departments of the German sports federations, appropriately applied pressure through financial support if any sports federations were unwilling to cooperate with the NADA, or simply to justify the use of tax money. For the first time in German sports history, in 2010, such controls led to claims for the return of financial support from the state from individual sports federations that were not able to explain exactly what they had done with the money, or that had directly or indirectly supported athletes or coaches who had doped or who were suspected of having done so. However, the message conveyed by the state to the sports organizations was, as mentioned, inconsistent. On the one hand, they expected outstanding achievements and many medals from the athletes and sports federations, but on the other hand, the state organs were suspecting and controlling them increasingly, because of doping. Finally, the most important consequence of recent anti-doping history in Germany was that the traditional relationship of mutual confidence between top-level sports and state, athletes, coaches, doctors, officials, politicians, journalists, and the public changed to one of distrust. One rather different and distinct consequence is the fact that an unknown but not insignificant number of parents seem to be increasingly wary of advising their children to become part of the sports system. Simultaneously, however, the same parents were often enthusiastic spectators of top-level sports events and unhappy if "their" athletes did not perform as expected.

The foundation of the NADA was certainly an important and useful step in the international direction of reducing doping according to the principles of the WADA. The state gained power and responsibility in sports and for the fight against doping. However, sports politicians and officials still refused to introduce a specific anti-doping law in Germany. "I warn against the call for more and stricter laws against doping," argued the minister of the interior,

Lothar de Maiziere, at the assembly of the German Olympic Sports Federation in 2009 in Duesseldorf. "I am not at all convinced that cheating in sport can be reduced more effectively by new laws. I believe that this cannot be the right way. In the long run, we would be cancelling criminal law into the field of sport and damaging its autonomy."[123]

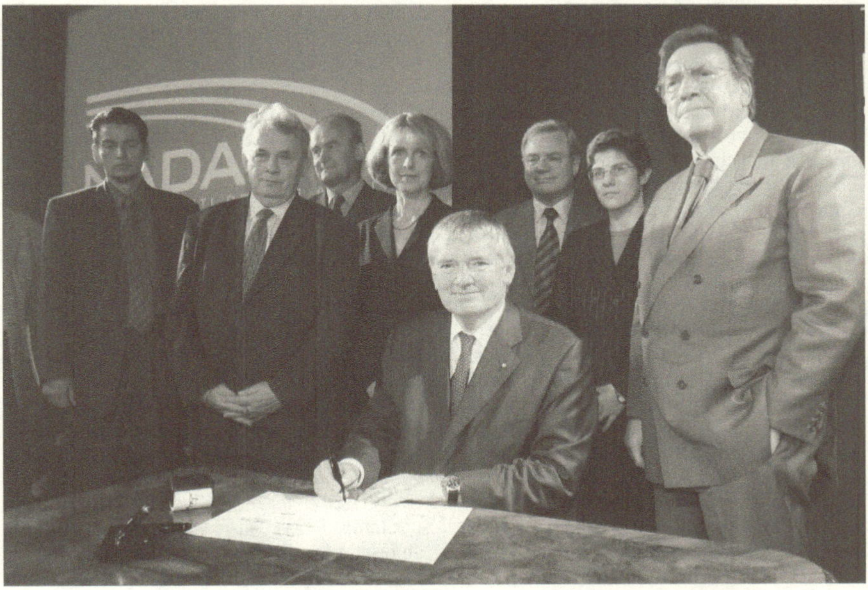

Figure 3.6. Foundation of the National Anti-Doping Agency (NADA) of Germany in Bonn, July 15, 2002. Minister of the Interior Otto Schily signs the contract in the presence of Manfred von Richthofen, then president of the DSB, and Walther Tröger, president of the NOC, as well as Annegret Kramp-Karrenbauer, chairperson of the sports ministers of the German counties, and Bärbel Dieckmann, mayor of Bonn, capital of the FRG until 1999/2000. *Source: Bundesregierung/ B 145 Bild-00004872/ Sepp Spiegl*

Nonetheless, after the elections in 2013, the new government of Social Democrats and Conservatives, with the same minister of the interior, included plans for a special anti-doping law in their coalition contract.[124]

NOTES

This chapter is based on Michael Krüger and Christian Becker, "Doping and Anti-Doping in the Process of German Reunification," *Sport in History* 34 (2014): 1–24, doi:10.1080/17460263.2014.897250.

1. The political background of sports during the Cold War is well researched and explained for an international audience in Mike Dennis and Jonathan Grix, *Sport under Communism: Behind the East German "Miracle,"* Global Culture and Sport (Basingstoke, Hampshire: Palgrave Macmillan, 2012); Thomas M. Hunt, *Drug Games: The International Olympic Commit-*

tee and the Politics of Doping, 1960–2008, Terry and Jan Todd Series on Physical Culture and Sports (Austin: University of Texas Press, 2011); Uta Andrea Balbier, *Kalter Krieg auf der Aschenbahn: Der deutsch-deutsche Sport, 1950–1972. Eine politische Geschichte,* Sammlung Schöningh zur Geschichte und Gegenwart (Paderborn: F. Schöningh, 2007); and Kay Schiller and Christopher Young, *The 1972 Munich Olympics and the Making of Modern Germany,* Weimar and Now 42 (Berkeley: University of California Press, 2010), in German as Kay Schiller and Christopher Young, *München 1972: Olympische Spiele im Zeichen des modernen Deutschland* (Göttingen: Wallstein, 2012), deal with German sports development in detail, especially the perspective of the 1972 Munich Olympics.

2. Willi Daume, interviewed by Richard Mandell, in Richard D. Mandell, *The Olympics of 1972: A Munich Diary* (Chapel Hill: University of North Carolina Press, 1991), 19.

3. The former president of the East German Gymnastics and Sports Association, Manfred Ewald, the most powerful sports organizer and sports politician in the GDR, argues in his memoirs that the GDR would have had the chance to be number one in world sports if the USSR had not boycotted the Los Angeles Olympics of 1984. Manfred Ewald and Reinhold Andert, *Manfred Ewald—Ich war der Sport: Wahrheiten und Legenden aus dem Wunderland der Sieger,* EP 526 (Berlin: Elefanten Press, 1994), 182.

4. See § 39, Absatz 2 of the treaty of the German unification. See http://www.gesetze-im-internet.de/einigvtr/art_39.html, accessed 13 June 2014.

5. The doping system of the GDR was uncovered and researched by various historians and commissions soon after the demise of the GDR. The most famous was the Eppelmann Commission, established by and named after its former chairman, Rainer Eppelmann, the last minister of defense of the GDR and a member of the first German parliament after unification. The report of this commission, which was set up by parliament, includes nine large volumes of papers by experts and contemporary witnesses. Volume 3 (III, 1, esp. 675–89) deals with sports and doping during the SED dictatorship. Deutscher Bundestag, ed., *Materialien der Enquete-Kommission "Aufarbeitung von Geschichte und Folgen der SED-Diktatur in Deutschland": (12. Wahlperiode des Deutschen Bundestages); Neue Bände in 18 Teilbänden*, III/I (Baden-Baden, Frankfurt am Main: Nomos-Verl.-Ges; Suhrkamp, 1995). Basic sources of information and documents for this purpose were from the Bundesamt für die Stasi-Unterlagen (BStU), the office that was founded in 1990 for the purpose of preserving the millions of secret documents from the secret service of the GDR (Stasi). The BStU was chaired by Joachim Gauck, current president of the Federal Republic of Germany. Concerning sports, see especially the booklet "MfS und Leistungssport" (1994), edited by the BStU. J. Ferstle, "World Conference on Doping in Sport," in *Doping in Elite Sport: Politics of Drugs in the Olympic Movement*, ed. Wayne Wilson and Edward Derse (Champaign, Ill.: Human Kinetics, 2001), 275–86.

6. Bundestags-Drucksache (Printings) 11/5784, Response of the Federal Government to the *Große Anfrage* (literally "major request") of members of the parliament of the Social Democratic Party (SPD), 1989, pp. 26, 29.

7. *Staatsdoping* is the title of a study by the historian Klaus Latzel about the VEB (Volkseigener Betrieb) Jenapharm, a factory producing doping substances (hormones, anabolics) especially for use in sports according to the Staatsplanthema 14.25, the governmental plan for using doping substances at all levels of GDR sports. See Klaus Latzel, *Staatsdoping: Der VEB Jenapharm im Sportsystem der DDR* (Cologne and Vienna: Böhlau, 2009). Brigitte Berendonk and Werner Franke were the first to detect the GDR doping system. Their famous and much imitated book, Brigitte Berendonk, *Doping Dokumente: Von der Forschung zum Betrug* (Berlin and New York: Springer-Verlag, 1991); Brigitte Berendonk, *Doping: Von der Forschung zum Betrug*, 2nd expanded ed., rororo Sport 8677 (Reinbek: Rowohlt, 1992), initiated substantial systematic research and study, also by journalists.

8. This scandal and others in Germany are discussed in Henk E. Meier and Marcel Reinold, "Dopingskandale in der alten Bundesrepublik: Öffentlicher Diskurs und sportpolitische Reaktionen," *Deutschland Archiv: Zeitschrift für das vereinigte Deutschland* 45, no. 2 (2012): 209–39.

9. Letter of Rudolf Seiters to Hans Hansen, 3 December 1991, German Olympic Sports Federation (DOSB) Archive.

10. Andreas Singler, *Doping und Enhancement: Interdisziplinäre Studien zur Pathologie gesellschaftlicher Leistungsorientierung*, Würzburger Beiträge zur Sportwissenschaft 6 (Göttingen: Cuvillier, 2012).

11. Andreas Singler and Gerhard Treutlein, "Doping in der Bundesrepublik Deutschland: Historische und soziologische Aspekte abweichenden Verhaltens im Spitzensport," in *Hormone und Hochleistung: Doping in Ost und West*, ed. Klaus Latzel and Lutz Niethammer (Cologne: Böhlau, 2008), 41–65.

12. Jutta Braun, "'Dopen für Deutschland': Die Diskussion im vereinten Sport, 1990–1992," in *Hormone und Hochleistung: Doping in Ost und West*, ed. Klaus Latzel and Lutz Niethammer (Cologne: Böhlau, 2008), 151–70.

13. See, for example, General Robertson in his so-called expertise in 1950 for the IOC, concerning the question of whether, when, and why Germany could again take part in the Olympic Games and become a member of the Olympic family. Annex 3 of the minutes of the IOC sessions in Copenhagen in 1950, IOC Archives.

14. See Hartmut Becker et al., *Die Gründerjahre des Deutschen Sportbundes: Wege aus der Not zur Einheit*, with the assistance of Ommo Grupe and Giselher Spitzer (Schorndorf: Karl Hofmann, 1990).

15. See Schiller and Young, *The 1972 Munich Olympics and the Making of Modern Germany*.

16. See Martin H. Geyer, "Der Kampf um nationale Repräsentation: Deutsch-deutsche Sportbeziehungen und die 'Hallstein-Doktrin,'" *Vierteljahreshefte für Zeitgeschichte*, no. 1 (1966).

17. This is a general result of our research project on doping in West Germany.

18. Carl Diem, *Wesen und Lehre des Sports,* Sportlehre 1 (Berlin: Weidmann, 1949).

19. This position of West German politicians and various administrations until the unification became clear and even obvious to the public through studying the "sports reports" of the federal government (*Sportberichte der Bundesregierung*), published since 1971 and after each election period.

20. We found from the Stasi archive that the organization had uncovered an internal report of the BND (Bundesnachrichtendienst, the West German secret service) containing detailed information about the doping system in the GDR. BStU, MfS ZAIG Nr. 11292.

21. Broadcasted 5 March1977, ZDF-Mediathek: www.zdf.de/ZDFmediathek/beitrag/video/1935254/, accessed 13 June 2014.

22. Berendonk, *Doping Dokumente*, 243. http://www.spiegel.de/spiegel/print/d-13499707.html, accessed 28 August 2014.

23. Spiegel 11 (1990). http://www.spiegel.de/spiegel/print/d-13498125.html (access 16/02/2015).

24. *Stern*, 8 November 1990.

25. *Spiegel* 52 (1990), 144.

26. *Stern*, 15 April 1991.

27. Berendonk, *Doping.*

28. John M. Hoberman, *Mortal Engines: The Science of Performance and the Dehumanization of Sport* (New York: Macmillan, 1992).

29. The report is documented at various places and archives, for example in the Carl and Liselott Diem Archive in Cologne, estate of August Kirsch, then director of the Bundesinstitut für Sportwissenschaft, folder 115. See also http://www.cycling4fans.de/uploads/media/1991_Bericht_der_Reiter-Kommission_01.pdf, accessed 18 February 2014.

30. Ibid., 10.

31. Ibid., 19.

32. Law of 24 August 2002, *Bundesgesetzblatt* 1:3410.

33. Manfred von Richthofen was the nephew of the famous "Red Baron," the World War I fighter pilot, and was president of the German Sportbund (DSB) from 1994 to 2006.

34. The commission presented its report in December 1991 after eleven meetings and hearings with forty-three persons, athletes, coaches, and officials. See DOSB Archive, folder "Anti-Doping-Kommissionen."

35. *Bundestagsdrucksache* (government printing), December 1999, 6.

36. Klaus Blume, *Die Dopingrepublik: Eine (deutsch-)deutsche Sportgeschichte* (Berlin: Rotbuch, 2012), 149; Daniel M. Rosen, *Dope: A History of Performance Enhancement in Sports from the Nineteenth Century to Today* (Westport, Conn. and London: Praeger, 2008), 85–89; Dennis and Grix, *Sport under Communism.* See also the magazine article "Der Traum vom Medaillenregen," *Spiegel,* 17 November 1997, 204.

37. This and other quotations about or from this debate can be found in Parlamentsarchiv Berlin, protocol of the ninth meeting of the parliamentary Commission for Sport, 18 September 1991.

38. Ibid.

39. Parlamentsarchiv Berlin, protocol of the tenth meeting of the parliamentary Commission for Sport, 25 September 1991.

40. Letter of the BMI to the sports federations, 27 September 1991, folder "Doping," DOSB Archive.

41. Peter Danckert, *Kraftmaschine Parlament: Der Sportausschuss und die Sportpolitik des Bundes,* Hauptsache Sport (Aachen: Meyer & Meyer, 2009), 173.

42. Parlamentsarchiv Berlin, protocol of the twelfth meeting of the parliamentary Commission for Sport, 6 November 1991, 6, 19–21.

43. Ibid., 28–29.

44. Ibid.

45. Ibid., 174–75.

46. Letter of Seiters to Hansen, 3 December 1991, folder "Doping," DOSB Archive.

47. The report can be downloaded from the website of the Canadian government: http://epe.lac-bac.gc.ca/100/200/301/pco-bcp/commissions-ef/dubin1990-eng/dubin1990-eng.htm, accessed 18 February 2014.

48. Barrie Houlihan, "Doping, Public Health and the Generalization of Interests," in *Elite Sport, Doping and Public Health*, ed. Verner Møller, Mike McNamee, and Paul Dimeo, (Odense: University Press of Southern Denmark, 2009), 41–54, esp. 43.

49. http://conventions.coe.int/treaty/ger/Treaties/Html/135.htm, accessed 18 February 2014.

50. Judith Amelie Schmidt, *Internationale Dopingbekämpfung: Grundlagen und nationalstaatliche Umsetzung,* Schriftenreihe Causa Sport 1 (Stuttgart, Zürich: Boorberg; Schulthess, 2009), 22.

51. Fabian Reissinger, *Staatliche Verantwortung zur Bekämpfung des Dopings*, Schriften zum Sportrecht 19 (Baden-Baden: Nomos-Verl.-Ges, 2010), 305.

52. Parlamentsarchiv Berlin, protocol of the meeting of the parliamentary Commission for Sport, 29 April 1992.

53. Dieter Baumann, *Lebenslauf: Mit aktuellem Beitrag zum Comeback*, 2nd expanded ed., Knaur 77668 (Munich: Droemer Knaur, 2003), himself describes in detail his *Lebenslauf* (CV), including his fight against doping and his personal doping case, which has never really been investigated and resolved. His autobiography includes, in the annex, the final sentence of his trial by the legal committee of the German Athletics Federation (DLV) from 13 July 2000, which in fact rendered a verdict of not guilty.

54. Lothar Gorris, Maik Großekathöfer, and Udo Ludwig, "Nur die ganz Dummen: Interview mit Werner Franke," *Der Spiegel*, 14 August 2006, http://www.spiegel.de/spiegel/print/d-48262955.html, accessed 20 July 2014.

55. Translated quotation from the report of the Projektgruppe Sonderprüfung Doping, 31 July 2007. The report can be downloaded on www.cycling4fans.de/index.php?id=5690, accessed 18 February 2014.

56. Udo Steiner, "Schutz des Sports: Verbands- oder Staatsaufgabe?" in *Wettkampfmanipulation und Schutzmechanismen* (Stuttgart: Boorberg, 2012), 45–52.

57. Charles L. Dubin, ed., *Commission of Inquiry into the Use of Drugs and Banned Practices Intended to Increase Athletic Performance* (Ottawa: Canadian Government Publication Centre, 1990), 553.

58. In his book, Richard W. Pound, *Inside Dope: How Drugs Are the Biggest Threat to Sports, Why You Should Care, and What Can Be Done about Them* (Mississauga, Ontario: Wiley & Sons Canada, 2006), Pound describes the dangerous phenomenon of doping from his perspective as WADA chair. See also an interview with Dick Pound in the German e-paper faz-

net, in which Pound criticizes the current anti-doping policies of the international sports federations and especially the insufficient financial support of the German anti-doping agency. http://www.faz.net/aktuell/sport/sportpolitik/doping/im-gespraech-doping-experte-pound-am-kampf-gegen-doping-ist-niemand-interessiert-12584625-p3.html, accessed 14 June 2014.

59. D. V. Hanstad, A. Smith, and Ivan Waddington, "Establishment of the World Anti-Doping Agency: A Study of the Management of Organisational Change and Unplanned Outcomes," *International Review for the Sociology of Sport* 43, no. 3 (2008): 227–49.

60. Barrie Houlihan, *Dying to Win: Doping in Sport and the Development of Anti-Doping Policy*, 2nd ed. (Strasbourg: Council of Europe Publications, 2002), 160.

61. For more detail, see Hanstad, Smith, and Waddington, "Establishment of the World Anti-Doping Agency," esp. 244.

62. Houlihan, "Doping, Public Health and the Generalization of Interests," 41–54, esp. 42–44.

63. P. Sperryn, ed., "Proceedings of the International Symposium on Anabolic Steroids in Sport: Special Issue of the Symposium in London," Special issue, *British Journal of Sport Medicine* 9, no. 2 (1975).

64. R. O. Keohane, "The Demand for International Regimes," *International Organization* 36, no. 2 (1982): 325–55; Stephen D. Krasner, *International Regimes,* Cornell Studies in Political Economy (Ithaca, N.Y.: Cornell University Press, 1983).

65. Europarat, Ein sauberer und gesunder Sport für das dritte Jahrtausend, Ordner 0717, 11/99–5/00, Nationale Verbindungen, Nationale Anti-Doping Agentur (NADA).

66. Hunt, *Drug Games*, 14ff.

67. Council of Europe, *Doping of Athletes: Reports of the Special Working Parties, Strasbourg, January 1963, Madrid, November 1963* (Strasbourg, 1964).

68. A. Röthel, "Neues Doping-Gesetz für Frankreich," *Sport und Recht (SpuRT)*, no. 1 (1999): 20–21; M. Krogmann, "Zur Dopinggesetzgebung im Ausland: Teil 1 1/99, Teil 2 2/99, Teil 3 4/99, Teil 4 1/2000," *Sport und Recht (SpuRT)*, 1999/2000.

69. Patrick Laure, "Zur Entwicklung von Dopingregeln und Antidoping-Gesetzen," in *Dopingprävention in Europa: Grundlagen und Modelle; Erstes internationales Expertengespräch 2005 in Heidelberg*, ed. Wolfgang Knörzer, G. Spitzer, and G. Treutlein (Aachen and Graz: Meyer & Meyer, 2006), 121–32, esp. 123.; C. Brissonneau and F. Depiesse, "Doping and Doping Control in French Sport," in *Doping and Doping Control in Europe: Performance Enhancing Drugs, Elite Sports and Leisure Time Sport in Denmark, Great Britain, East and West Germany, Poland, France, Italy*, ed. Giselher Spitzer, Edition Sport & Freizeit 15 (Aachen: Meyer & Meyer, 2006), 145–67.

70. Schmidt, *Internationale Dopingbekämpfung*, 24.

71. Hanstad, Smith, and Waddington, "Establishment of the World Anti-Doping Agency," 245.

72. Schmidt, *Internationale Dopingbekämpfung*, 70.

73. Ibid., 77.

74. J. Hoberman, "Doping, Gambling, and the Decline of the IOC," *Georgetown Journal of International Affairs* 13, no. 2 (2012).

75. Houlihan, *Dying to Win*, 140.

76. Ferstle, "World Conference on Doping in Sport," 275–86.

77. The political scholars Volker Rittberger and H. Boekle, "Das International Olympische Komitee: Eine Weltregierung des Sports?" in *Olympischer Sport: Rückblick und Perspektiven*, ed. Ommo Grupe (Schorndorf: Hofmann, 1997), 127–57, named the IOC as "Weltregierung des Sports" (world government of sport), but with a question mark.

78. The Tour de France scandals have been broadly researched by various scholars, esp. Hanstad, Smith, and Waddington, "Establishment of the World Anti-Doping Agency," 228–31; also Ivan Waddington, *Sport, Health and Drugs: A Critical Sociological Perspective* (London and New York: E & FN Spon, 2000), 153–69; and J. Hoberman, "How Drug Testing Fails: The Politics of Doping Control," in *Doping in Elite Sport: Politics of Drugs in the Olympic Movement*, ed. Wayne Wilson and Edward Derse (Champaign, Ill.: Human Kinetics, 2001), 241–74.

79. J. MacAloon, "Doping and Moral Authority: Sports Organizations Today," in *Doping in Elite Sport: Politics of Drugs in the Olympic Movement*, ed. Wayne Wilson and Edward Derse (Champaign, Ill.: Human Kinetics, 2001), 205–24, esp. 206.

80. Some investigative German journalists have accused the IOC of corruption, for example, Thomas Kistner, "So korrupt ist das IOC" (How corrupt is the IOC), *Cicero*, 15 May 2008, http://www.cicero.de/weltb%C3%BChne/so-korrupt-ist-das-ioc/38707, accessed 17 June 2014.

81. J. Ferstle, "World Conference on Doping in Sport," 275–86, esp. 279; Hunt, *Drug Games*, 106; J. Hoberman, *Testosterone Dreams: Rejuvenation, Aphrodisia, Doping* (Berkeley: University of California Press, 2005), 260–62.

82. Hanstad, Smith, and Waddington, "Establishment of the World Anti-Doping Agency," 229.

83. Ibid., 234ff.; Anita DeFrantz, "Which Rules? International Sport and Doping in the 21st Century," *Houston Journal of International Law* 31, no. 1 (2008): 1–26; D. Oswald, "A Lesson to the Moralizers," *Olympic Review* 26 (1999): 21–23.

84. Sarah Teetzel, "The Road to WADA: Seventh International Symposium for Olympic Research (S. 213–224)," unpublished manuscript, http://library.la84.org/SportsLibrary/ISOR/ISOR2004t.pdf, accessed 18 June 2014.

85. Hanstad, Smith, and Waddington, "Establishment of the World Anti-Doping Agency," 236ff.

86. Duncan Mackay, "Banks Says No to New Initiative to Fight Drugs," *Guardian*, 3–5 February 1999; Jere Longman, "IOC Makes Changes, but Trust Becomes Issue," *New York Times*, 19 March 1999; Hunt, *Drug Games*, 107.

87. IOC, Minutes of the IOC, 17–18 March 1999; P. L. Montgomery, "I.O.C. Falters In Doping Bids As Summit Ends," *New York Times*, 5 February 1999. The history of the WADA, including the Lausanne conference, is well documented by the WADA itself. See http://www.wada-ama.org/en/About-WADA/History/WADA-History/, accessed 18 June 2014. See also the documents on the website of the Council of Europe: https://wcd.coe.int/ViewDoc.jsp?id=402791, accessed 18 June 2014.

88. World Anti-Doping Agency (WADA), *Cape Town Declaration on Anti-Doping in Sport*, http://www.wada-ama.org/rtecontent/document/capetowndeclaration.pdf, accessed 18 June 2014.

89. Hanstad, Smith, and Waddington, "Establishment of the World Anti-Doping Agency"; IOC, Minutes of the 115th IOC Session, Prague, 2–4 July 2003, 54.

90. World Anti-Doping Agency (WADA), World Anti-Doping Code (WADC).

91. WADA, http://www.wada-ama.org/rtecontent/document/qa_strict_liability.pdf, accessed 21 June 2014.

92. The UNESCO documents can be downloaded from UNESCO, *Records of the General Conference. 33rd Session. Paris, October, 3rd–21st. Volume I Resolutions* (2005), http://unesdoc.unesco.org/images/0014/001428/142825e.pdf, accessed 18 June 2014; Scott R. Jedlicka and Thomas M. Hunt, "The International Anti-Doping Movement and UNESCO: A Historical Case Study," *International Journal of the History of Sport* 30, no. 13 (2013): 1523–35, doi:10.1080/09523367.2013.823404.

93. UNESCO, *UNESCO Media Services: Meeting of States Parties to the International Convention against Doping Sport* (2011).

94. Clemens Prokop, "Probleme einer nationalen Anti-Doping-Agentur," in *Dopingforum: Aktuelle rechtliche und medizinische Aspekte*, ed. Volker Röhricht and Klaus Vieweg, Recht und Sport Sonderband (Stuttgart and Munich: Richard Boorberg Verlag, 2000), 77–85, esp. 77.

95. Deutscher Olympischer Sportbund (DOSB), minutes of the 64th meeting of the chair of the DSB, September 3rd, Berlin, Annex 1 of Top 16.

96. Bundesministerium des Inneren (BMI), *Sportberichte der Bundesregierung* (Bonn, Berlin, 1973–2010), ninth report (1999), 50.

97. Holger Niese, "Stiftung National Anti-Doping Agentur," in *Schiedsgerichtsbarkeit im Sport*, ed. Ulrich Haas, Recht und Sport 31 (Stuttgart: Boorberg, 2003), 61–74, esp. 70.

98. Bundesinstitut für Sportwissenschaft (BISp) Archive, folder 0717, NADA 2000–2005. Bundesministerium des Inneren (BMI), *Sportförderung des Bundes* (1970ff.), Zwischenbericht Projektgruppe Sonderprüfung Doping 2007, 31 July 2007.

99. Bundesministerium des Inneren (BMI), *Sportberichte der Bundesregierung* (Bonn, Berlin, 1973–2010), eleventh report (2006), 55.

100. Holger Niese, "Stiftung National Anti-Doping Agentur," 61–74, 68ff.; see also the regular reports of the NADA, http://www.nada.de/de/home#.U6LojhAWe4c, accessed 18 June 2014.

101. Bundesinstitut für Sportwissenschaft (BISp) Archives, folder 0717, NADA, Urkunde über die Errichtung "Stiftung Nationale Anti-Doping Agentur," 15 July 2002.

102. C. Weber, "Die Stiftung Nationale Anti-Doping Agentur," in *Persönlichkeitsrechte im Sport*, ed. Martin Nolte, Recht und Sport 36 (Stuttgart: Boorberg, 2006), 71–85, esp. 79.

103. Nationale Anti-Doping Agentur (NADA), report 2009, 6.

104. Werner Pitsch, Eike Emrich, and Michael Klein, "Zur Häufigkeit des Dopings im Leistungssport: Ergebnisse eines www-surveys," *Leipziger Sportwissenschaftliche Beiträge* 46, no. 2 (2005): 63–77.

105. Thomas Kistner, "Anti-Doping-Organisation: Unterfinanziert und überfordert," *Süddeutsche Zeitung*, 12 October 2006.

106. The German press, mainly containing the work of investigative journalists like Thomas Kistner of the *Süddeutsche Zeitung* (SZ), reported often and intensively about this crisis of anti-doping, for example in http://www.sueddeutsche.de/sport/verbaende-in-der-doping-krise-zehn-punkte-gegen-den-betrug-1.862587, accessed 20 June 2014.

107. http://www.faz.net/aktuell/sport/sportpolitik/doping/im-gespraech-doping-experte-pound-am-kampf-gegen-doping-ist-niemand-interessiert-12584625.html, accessed 20 June 2014.

108. "Abschlussbericht der Expertenkommission zur Aufklärung von Dopingvorwürfen gegenüber Ärzten der Abteilung Sportmedizin des Universitätsklinikums Freiburg," Cologne, 23 March 2009 und nach redaktioneller Überarbeitung bis zum 12 May 2009, http://www.danieldrepper.de/wp-content/uploads/2010/11/Abschlussbericht-Freiburg.pdf, accessed 20 June 2014.

109. Bundesministerium des Inneren (BMI), *Sportförderung des Bundes* (1970ff.), Abschlussbericht Projektgruppe Sonderprüfung Doping (19 December 2007), http://www.bmi.bund.de/SharedDocs/Downloads/DE/Broschueren/nichtinListe/2007/Abschlussbericht_Doping.pdf?
__blob=publicationFile, accessed 20 June 2014.

110. Ibid., esp. 7–8.

111. Ibid., 9.

112. Parlamentsarchiv (PA), printings 14/1867 und 1470, Doping im Spitzensport und Fitnessbereich, http://dipbt.bundestag.de/doc/btd/14/010/1401032.pdf and http://dipbt.bundestag.de/doc/btd/14/044/1404470.pdf, p. 8–9. Accessed 20 June 2014.

113. Bundesministerium des Inneren (BMI), *Sportberichte der Bundesregierung* (Bonn, Berlin, 1973–2010), tenth report (2002), 62.

114. Bundesministerium des Inneren (BMI), *Sportförderung des Bundes* (1970ff.), department SH I 1 – 371600/2, 2001.

115. Deutscher Olympischer Sportbund (DOSB), Abschlussbericht der Rechtskommission gegen Doping im Sport (ReSpoDo) zu möglichen gesetzlichen Initiativen für eine konsequente Verhinderung, Verfolgung und Ahndung des Dopings im Sport, https://www.dosb.de/fileadmin/fm-dosb/downloads/dosb/endfassung_abschlussbericht.pdf, accessed 21 June 2014. C. Weber, "Die Stiftung Nationale Anti-Doping Agentur," 71–85, esp. 77.

116. Deutscher Olympischer Sportbund (DOSB), Abschlussbericht der Rechtskommission gegen Doping im Sport (ReSpoDo) zu möglichen gesetzlichen Initiativen für eine konsequente Verhinderung, Verfolgung und Ahndung des Dopings im Sport, https://www.dosb.de/fileadmin/fm-dosb/downloads/dosb/endfassung_abschlussbericht.pdf, accessed 21 June 2014.

117. Parlamentsarchiv (PA), printings 16/17, 2006, Öffentliche Anhörung von Sachverständigen zum Thema Doping, https://www.dosb.de/de/service/sport-mehr/news/detail/

news/protokoll_der_17_sitzung_des_sportausschusses_zum_thema_doping/, accessed 21 June 2014.

118. Bundesministerium des Inneren (BMI), *Sportförderung des Bundes* (1970ff.), Abschlussbericht Projektgruppe Sonderprüfung Doping (19 December 2007), http://www.bmi.bund.de/SharedDocs/Downloads/DE/Broschueren/nichtinListe/2007/Abschlussbericht_Doping.pdf?__blob=publicationFile, accessed 20 June 2014.

119. Parlamentsarchiv (PA), Plenarprotokoll 16/67, Deutscher Bundestag, Stenographischer Bericht 67. Sitzung, Berlin, 23 November 2006, http://dip21.bundestag.de/dip21/btp/16/16067.pdf, p. 6670A. Accessed 21 June 2014.

120. Peter Danckert, *Kraftmaschine Parlament: Der Sportausschuss und die Sportpolitik des Bundes,* Hauptsache Sport (Aachen: Meyer & Meyer, 2009), 28; Deutscher Olympischer Sportbund (DOSB), *Anti-Doping Aktionsplan: Zehn Punkte für Sport und Staat.*

121. D. V. Hanstad, "Anti-Doping Policies in Sport: Elite Level Athletes & Whereabouts Information," *Sport & EU Newsletter* 2 (March 2007): 3–4; Hanstad, Smith, and Waddington, "Establishment of the World Anti-Doping Agency," 247.

122. Martin Nolte, "Dopingbekämpfung in Deutschland: Prototyp einer Verantwortungsteilung von Staat und Gesellschaft," in *Die Freiheit des Menschen in Kommune, Staat und Europa: Festschrift für Edzard Schmidt-Jortzig,* ed. Utz Schliesky (Heidelberg and Hamburg: Müller, 2011), 771–82.

123. Bundesministerium des Inneren (BMI), *Sportförderung des Bundes* (1970ff.), BMI-Nachrichten, 5 December 2009, Rede von Bundesinnenminister Thomas de Maiziere auf der 5. Mitgliederversammlung des Deutschen Olympischen Sportbundes (DOSB) am 5. Dezember 2009 in Düsseldorf (Speech of the Federal Minister of the Interior at the General Convention of the DOSB on 5 December 2009 in Düsseldorf), http://www.dosb.de/fileadmin/Bilder_allgemein/Veranstaltungen/Mitgliederversammlung_Duesseldorf_2009/Protokoll_5__Mitgliederversammlung_Duesseldorf_05_12_2009.pdf, accessed 21 June 2014.

124. "Deutschlands Zukunft gestalten," coalition agreement between CDU, CSU, and SPD.18. Legislaturperiode (2013), http://www.bundesregierung.de/Content/DE/_Anlagen/2013/2013-12-17-koalitionsvertrag.pdf;jsessionid=6EEB0CAED545A800026EA735341A4DC7.s3t2?__blob=publicationFile&v=2, p. 138. Accessed 21 June 2014.

Conclusion

THE GERMAN STORY OF DOPING: A RELEVANT ELEMENT OF THE OVERALL SPORTS PROCESS

Doping and anti-doping in Germany are part of the global doping story. Additionally, doping is an integral part of the sports process. Enhancing performance by more than natural means is an invention of neither modern sports nor German physical culture and sports. The history of sports is inextricably connected to drug use. Since antiquity, athletes have used every opportunity to enhance their performance, cope with the enormous physical stress of their agons, and, finally, to recuperate from injuries of all kinds. It seems to be an anthropological characteristic to take drugs to feel better, achieve more, have fun, promote good health, and ease frustration and aggression, for sports or whatever. Getting high and feeling better are closely connected. The boundary between feeling invincible and feeling dejected is fluid.

Depending on the sophistication and quality of technical and scientific methods for producing drugs, people have always used them for various reasons and mostly for enhancing performance. Such behavior is not necessarily regarded as immoral or forbidden. Actually, taking drugs can best be described as partly forbidden. The same drug can be useful, dangerously addictive, and performance enhancing. In some parts of modern society—in the working world, cultural life, and leisure—drugs are more or less accepted. Modern pharmaceutical industries produce huge amounts of various drugs for the treatment of diseases, which can also be used in principle by healthy individuals. Some artists, musicians, and authors are unable to perform without certain drugs or stimulants (or at least they believe so), ranging from caffeine to cocaine and heroin. Alcohol is an accepted mass drug in most countries of the civilized world, even though the addictive and often serious consequences of alcohol abuse are well known and scientifically validated. An increasing part of the population, including older people, is addicted to a variety of medications and pills.

Apart from the transport sector, sports constitute the only sphere of civilized society governed by comparatively strict bans on the use of drugs. The situation in sports is rather complicated, because athletes, especially in top-level sports, can perform optimally only through performance-enhancing means like intensive and elaborate training activities and equally intensive health care. The latter without drugs in any shape or form seems to be impossible, at least in top-level sports. Nonetheless, taking special substances to enhance performance in sports is defined as forbidden doping by all sports authorities and, in some countries, also by state laws.

The process of defining doping as illegal and contrary to the spirit of sports according to the rules of sports federations or other authorities took place in the twentieth century, beginning with the rules of the marathon race at the London Olympics in 1908 and developing up to the current World Anti-Doping Code (WADC). Predecessors of this anti-doping process were the horse races in Britain since the seventeenth century, when horses were doped either to enhance their performance or to weaken the performance of other horses, in order to manipulate the bets. The doping and anti-doping process is as long as the contemporary development of sports, but no longer than about a hundred years. Physical activities related to former or different physical cultures than contemporary sports had no idea of doping or of doping bans, in the sense that performance-enhancing drugs should be forbidden.

The kind of negative doping used in animal sports, as in horse racing since the seventeenth century, was widely unknown in contemporary human sports. The only curious case of negative doping in German sports was discussed in 1952, when the sports doctor and athletics coach Martin Brustmann doped his rowing team with testoviron in order to enhance its performance, although in fact it did the converse. However, what Brustmann did was not deliberate negative doping like that of horses in England. He never wanted to weaken anybody, but rather failed to dope positively.

The German single sculler Peter Michael Kolbe faced the same experience twenty-five years later at the Olympic Games in Montreal. He did not dope, but he did receive (with his agreement) special injections designed to enhance his performance. The substances in the injection were not included in the IOC's doping list. They tested scientifically as ones that were not forbidden by definition, but they were intended to help Kolbe win a gold medal. In fact, he and his doctors—and, in the background, the German medical scientists—all failed. Kolbe's strength declined unexpectedly and rapidly in the last meters of the race.

Both cases were early attempts to take performance-enhancing substances, the first inspired by a doctor who was willing to take risks and apply means with only a low level of scientific and practical knowledge about the effects and side effects. The other was a failed attempt of West German sports officials and sports doctors to apply means that seemed familiar (enough) from East German athletes. However, the West German sports doctors and athletes like Kolbe actually had no idea how to deal with these drug cocktails. Kolbe's tactics in the race were completely wrong or at least incompetent and in fact not coordinated with the drugs he had taken, which were indeed not "doping," according to the doping list at that time.

EXPLANATIONS FOR THE DOPING AND ANTI-DOPING PROCESS

These stories explain several aspects of the doping and anti-doping processes in Germany and worldwide.

First, the anti-doping rule at the marathon race in London in 1908 was apparently motivated by concerns about the health of the athletes in the face of such a demanding event like a marathon and the ethos of amateur sport. Contemporaries were aware of the old story of the soldier running from Marathon to Athens in 490 BCE who died after the run and—most relevant—after conveying the news of the victory. It was hoped that the London race of 1908 would not end with such a disaster, which—and this was another reason for the official ban of doping at the marathon race of London in 1908—was not unknown in professional sports or animal sports like horse races. International amateur sports festivals, which the Olympics indeed were, made a clear distinction between professional and amateur sports. The early anti-doping rules of the IOC can therefore be connected to the Olympic spirit of amateur sports. A true modern athlete is an amateur who loves the game for its own sake and not for money or any other personal gain. An ideal amateur athlete is neither motivated nor pressured to take drugs to enhance performance or to win by any form of dishonesty. By contrast, in professional sports, both drug taking and cheating were rampant. Gentlemen were familiar with the world of professional sports, including animal sports like horse races, and their side effects, which were regarded as morally unacceptable. The bifurcation of professional and amateur sports was part of the social segregation of the upper classes from the lower-middle and working classes, and their respective sports. Part of the ideology of creating a socially distinct concept of Olympic sport was that of amateurism, including the moral stand that an amateur athlete does not use drugs.

Second, stimulants were originally the most relevant and well-known drugs in Germany as well as internationally. Therefore, the Brustmann case was surprising in some respects for all involved actors. The drug from Dr. Brustmann did not enhance achievement in the race, but the exact opposite. Brustmann had tested a hormonal substance that had theoretically been familiar to scientists since the 1930s, but its true effects and side effects were in fact unknown and controversial. Brustmann used and applied testoviron like a stimulant drug, which was actually counterproductive. However, he was nonetheless a pioneer of modern anabolic-steroid doping, which became popular among athletes in the 1960s and beyond. Although Brustmann failed miserably in 1952, his successors later applied similar drugs successfully in training, but not immediately before competitions.

Third, defining, testing, and sanctioning doping changed significantly between the days of Brustmann and those of Kolbe. At the beginning of the twentieth century, and after World War II, the amateur sports community, with the IOC at the apex, and the international sports federations were convinced that taking drugs in amateur sports was not a real problem or contrary to the spirit of amateur sport. Therefore, the first rules against doping in the Olympic charter and in the regulations of the sports federations indeed mentioned doping and banned it from amateur sports, which were also Olympic sports. However, one could say that doping was "banned" morally, but not punished in any way.

In Germany, the first definition of doping, initiated by the West German Sports Doctors Association in 1952 and adopted by the German Sports Federation, the umbrella organization of German sports, included mostly moral and ideal categories of people. The intention to dope, and thus to dupe one's opponents and to jeopardize one's own health, was defined as doping and forbidden. This definition accorded with the spirit of amateur sport: an Olympic athlete plays the games, including the Olympic Games, for his own sake and is therefore not at all pressured to cheat or to take any substances that could affect his health. Such amateurs do not rely existentially on sporting success, as professionals do. Neither do they rely on artificial drugs or any other forbidden means of enhancing performance. Performance is only dependent on willpower, character, talent, effort, individual resources, and, finally, *natural* training. However, training was indeed not originally inherent to the habitus of a true gentleman or sportsman. What a sportsman can do was regarded as his individual achievement and not the result of any additional means or support. Logically, doping could only be an exception with respect to those athletes who were not aware of the true spirit of Olympic amateur sport.

This argument was supported by the political environment after World War II and the defeat of the Nazi regime. Both parts of Germany wanted to become members of the Olympic family as soon as possible. Therefore, they attempted to revive the Olympic amateur spirit, at least on the surface. Germany, which had been a major player in Olympic history before, should get back to the Olympics. Both East and West Germany consequently accepted and praised the ideology of Olympic amateur sport. However, East and West were motivated differently, the one by the concept of free Western sport, and the other by that of socialist state sport. In addition, the West Germans of the Federal Republic of Germany (FRG), supported by the Western Allied Forces, rejected any influence of the state in sports and sports organizations, mainly the sports clubs, associations, and federations. They should be completely independent of the state. The autonomy of sport was a major dogma of the "free" sport of West Germany, similar to the relationship between sports and politics in Great Britain or the United States of America. Sports should be part of civil society, but not a responsibility of the state.

By contrast, East German athletes of the German Democratic Republic (GDR) had a political mission to be better than the West. They were under pressure to contribute to the political legitimation of the communist regime. Athletes of the GDR were in fact *Staatsamateure*—amateur in name, but really working and competing for the socialist state. They were paid by the state and completely dependent on their coaches, officials, and sports politicians. They could not even make their own decisions, whereas West German athletes as well as other athletes of the free West could do just that. In fact, they were thoroughly dependent on the sports process. This process was also characterized as one of "totalization" of top-level sports, which means the increasing incapacitation of athletes because of various external constraints, coaches, expert knowledge, medical care, and financial support. Athletes in fact degenerated to small cogs in the machinery of top-level sports. In addition, West German athletes were also dependent on the authorities of the federations. If they were not willing to comply with their rules, they could be banned from the team.

In contrast to that very real development, West German sports officials invented the notion (or type) of the "mature athlete" as an idol of West German Olympic amateur sport, in order to withstand these constraints and develop a counterpart to the dependent "diplomats in track suits" of the East.

RELEVANCE OF THE COLD WAR

The Cold War between East and West Germany was in general highly relevant to sports and doping development in both German states. A common and traditional definition of doping based on moral arguments could no longer be maintained during the Cold War and in the face of the totalization of top-level sports. This became evident to sports officials both in Germany and internationally. In consequence, in the 1960s, the definition of doping became more realistic. Doping and anti-doping experienced a real-world change, in that a list of forbidden drugs and substances was declared as doping and therefore punished, mostly by the perpetrators being banned from competitions. In consequence, athletes had to be controlled, and their urine and blood tested by experts on the basis of valid scientific methods. Anti-doping had to be administrated, and it became professionalized, scientific, and bureaucratized—parallel to the process of "sportization" in general.

Scientists and sports doctors played a major and very specific role in both the doping and anti-doping process, and again both internationally and in Germany. They have always been interested in acquiring more, and more precise, expertise about the limits of physical achievement. However, sports are by no means the only field of endeavor to experience such limits. Traditionally, scientists had researched these problems of physical stress in the context of work or soldiers in the military. Since the beginning of the twentieth century, and in Germany, at least since the opening of the Kaiser Wilhelm Institut für Arbeitsphysiologie (Kaiser Wilhelm Institute for Work Physiology) in Berlin in 1913 (and subsequently in Dortmund), such tests of human physical achievement were conducted systematically. Far from coincidentally, the German Sports Doctors Association (Deutscher Sportärztebund, DSÄB) had been founded in 1912, after a scientific congress and exhibition on hygiene in Dresden in 1911.

Doctors can be divided into those who are in fact scientists working on scientifically established knowledge about human health and disease on the one hand, and on the other hand, doctors who look after real patients. Sometimes an individual doctor combines both science and direct health care. Most of the sports doctors at the beginning of modern sports science did both. However, a dilemma soon became apparent to sports doctors involved with top-level sports with respect to constantly increasing the physical achievements of athletes. Should they support the athletes in their desire for ever-greater achievements, or should they care for athletes only in cases of injury or disease? In their role as scientists, they were more interested in the physical limits of athletes, but as doctors, they were obliged, according to their professional oath, to care for the health and well-being of their patients. This oath implied quite clearly that medication (or any drugs) was allowed only for the treatment of disease, and *not* for performance enhancement.

This dilemma was one of the main reasons why the German Sports Doctors Association was the first in Germany after World War II to initiate a fundamental debate about doping in sports and finally to propose a definition of doping in order to ban it from both sports and the realm of medical responsibility. Neither athletes nor sports doctors should be compromised by doping issues in the future. This doping definition was successful with regard to the moral ban on doping but not at all in terms of true controls, tests, and a practical ban on doping, including sanctioning those who had really doped. Such a system of testing and controlling has developed from the 1960s to today, culminating in the WADA as a worldwide administration of sports and political members against doping.

In communist East Germany, numerous sports scientists and sports doctors worked toward the progress of top-level sports. Scientific support for and monitoring of top-level sports was one explanation of the *Sportwunder DDR*, the miraculous success of the small GDR, which became one of the leading sporting nations of the world, close to the United States and the USSR, at least measured by the number of medals at the Olympic Games. Technological research and progress was part of their concept of a new, modern, socialist world, imitated by the USSR in order to overcome the capitalist West. Sports doctors of the GDR invented and implemented the doping program of the state, including a systematic scientific research program for doping substances and their production in the state pharmaceutical factory Jenapharm, exclusively for use in top sports. In fact, this entailed the controlled administration of testing to the athletes, from young and talented newcomers to successful winners of world records and Olympic medals.

The Doping-Control Laboratory in Kreischa, accredited and recommended by the IOC, supervised the doping system of the GDR in order to keep secret the sports-related cheating by the GDR state. The high level and public acknowledgment of GDR sports science and sports doctors was demonstrated by the fact that a special degree, *Facharzt Sportmedizin*, was introduced in 1956 in the GDR. In addition, a systematic service for sports medicine, the Sportmedizinische Dienst (SMD), was established in 1963, and was very much part of the GDR sports miracle. In fact, the main job of the SMD was that of implementing and controlling doping. Instead of the multiple constraints by the SED state, doctors who supported doping acted against both the law of the GDR and the universal ethos of doctors according to the Hippocratic oath.

While the involvement of the medical service and the sports doctors in the GDR in the state doping program violated fundamental ethical standards both of sport and of doctors, the situation of sports doctors in West Germany was quite differentiated and varied. On the one hand, scientists and doctors worked together with their international colleagues on the progress of sports science and sports medicine. Numerous West German sports doctors even looked respectfully and enviously across the Iron Curtain at the ideal conditions of work and sports science in the GDR. Furthermore, East and West German sports doctors—as well as coaches and sports officials—knew each other very well from meetings, conferences, and competitions. Some of the older ones even had common ties from the Nazi period. The story is told that at the height of the Cold War between East and West, when the highest-ranking leader in GDR sports, Manfred Ewald, and the president of the West German Deutscher Sportbund, Willi Weyer, met for consultations about the internal German sports relationship, Weyer remembered their common past as young officers in the Hitler Youth, the mass organization of the Nazi party. This was in fact very damning for Ewald, who was regarded as a hard-core communist in the GDR. Of course, other similar cases of scientists and sports doctors in the East and West were known. Interestingly, the common past was one of the reasons why the German reunification succeeded comparatively well after forty years of separation.

However, sports doctors and scientists in the West were neither pressured nor controlled by the state. They were merely obliged to follow their consciences, their professional oath as doctors, and the spirit of Olympic sport. We could not find any document indicating that an athlete, sports official, or sports doctor was under pressure by politicians or the state administration to dope, break the rules of sports, or violate the Hippocratic oath. Another question worth asking is whether athletes and coaches, politicians, and sports officials were really interested in keeping to these rules and controlling compliance. Yet all participants were acutely aware of the dilemma of international top-level sports, between fair play on the one hand and striving for excellence and success on the other. The system of fair sports indeed fails when a majority, or at least a critical mass of participants, does not keep to the rules. For athletes to set records and win competitions through achievements that are simply not possible without "additional support" in the form of doping, and for the sports community to accept this as normal and fair play, is no longer acceptable. This dilemma in fact emerged in the 1970s. A leading German sports doctor argued in the 1960s that a shot-putter may be able to reach a distance of fifteen or sixteen meters through his own natural means, the best techniques, and intensive training, but not twenty-one or twenty-two meters. However, top athletes have been achieving much *more* than twenty meters for many years. It thus seems unrealistic to believe that such performances were achieved without doping. In some disciplines of heavy athletics, world records have not been broken for many years, especially since the peak years of anabolic doping in the 1970s. This implies at least a high probability of anabolic doping in the 1960s and 1970s.

At the peak of the Cold War on the track in the late 1960s and 1970s, anabolic steroids were being widely used by Olympic athletes. East German sports doctors did not refer to the application of these "blue pills" as doping, but as "sustaining means." Some West German sports doctors regarded the East German system of sports medical support in any case as optimal. Analogously to the "sustaining means" concept, they invented that of "substitution." Anabolic steroids were legitimized for administration to top-level athletes on the basis of their extraordinary need for hormones—as well as minerals, dietary supplements, and so on—during and after training and competitions. The base levels of these substances should be substituted, that is "replaced," due to wear and tear! This substitution was also declared a matter of preventive health care for athletes. These doctors really believed or at any rate argued that they were merely acting for the health and well-being of the athletes, whom they in fact regarded as special patients. However, the theory of "sustaining means" and "substitution" had never been scientifically proved.

An ongoing issue of doping and its control revolves around the empirical validation of doping in sport. This problem is similar to that concerning statistics on criminality, economic fraud, or deviant behavior in general. Until now, despite some impressive achievements and large sums of money being invested in the doping-control system, the number of positively tested athletes remains very low indeed, about 2 or 3 percent for many years. This could be interpreted as a success of the elaborate control system, but there may be other reasons. One is undoubtedly the definition of doping by means of a list of forbidden drugs and substances. This kind of enumerative definition of doping is less a moral warning than a motivation to find alternative ways of enhancing performance and new, unlisted substances. Similar to taxpayers who look together with their tax accountants for the best ways to avoid taxes or fiscal offenses, top-level athletes find ways with their coaches, doctors, and advisers to be successful without violating the doping rules. However, they still violate the spirit of sport and fair play.

The German cases of the Kolbe injection and the air clyster affair in the 1970s were just such officially permitted alternatives, which were discussed in public and both of which ultimately failed. The most common attempts at performance enhancing in top-level sports without breaking the rules were, however, mostly scientifically based searches for new substances not yet listed. This race on both sides of biochemical or pharmaceutical science and sports doctors, between those who had to control for listed substances and the others who tried to find out and test new effective means not yet listed, is generally true for the history of doping. When amphetamines were banned according to the first doping lists in the 1960s, anabolic steroids were applied. These drugs had not been developed for sport at all, but were subsequently tested and used by athletes and sport doctors. For a long time, until the late 1970s, the effects and side effects of these drugs were highly controversial. In addition, the testing of these substances was difficult and not really valid, and, finally, when such tests could be conducted, the timing of doping could be varied so that it was effective in competitions but would not test positively at competition controls.

The GDR sports medical system and service were the worldwide champions in developing such perfidious techniques. Aside from one female athlete, no other GDR athlete ever tested positive for anabolic steroids, although everybody knew with complete certainty that these athletes were being systematically and intensively doped with anabolic steroids.

In West Germany and the Western world, where anabolic doping was also practiced, but less professionally, this dilemma—or perhaps more correctly, serious or even deadly problem—became apparent to everybody as a result of the scandal over the death of the West German heptathlete Birgit Dressel. She was in fact doped, but in the unsystematic and chaotic way that West German top-level sports generally worked, compared to the highly organized system of the GDR. Dozens of doctors treated her for a long time with hundreds of drugs, but there was no interaction or coordination between them. Therefore, Birgit Dressel died not primarily because of forbidden anabolic doping, but in a sense because of her own behavior, which may be compared to that of a drug addict or a junkie, albeit in the world of sports. Therefore, she was not a true victim, although her death could also be associated with the unsatisfactory system of West German top sport, with its total lack of viable controls on drugs for athletes.

In consequence, after the death of Dressel, doping controls and consistent anti-doping policies were not only stressed, but became a crucial demand, in order to improve the sports system—shortly before the end of the GDR—according to the concept of GDR sports. The sports officials of the FRG asked for more money for sports doctors, medical support, coaches, and the federations, but they were not interested in sanctioning doping by reducing financial support for doping-enhancing federations, coaches, and athletes.

Far too late, out-of-competition controls for anabolic doping were introduced in the 1980s. However, the same hopeless race between dopers and controllers started with the next generations of doping substances and methods: EPO, hormonal doping, and genetic doping, including all manner of varieties to avoid contravening the doping list. The race can be compared metaphorically to the German fairy tale of the hedgehogs and the rabbit, who bet on who is faster. The rabbit is convinced that he can run faster than a hedgehog. He runs across the field, but when he reaches the finish line, a hedgehog appears and calls, "I am here," and when the rabbit repeats the race back in the other direction, the other hedgehog calls out again. In the end, the honest rabbit runs until he dies of exhaustion, outwitted by the clever but dishonest hedgehogs. This story can be applied extremely well to modern sports.

This fatalistic and pessimistic fairy tale is symptomatic of the history of doping in at least two respects. First, sports along these lines are not fair at all and cheating seems to be inherent to this system of top-level sports. Second, races between differently talented, trained, and doped athletes cannot be fair by definition. Clever athletes and teams finish first, not honest ones. Of course, the rabbit is not without blame either. He agrees to an unfair race and is too stupid to see through the dirty tactics of the hedgehogs. Finally, he pays a high price for his naïveté. In addition, there is no independent umpire who could ensure a fair competition.

CHANGES TO THE RELATIONSHIP BETWEEN STATE AND SPORT

Step by step, the West German concept of free, autonomous sport changed to a system of state-sponsored sport similar to that in the GDR—minus the political and ideological context. The traditional concept of the autonomy of sport had in some way been comfortable for both state and sport. The sports organizations could do what and how they wanted. They were commended and praised by state politicians for their mostly voluntary work for state, nation, and society. For many years, top-level sports were supported by state money, lobbied by a grand coalition of sporting friends in the German parliaments. Politicians and federal administrations were not really concerned about how exactly the money for sports was spent. The German public agreed with the increasing support of top-level sports by tax-financed means. However, this agreement changed analogously to the process of doping and anti-doping in German and international sports. The state then had to take more responsibility for sports policies and to protect the ethos of fair sport.

West German politicians and sports officials hesitated for a long time to acknowledge the new realities of national, inter-German, and international interdependence and development of sport. For a long time, they attempted to maintain the balancing act between the autonomy of sport and the need for state sponsorship. They did not realize sufficiently and early enough that state authorities must also take responsibility for the problems or negative effects of developments in national and international sport.

In fact, European and international initiatives against doping since the early 1960s had pushed the Germans to be more active in their anti-doping policies. Neither German sports officials nor politicians wished to remain isolated from the mainstream of Western sports policies, including anti-doping strategies. Therefore, on the one hand, West German athletes should take part successfully at international sporting events and competitions. On the other hand, the German sports federations followed, mostly very closely, the anti-doping initiatives of the international sports organizations, led by the IOC, and German sports politicians also followed the initiatives of the European Council and UNESCO. German sport would not risk international isolation, according to the guidelines of German foreign policy.

Finally, German politicians were even mainly responsible for political initiatives supporting the foundation of the WADA in 1999. The WADA and, in consequence, the NADA foundations, signaled a paradigmatic benchmark in the relationship between state and sport at both national and international levels. The dogma of nonpolitical sport could definitely be overcome at last. The IOC at the international level and German sport at the national level admitted that politicians and states had a decisive role to play in sports policies in general and in anti-doping policies in particular. In addition, states, governments, and politicians accepted that sports are far more than a fun leisure-time activity, but also a significant component of power in international and national politics.

However, the vision of a civilized and autonomous sports sphere was still alive. German sports organizations and their representatives were seriously motivated to define the ethical fundaments of modern top-level sports in Germany. However, it took a long time for them to accept the realities of doping and act accordingly. During numerous hearings, conferences, and meetings, they discussed doping and anti-doping in the context of modern sporting developments. Until now, they remain convinced that the free and autonomous German sports movement can overcome the serious problems of doping and anti-doping by means of internal activities and measures like declarations, discussions, recommendations, guidelines, rules of compliance, and so on.

A remarkable part of these achievements in anti-doping policies was the updating of the Declaration of Principles for Top Sport of 1977. This paper was originally a commitment to top-level sports, but not in all respects. Despite the various sporting and political stresses and pressures, sports should be a human endeavor in the interest of the athletes, including their health and well-being. Therefore, doping of all kinds must be banned and prevented. Second, athletes were neither regarded as objects of top-level sports nor as victims of doping, but as responsible and mature athletes and adults. These young men and women earn appreciation and support for their high performance and for their nations. However, they are expected to do so without doping.

In principle, nobody can disapprove of this concept and image of an athlete of free sport in a free civil society. These principles of top-level sports in the Federal Republic of Germany can also be considered as a clear and desirable alternative to the concept of top-level sports in the GDR, including its system of state doping. The Western alternative did not imply, however, the ability to reduce doping in the Federal Republic consistently and effectively. By contrast, state and sports officials, as well as coaches and athletes, often differed considerably in terms of actions and words. Win at all costs was too often the real motto of all participants in the doping and anti-doping game. Neither athletes nor sports organizations, state authorities, and politicians really wanted to sacrifice sporting success in favor of doping-free and fair sport.

The end of the Cold War on the track in the context of the breakdown of the Soviet Union and the GDR paved the way for new initiatives against doping in sports. That is probably true at least for long-term developments. However, immediately after German reunification, a large number of German sports representatives, coaches, and doctors hoped, as did the German public and media, that the unification of two powerful sports states would constitute a unique chance for sports in Germany to become number one in the world. However, the heritage of the GDR included not only the positive parts of the system, but also the negative system of doping. This heritage did indeed challenge the largely successful German reunification. The doping case of Kathrin Krabbe immediately after the constitution of a unified Germany made clear to everybody that one plus one did not always make two, neither in politics nor in sports. The pessimistic bill of the reunification of German sports was in fact the combination of two different doping systems, which were both successful in their own way and also lacked integrity in their own way.

This conclusion should not, however, end on too pessimistic a note. Over time, the public debate on doping and the implementation of various means and instruments of reducing doping have become relevant parts of the sports process, both in Germany and worldwide. As mentioned above, the foundation of the WADA and the numerous NADAs, including in Germany, have raised hopes that the right course has now been set for a future in sports with less doping. Such hopes would, though, be unrealistic if implying that the doping problem could be resolved completely.

Pierre de Coubertin once asked for an alternative to the Olympic movement between "*Markt oder Tempel*"—the market or the temple, which means professional sports ruled by money (and drugs) or rather sports (without money and drugs) as a means for achieving peace and benefiting mankind. The sportsmen and sportswomen of the world arguably needed to choose between these two extremes. However, this was and is not really the case. The difference between amateur and professional sports does not exist anymore. Today, the alternative is simply that between more or less doping-free sports, which are able to harness the human functions of performance sports for education and society, or doped sports, which undermine the process of humanistic sportization. Less doping undoubtedly contributes to more civilized sports but also implies more doping controls, more testing, and a negative vision of athletes with little privacy. The complete control of sports and athletes is clearly also a dark side of the sports process.

Bibliography

ARCHIVES

Archiv Willi Daume in der Deutschen Olympischen Akademie, Frankfurt am Main
Bundesarchiv Berlin und Koblenz
Bundesinstitut für Sportwissenschaft, Bonn
Bundesnachrichtendienst, Pullach
Bundesverband Deutscher Gewichtheber, Leimen
Carl und Liselott Diem-Archiv, Cologne
Der Bundesbeauftragte für die Unterlagen des Staatssicherheitsdienstes der ehemaligen Deutschen Demokratischen Republik (BStU), Berlin
Deutsche Sporthochschule, Cologne
Deutscher Leichtathletik-Verband, Darmstadt
Deutscher Olympischer Sportbund (DOSB), Frankfurt am Main
Deutscher Ruder-Verband, Hannover
Deutscher Schwimm-Verband, Kassel
International Olympic Committee Library and Archives, Lausanne
Internationales Dopingarchiv, Weinheim (now Berlin)
Nationale Anti-Doping Agentur (NADA), Bonn
Parlamentsarchiv, Berlin
Universitätsarchiv Freiburg

200 Jahre Turnbewegung—200 Jahre soziale Verantwortung. Frankfurt am Main: DTB, 2011.

"Abschlussbericht der Expertenkommission zur Aufklärung von Dopingvorwürfen gegenüber Ärzten der Abteilung Sportmedizin des Universitätsklinikums Freiburg." Unpublished manuscript.

Acker, Helmut, ed. *Rekorde aus der Retorte: Leistungssteigerung im modernen Hochleistungssport*. Stuttgart: Deutsche Verlags-Anstalt, 1972.

Alfes, H., J. C. D. Reisch, and H. Möllmann. "Der Nachweis von zentralstimulierenden Arzneimitteln (Dopingmitteln) durch die Gaschromatographie." *Sportarzt und Sportmedizin*, no. 11 (1968): 492–96.

Ariens, E. J. "Organisation et résultats du contrôle antidoping." In *Doping: Proceedings of an International Seminar Organized at the Universities of Ghent and Brussels, May 1964, by the Research Committee of the International Council of Sport and Physical Education (U.N.E.S.C.O.)*, edited by A. F. de Schaepdryver, 27–50. Oxford: Pergamon Press, 1965.

Asbell, Bernard. *Die Pille und wie sie die Welt veränderte*. Frankfurt am Main: Fischer-Taschenbuch-Verlag, 1998.

Asmuth, Christoph. "Dopingdefinitionen—Von der Moral zum Recht." In *Was ist Doping? Fakten und Probleme der aktuellen Diskussion*, edited by Christoph Asmuth, 13–32. Brennpunkt Doping 1. Bielefeld: transcript, 2010.

Balbier, Uta A. *Kalter Krieg auf der Aschenbahn: Der deutsch-deutsche Sport, 1950–1972; Eine politische Geschichte*. Paderborn: F. Schöningh, 2007.

Baring, Arnulf, and Manfred Görtemaker. *Machtwechsel: Die Ära Brandt-Scheel*. Stuttgart: Deutsche Verlags-Anstalt, 1982.

Baumann, Dieter. *Ich laufe keinem hinterher*. Cologne: Kiepenhauer & Witsch, 1995.

———. *Lebenslauf: Mit aktuellem Beitrag zum Comeback*. 2nd expanded ed. Munich: Droemer Knaur, 2003.

Beamish, Rob, and Ian Ritchie. *Fastest, Highest, Strongest: A Critique of High-Performance Sport*. New York: Routledge, 2006.

———. "From Chivalrous 'Brothers in Arms' to the Eligible Athlete: Changed Principles and the IOC's Banned Substance List." *International Review for the Sociology of Sport* 39, no. 4 (2004): 355–71.

Becker, Frank. *Den Sport gestalten: Carl Diems Leben (1882–1962)*. Duisburg: Universitätsverlag Rhein-Ruhr, 2009–2010.

Becker, Hartmut, et al., eds. *Die Gründerjahre des Deutschen Sportbundes: Wege aus der Not zur Einheit*. Schorndorf: Karl Hofmann, 1990.

Becker, Howard S. *Outsiders: Studies in the Sociology of Deviance*. New York: Free Press, 1997. Original published 1963.

Beckett, A. H, G. T. Tucker, and A. C. Moffat. "Routine Detection and Identification in Urine of Stimulants and Other Drugs, Some of Which May Be Used to Modify Performance in Sport." *Journal of Pharmacy and Pharmacology* 19 (1967): 273–94.

Berendonk, Brigitte. *Doping Dokumente: Von der Forschung zum Betrug*. 2nd expanded ed. Reinbek: Rowohlt, 1992.

Bernett, Hajo. *Guido von Mengden: "Generalstabschef" des deutschen Sports*. Turn- und Sportführer im Dritten Reich 5. Berlin: Bartels & Wernitz, 1976.

Berryman, Jack W., and Roberta J. Park, eds. *Sport and Exercise Science: Essays in the History of Sports Medicine*. Urbana: University of Illinois Press, 1992.

Bette, Karl-Heinrich, and Uwe Schimank. *Doping im Hochleistungssport: Anpassung durch Abweichung*. Frankfurt am Main: Suhrkamp, 2006.

Bliesener, J. "Zur Frage des Doping: Mit Hilfe von Umfragen und zum Teil eigenen Beobachtungen im Radsport." Thesis, Sporthochschule Cologne, 1959.

Blume, Klaus. *Die Dopingrepublik: Eine (deutsch-)deutsche Sportgeschichte*. Berlin: Rotbuch, 2012.

Boyes, S. "The International Olympic Committee, Transnational Doping Policy and Globalisation." In *Drugs and Doping in Sports*, edited by John O'Leary, 167–79. London: Routledge-Cavendish, 2001.

Braun, Jutta. "'Dopen für Deutschland': Die Diskussion im vereinten Sport, 1990–1992." In *Hormone und Hochleistung: Doping in Ost und West*, edited by Klaus Latzel and Lutz Niethammer, 151–70. Cologne: Böhlau, 2008.

———. "'Republikflucht' und 'Fluchthelfer': Ein verdrängtes Kapitel deutsch-deutscher Sportbeziehungen." In *Vergessen, verdrängt, abgelehnt—Zur Geschichte der Ausgrenzung im Sport: Tagungsbericht der 10. Hoyaer Tagung zur Sportgeschichte vom 10. bis 12. Oktober 2008*, edited by Arnd Krüger, 106–16. Berlin: Lit-Verlag, 2009.

Braun, Jutta, René Wiese, and Claudia de la Garza. *ZOV Sportverräter: Spitzenathleten auf der Flucht; Begleitbuch zur Ausstellung; Eine Ausstellung des Zentrums Deutsche Sportgeschichte Berlin-Brandenburg e.V. (ZdS) in Zusammenarbeit mit der Künstlerin Laura Soria und der Ausstellungsagentur Exhibeo*. With the assistance of Gloria Fochs. Berlin: Zentrum Deutsche Sportgeschichte Berlin-Brandenburg, 2011.

Brissonneau, C., and F. Depiesse. "Doping and Doping Control in French Sport." In *Doping and Doping Control in Europe: Performance Enhancing Drugs, Elite Sports and Leisure Time Sport in Denmark, Great Britain, East and West Germany, Poland, France, Italy*, edited by Giselher Spitzer, 145–67. Aachen: Meyer & Meyer, 2006.

Brüggemeier, Franz-Josef. "Das Wunder von Bern. The 1954 Football World Cup, the German Nation and Popular Histories". In *Popular Historiographies in the 19th and 20th Centuries. Cultural Meanings, Social Practices*, edited by Sylvia Paletschek, 188–200. Oxford: Berghahn (New German Historical Perspectives, 4), 2011.

———. *Fußball—Mehr als ein Spiel.* Informationen zur politischen Bildung 290. Munich: Franzis-Verlag, 2006.

Brustmann, Martin. "Erfahrungen mit der Verabreichung von Zellaufbaustoffen beim Körpertraining." *Arzt und Sport: Mitteilungen des deutschen Sportärzte-Bundes* 12, no. 23 (1936): 93–95.

Bundesminister des Inneren (BMI). *Sportberichte der Bundesregierung*. Bonn, Berlin, 1973–2010.

Bundesminister des Inneren (BMI). *Sportförderung des Bundes*. 1970ff.

Coubertin, Pierre de, and Norbert Müller. *Olympism: Selected Writings*. Lausanne: International Olympic Committee, 2000.

Council of Europe. *Doping of Athletes: Reports of the Special Working Parties, Strasbourg, January 1963, Madrid, November 1963*. Strasbourg, 1964.

Court, Jürgen, ed. *Jahrbuch 2011 der Deutschen Gesellschaft für Geschichte der Sportwissenschaft e.V.* Berlin: Lit-Verlag, 2012.

Danckert, Peter. *Kraftmaschine Parlament: Der Sportausschuss und die Sportpolitik des Bundes*. Hauptsache Sport. Aachen: Meyer & Meyer, 2009.

Daume, Willi. *Deutscher Sport, 1952–1972*. Munich: ProSport, 1973.

Decker, Wolfgang. *Sport in der griechischen Antike: Vom minoischen Wettkampf bis zu den Olympischen Spielen*. Hildesheim: Arete, 2012.

DeFrantz, Anita. "Which Rules? International Sport and Doping in the 21st Century." *Houston Journal of International Law* 31, no. 1 (2008): 1–26.

Dennis, Mike. "Securing the Sports 'Miracle': The Stasi and East German Elite Sport." *International Journal of the History of Sport* 29, no. 18 (2012): 2551–74.

Dennis, Mike, and Jonathan Grix. *Sport under Communism: Behind the East German "Miracle."* Basingstoke, Hampshire: Palgrave Macmillan, 2012.

Deutscher Bundestag. "Humanität im Spitzensport: Öffentliche Anhörung des Sportausschusses des Deutschen Bundestags am 14. Oktober 1987 in Bonn." Unpublished manuscript.

———, ed. Materialien der Enquete-Kommission "Aufarbeitung von Geschichte und Folgen der SED-Diktatur in Deutschland": (12. Wahlperiode des Deutschen Bundestages); neuen-eun? Bände in 18 Teilbänden. 1st ed. III/I. Baden-Baden and Frankfurt am Main: Nomos-Verlags-Gesellschaft; Suhrkamp, 1995.[2 Verlage?]

Deutscher Fechterbund (F.I.E.). *Kampfregeln des Internationalen Fechterbundes (F.I.E.)*. Krefeld: Verlag van Acken, 1950.

Deutscher Leichtathletik-Verband. *Amtliche Leichtathletik-Bestimmungen*. 1957ff.

Deutscher Sportbund, ed. *Berichte des Präsidiums*. 3 vols.

———, ed. *Grundsatzerklärung für den Spitzensport: 17. Sitzung des Hauptausschusses des Deutschen Sportbundes am 11. Juni in Baden-Baden*. 1977.

———. *Rahmen-Richtlinien zur Bekämpfung des Dopings: Beschlossen am 26. September 1970 durch den Hauptausschuss des DSB in Mannheim.*

———, ed. *Sportmedizin und Gesundheitserziehung*. Frankfurt am Main: Limpert, 1954.

Deutscher Sportbund, et al., eds. *Training, Leistung, Gesundheit: Vorträge und Referate anlässlich des Sportärztekongresses Berlin 1952*. Frankfurt am Main: Limpert, 1953.

Diem, Carl. *Weltgeschichte des Sports*. 2nd ed. 2 vols. Stuttgart: Cotta, 1967.

———. *Wesen und Lehre des Sports*. 4th ed. Berlin: Weidmann, 1964. Originally published 1949.

Dimeo, Paul. *A History of Drug Use in Sport, 1876–1976: Beyond Good and Evil*. New York and London: Routledge, 2007.

Donati, S. "Doping and Anti-Doping Fight in Italian Sport." In *Doping and Doping Control in Europe: Performance Enhancing Drugs, Elite Sports and Leisure Time Sport in Denmark, Great Britain, East and West Germany, Poland, France, Italy*, edited by Giselher Spitzer, 17–56. Aachen: Meyer & Meyer, 2006.

Donike, Manfred. "Der Dopingnachweis mit Hilfe chromatographischer Methoden." *Sportarzt und Sportmedizin*, no. 2 (1966): 81–86.

———. "Dopinganalytik bei Olympischen Spielen." In *Rekorde aus der Retorte: Leistungssteigerung im modernen Hochleistungssport*, edited by Helmut Acker, 46–52. Stuttgart: Deutsche Verlags-Anstalt, 1972.

———. "Zum Problem des Nachweises der anabolen Steroide: Gas-chromatographische und massenspezifische Möglichkeiten." *Sportarzt und Sportmedizin*, no. 1 (1975): 1–6.

Dubin, Charles L., ed. *Commission of Inquiry into the Use of Drugs and Banned Practices Intended to Increase Athletic Performance*. Ottawa: Canadian Government Publications Centre, 1990.

Eggers, Erik. "Der Sportarzt Martin Brustmann, das Rudern und das Testoviron—Über die Anfänge des Hormondopings im deutschen Leistungssport vor den Olympischen Spielen 1952 in Helsinki." In *Jahrbuch 2011 der Deutschen Gesellschaft für Geschichte der Sportwissenschaft e.V.*, edited by Jürgen Court, 227–44. Berlin: Lit-Verlag, 2012.

Elias, Norbert. *Was ist Soziologie? Grundfragen der Soziologie*. 10th ed. Weinheim: Juventa-Verlag, 2004.

———. *What Is Sociology? European Perspectives*. New York: Columbia University Press, 1978.

Elias, Norbert, and Eric Dunning. *Quest for Excitement: Sport and Leisure in the Civilizing Process*. Oxford: Basil Blackwell, 1993.

Emrich, Eike, and Werner Pitsch, eds. *Sport und Doping: Zur Analyse einer antagonistischen Symbiose*. Frankfurt am Main: Lang, 2009.

Engelhardt, E. "Ernährungsprobleme im Sport." In *Training, Leistung, Gesundheit: Vorträge und Referate anlässlich des Sportärztekongresses Berlin 1952*, edited by Deutscher Sportbund, 103–5. Frankfurt am Main: Limpert, 1953.

Europarat: 9. Sportministertreffen des Europarats: "Ein sauberer und gesunder Sport für das dritte Jahrtausend." Pressburg, Slowakei, 30.-31. Mai 2000. Resolution Nr. 1/2000 zur Dopingbekämpfung. BISp-Archiv. Ordner 0717 Nationale Verbindungen. Nationale Anti-Doping Agentur (NADA). 11/99-5/00, o.P.

Ewald, Manfred, and Reinhold Andert. *Manfred Ewald—Ich war der Sport: Wahrheiten und Legenden aus dem Wunderland der Sieger*. Berlin: Elefanten Press, 1994.

Ferstle, J. "World Conference on Doping in Sport." In *Doping in Elite Sport: The Politics of Drugs in the Olympic Movement*, edited by Wayne Wilson and Edward Derse, 275–86. Champaign, Ill.: Human Kinetics, 2001.

Fischbach, E. "Zum Kapitel 'Doping.'" *Sportmedizin* 9 (1955): 145–46.

Francis, Dick. *Doping: Roman*. Zurich: Diogenes, 2000.

———. *For Kicks*. Large Print. [S.l.]?: Ulverscroft, 1973.

Friedrich, Franz. *Sport und Körper: Die biologischen Grundlagen der Leibeserziehung*. 4th ed. Munich: Ehrenwirth, 1950.

Gabler, Hartmut, and Ulrich Göhner, eds. *Für einen besseren Sport: Themen, Entwicklungen und Perspektiven aus Sport und Sportwissenschaft*. Tübingen: Institut für Sportwissenschaft der Universität Tübingen, 1990.

Gamper, Michael, Jan Mühlethaler, and Felix Reidhaar, eds. *Doping: Spitzensport als gesellschaftliches Problem*. Zurich: NZZ Verlag, 2000.

Gerschler, Woldemar. "Diskussionsbemerkungen eines erfahrenen Trainers." In *Training, Leistung, Gesundheit: Vorträge und Referate anlässlich des Sportärztekongresses Berlin 1952*, edited by Deutscher Sportbund. Frankfurt am Main: Limpert, 1953, 179–182.

Geyer, Martin H. "Der Kampf um nationale Repräsentation: Deutsch-deutsche Sportbeziehungen und die 'Hallstein-Doktrin.'" *Vierteljahreshefte für Zeitgeschichte*, no. 1 (1966): 55–86.

Gieseler, Karlheinz, ed. *Der Sport in der Bundesrepublik Deutschland*. Ämter und Organisationen der Bundesrepublik Deutschland 35. Bonn: Boldt, 1972.

———. "Soziale Hilfen für den Spitzensport." In *Berichte des Präsidiums*, edited by Deutscher Sportbund, 143–45.

Gilbert, B. "Drugs in Sport: Part 1: Problems in a Turned On World." *Sports Illustrated*, June 23, 1969.

Gleaves, John. "'Enhancing the Odds': Horse Racing, Gambling and the First Anti-Doping Movement in Sport, 1889–1911." *Sport in History* 32, no. 1 (2012): 26–52.

Gleaves, John, and Matthew Llewellyn. "Sport, Drugs and Amateurism: Tracing the Real Cultural Origins of Anti-Doping Rules in International Sport." *International Journal of the History of Sport* 31, no. 8 (2014): 839–53.

Gorris, Lothar, Maik Großekathöfer, and Udo Ludwig. "Nur die ganz Dummen: Interview mit Werner Franke." *Der Spiegel*, August 14, 2006. http://www.spiegel.de/spiegel/print/d-48262955.html.

Grupe, Ommo. "33 Jahrgänge 'Sportwissenschaft,'" *Sportwissenschaft*, no. 35 (2005): 336–38.

———. *Bewegung, Spiel und Leistung im Sport: Grundthemen der Sportanthropologie*. Schorndorf: K. Hofmann, 1982. Manuscript in the DOSB Archives.

———. "Der Athlet im Mittelpunkt: Einführung in die Grundsatzerklärung." In *Grundsatzerklärung für den Spitzensport: 17. Sitzung des Hauptausschusses des Deutschen Sportbundes am 11. Juni in Baden-Baden*, edited by Deutscher Sportbund. 1977.

———, ed. *Olympischer Sport: Rückblick und Perspektiven*. Schorndorf: Hofmann, 1997.

———, ed. *Sport in the Modern World—Chances and Problems: Papers, Results, Materials; Scientific Congress, Munich, August 21 to 25, 1972*. Berlin: Springer, 1973.

———. "Was erwartet der Sport von der Sportmedizin?" Special issue, *Der Sportarzt* (1959).

Guttmann, Allen. *From Ritual to Record: The Nature of Modern Sports*. Updated, with a new afterword. New York: Columbia University Press, 2004.

———. *The Olympics: A History of the Modern Games*. Illinois History of Sport. Urbana: University of Illinois Press, 1992.

Haas, Ulrich, ed. *Schiedsgerichtsbarkeit im Sport*. Stuttgart: Boorberg, 2003.

Hanekopf, Günter, ed. *XVI. Weltkongress für Sportmedizin 1966 in Hannover 12. bis 16. Juni 1966: Kongressbericht: Generalthema: Funktionsminderung und Funktionsertüchtigung im modernen Leben*. Cologne: Deutscher Ärzte Verlag, 1966.

Hanstad, D. V. "Anti-Doping Policies in Sport: Elite Level Athletes & Whereabouts Information." *Sport & EU Newsletter* 2 (March 2007): 3–4.

Hanstad, D. V., A. Smith, and Ivan Waddington. "Establishment of the World Anti-Doping Agency: A Study of the Management of Organisational Change and Unplanned Outcomes." *International Review for the Sociology of Sport* 43, no. 3 (2008): 227–49.

Hartmann, Robert. "Das Trauma Anabolika." *Leichtathletik* 47: 1660–61.

Haug, Tanja. *Doping: Dilemma des Leistungssports*. Hamburg: Merus-Verlag, 2006.

Havemann, Nils. *Fußball unterm Hakenkreuz: Der DFB zwischen Sport, Politik und Kommerz*. Frankfurt: Campus-Verl, 2005.

———. *Samstags um halb vier: Die Geschichte der Fußballbundesliga*. Berlin: Siedler, 2013.

Heinilä, Kalevi. "Citius—altius—fortius: The Olympic 'Contribution' to the Professionalization of Sport?" In *Sport in the Modern World—Chances and Problems: Papers, Results, Materials; Scientific Congress, Munich, August 21 to 25, 1972*, edited by Ommo Grupe, 351–55. Berlin: Springer, 1973.

———. *The Totalization Process in International Sport: Toward a Theory of the Totalization of Competition in Top-Level Sport*. Jyväskylä: University of Jyväskylä, 1982.

Henne, Kathryn. "The Emergence of Moral Technopreneurialism in Sport: Techniques in Anti-Doping Regulation, 1966–1976." *International Journal of the History of Sport* 30 (2013): 1–18.

Heydn, G. "'Luftduschen' nutzen nichts." *Der Deutsche Schwimmsport*, no. 6 (1977): 140.

Hilpert, Horst. *Sportrecht und Sportrechtsprechung im In- und Ausland*. Berlin: de Gruyter Recht, 2007.

Hoberman, J. "Doping, Gambling, and the Decline of the IOC." *Georgetown Journal of International Affairs* 13, no. 2 (2012), 135–142.

———. "The Early Development of Sports Medicine in Germany." In *Sport and Exercise Science: Essays in the History of Sports Medicine*, edited by Jack W. Berryman and Roberta J. Park, 233–82. Urbana: University of Illinois Press, 1992.

———. "How Drug Testing Fails: The Politics of Doping Control." In *Doping in Elite Sport: The Politics of Drugs in the Olympic Movement*, edited by Wayne Wilson and Edward Derse, 241–74. Champaign, Ill.: Human Kinetics, 2001.

———. *Mortal Engines: The Science of Performance and the Dehumanization of Sport*. New York: Macmillan, 1992.

———. *Sterbliche Maschinen: Doping und die Unmenschlichkeit des Hochleistungssports*. Aachen: Meyer & Meyer, 1994.

———. *Testosterone Dreams: Rejuvenation, Aphrodisia, Doping*. Berkeley: University of California Press, 2005.

Holzweissig, Gunter. *Sport und Politik in der DDR*. Berlin: Holzapfel, 1988.

Houlihan, Barrie. "Doping, Public Health and the Generalization of Interests." In *Elite Sport, Doping and Public Health*, edited by Verner Møller, Mike McNamee, and Paul Dimeo, 41–54. Odense: University Press of Southern Denmark, 2009.

———. *Dying to Win: Doping in Sport and the Development of Anti-Doping Policy*. 2nd ed. Strasbourg: Council of Europe Publications, 1999/2002.

———. "The World Anti-Doping Agency and the Campaign against Doping in Sport in Europe." *European Yearbook*. In *Council of Europe Handbook 1998*, Council of Europe Publishing (1998): pp. 8–21

———. "The World Anti-Doping Agency: Prospects for Success." In *Drugs and Doping in Sport: Socio-Legal Perspectives*, edited by John O'Leary. London: Cavendish, 2001, 125–145.

Hübner, Emanuel. *Planung, Bau und Nutzung des Olympischen Dorfes von 1936*. Paderborn: Schöningh, 2014. Forthcoming.

Hunt, Thomas M. *Drug Games: The International Olympic Committee and the Politics of Doping, 1960–2008*. Austin: University of Texas Press, 2011.

International Olympic Committee, ed. *Final Research Report of the IOC Postgraduate Research Grant Program, 2011*. http://doc.rero.ch/record/29383?In=fr, 2012. Accessed 20 August 2014.

———. *Le Mouvement olympique de lavenir: Thème 3. XIe Congrès olympique à Baden-Baden, 1981*. Lausanne: CIO, 1982.

———. *Minutes of the IOC. Meeting of the 108th IOC Session*.

Jedlicka, Scott R., and Thomas M. Hunt. "The International Anti-Doping Movement and UNESCO: A Historical Case Study." *International Journal of the History of Sport* 30, no. 13 (2013): 1523–35.

Jütte, Robert. "Zur Geschichte des Dopings." *Geschichte in Wissenschaft und Unterricht* 5/6 (2008): 308–22.

Katzer, Nikolaus. "Am Rande der Vollkommenheit: Aspekte einer Geschichte sowjetischer Körperoptimierung." In *Hormone und Hochleistung: Doping in Ost und West*, edited by Klaus Latzel and Lutz Niethammer, 205–30. Cologne: Böhlau, 2008.

———. "Körperkult und Bewegungszwang: Zur gesellschaftlichen Dynamik des frühen sowjetischen Sportsystems." In *Der deutsche Sport auf dem Weg in die Moderne: Carl Diem und seine Zeit*, edited by Michael Krüger, 257–84. Berlin and Münster: Lit-Verlag, 2009.

Keohane, R. O. "The Demand for International Regimes." *International Organization* 36, no. 2 (1982): 325–55.

Keul, Josef. "Freiwillige Dopingkontrolle während des Trainings empfohlen." *NOK-Report*, no. 3 (1987): 16.

Kistner, Thomas. "Anti-Doping-Organisation: Unterfinanziert und überfordert." *Süddeutsche Zeitung*, October 12, 2006.

Klaus, E. J. "Sporthygienische Fragen." In *Sportmedizin und Gesundheitserziehung*, edited by Deutscher Sportbund, 31–41. Frankfurt am Main: Limpert, 1954.

Kleffel, W. "Wunderpillen endgültig verboten." *Die Zeit*, no. 47 (1952).

Knabe, Hubertus. *Honeckers Erben: Die Wahrheit über die Linke*. Berlin: Propyläen, 2009.

Knörzer, Wolfgang, G. Spitzer, and G. Treutlein, eds. *Dopingprävention in Europa: Grundlagen und Modelle; Erstes internationales Expertengespräch 2005 in Heidelberg*. Aachen and Graz: Meyer & Meyer, 2006.

Koch, Alfred. "Der Präsident des Deutschen Sportärztebundes zum Kongreß 1954." *Sportmedizin*, no. 9 (1954): 257–58.

———, ed. *Präventive Medizin und Leibesübungen in der Jugend: Vorträge und Referate anläßlich des Deutschen Sportärztekongresses 1955 in Augsburg*. Freiburg im Breisgau: Tries, 1956.

———. *Sportmedizin*. Therapie und Praxis 17. Vienna and Innsbruck: Urban & Schwarzenberg, 1958.

Koch, Alfred, Hanns Hoske, and J. M Hammacher. "Vom Wirken des Sportarztes." In *Sportmedizin und Gesundheitserziehung*, edited by Deutscher Sportbund, 15–29. Frankfurt am Main: Limpert, 1954.

Kohlhaas, M. "Gesetzliche Grundlagen für ein Verbot von 'Doping.'" *Sportarzt und Sportmedizin* 17, no. 2 (1966): 64–81.

Krasner, Stephen D. *International Regimes*. Cornell Studies in Political Economy. Ithaca, N.Y.: Cornell University Press, 1983.

Krogmann, M. "Zur Dopinggesetzgebung im Ausland: Teil 1 1/99, Teil 2 2/99, Teil 3 4/99, Teil 4 1/2000." *Sport und Recht (SpuRT)*, 1999/2000.

Krüger, Arnd. *Sport und Politik: Von Turnvater Jahn zum Staatsamateur*. Hannover: Fackelträger-Verlag, 1975.

———, ed. *Vergessen, verdrängt, abgelehnt—Zur Geschichte der Ausgrenzung im Sport: Tagungsbericht der 10. Hoyaer Tagung zur Sportgeschichte vom 10. bis 12. Oktober 2008*. Schriftenreihe des Niedersächsischen Instituts für Sportgeschichte Hoya e.V. Berlin: Lit-Verlag, 2009.

Krüger, Michael. "60 Jahre Sport in Deutschland." *Sportwissenschaft* 39, no. 3 (2009): 237–50.

———, ed. *Der deutsche Sport auf dem Weg in die Moderne: Carl Diem und seine Zeit*. Berlin and Münster: Lit-Verlag, 2009.

———. "Doping im Radsport—Zivilisationstheoretische Anmerkungen zu einer langen Geschichte." *Sport und Gesellschaft*, no. 3 (2006): 324–52.

———. "The German Workers' Sport Movement between Socialism, Workers' Culture, Middle-Class Gymnastics and Sport for All." *International Journal of the History of Sport* 31, no. 9 (2014): 1098–1117. doi:10.1080/09523367.2014.882327.

———. "The History of German Sports Clubs between Integration and Emigration." *International Journal of the History of Sport* 30, no. 14 (2013): 1586–1603.

———. *Leibesübungen im 20. Jahrhundert: Sport für alle*. 2nd ed. Schorndorf: Hofmann, 2005.

———. "Die Neugründung des Deutschen Turner-Bundes 1950." In *200 Jahre Turnbewegung—200 Jahre soziale Verantwortung*, 118–22. Frankfurt: DTB, 2011.

———. "Ruhmsucht und Rekordfimmel: Zur Geschichte der Leistung im Sport." In *Für einen besseren Sport: Themen, Entwicklungen und Perspektiven aus Sport und Sportwissenschaft*, edited by Hartmut Gabler and Ulrich Göhner, 343–62. Tübingen: Institut für Sportwissenschaft der Universität Tübingen, 1990.

———. "Vorbild DDR? Neuorientierung im westdeutschen Sport." In *Wir gegen uns: Sport im geteilten Deutschland*, edited by Anne Martin, 98–107. Darmstadt: Primus-Verlag, 2009.

Krüger, Michael, and Christian Becker. "Doping and Anti-Doping in the Process of German Reunification." *Sport in History* 34 (2014): 1–24.

Krüger, Michael F., Stefan Nielsen, and Christian Becker. "The Munich Olympics 1972: Its Impact on the Relationship between State, Sports and Anti-Doping Policy in West Germany." *Sport in History* 32, no. 4 (2012): 526–49.

Lames, Martin. "Leistungsentwicklung in der Leichtathletik: Ist Doping als leistungsfördernder Effekt identifizierbar?" *dvs-informationen* 17, no. 4 (2002): 15–22.

Latzel, Klaus. *Staatsdoping: Der VEB Jenapharm im Sportsystem der DDR*. Cologne and Vienna: Böhlau, 2009.

Latzel, Klaus, and Lutz Niethammer, eds. *Hormone und Hochleistung: Doping in Ost und West*. Cologne: Böhlau, 2008.

Laure, Patrick. *Le dopage: Pratiques corporelles*. Paris: Presses Universitaires de France, 1995.

———. “Zur Entwicklung von Dopingregeln und Antidoping-Gesetzen.” In *Dopingprävention in Europa: Grundlagen und Modelle; Erstes internationales Expertengespräch 2005 in Heidelberg*, edited by Wolfgang Knörzer, G. Spitzer, and G. Treutlein, 121–32. Aachen and Graz: Meyer & Meyer, 2006.

Lendle, L. “Stimulantio—Excitantia (Dopingmittel).” *Sportmedizin*, no. 1 (1957): 22–26.

Lenk, Hans. *Leistungssport: Ideologie oder Mythos? Zur Leistungskritik und Sportphilosophie*. Stuttgart: Kohlhammer, 1972.

———. *Werte, Ziele, Wirklichkeit der modernen Olympischen Spiele*. 2nd ed. Schorndorf: Hofmann, 1972.

Longman, Jere. “IOC Makes Changes, but Trust Becomes Issue.” *New York Times*, March 19, 1999.

MacAloon, John J. “Doping and Moral Authority: Sports Organizations Today.” In *Doping in Elite Sport: The Politics of Drugs in the Olympic Movement*, edited by Wayne Wilson and Edward Derse, 205–24. Champaign, Ill.: Human Kinetics, 2001.

Mackay, Duncan. “Banks Says No to New Initiative to Fight Drugs.” *Guardian*, February 5, 1999.

Mandell, Richard D. *The Olympics of 1972: A Munich Diary*. Chapel Hill: University of North Carolina Press, 1991.

Martin, Anne, ed. *Wir gegen uns: Sport im geteilten Deutschland*. Darmstadt: Primus-Verlag, 2009.

Martin, David E., and Roger W. H. Gynn. *The Olympic Marathon*. Champaign, Ill.: Human Kinetics, 2000.

Meier, Henk E., and Marcel Reinold. “Dopingskandale in der alten Bundesrepublik: Öffentlicher Diskurs und sportpolitische Reaktionen.” *Deutschland Archiv: Zeitschrift für das vereinigte Deutschland* 45, no. 2 (2012): 209–39.

———. “Performance Enhancement and Politicisation of High-Performance Sport: The West German ‘Air Clyster’ Affair of 1976.” *International Journal of the History of Sport* 30, no. 12 (2013): 1351–73.

Mengden, Guido V. “Beiträge zur Geschichte des Deutschen Sportbundes.” *Jahrbuch des Sports, 1959–1962* (1962).

Møller, Verner. *The Ethics of Doping and Anti-Doping: Redeeming the Soul of Sport?* Ethics and Sport. London: Routledge, 2010.

———. “Knud Enemark Jensen’s Death during the 1960 Rome Olympics: A Search for the Truth?” *Sport in History* 25 (2005): 452–71.

Møller, Verner, Mike McNamee, and Paul Dimeo, eds. *Elite Sport, Doping and Public Health*. Odense: University Press of Southern Denmark, 2009.

Montgomery, P. L. “I.O.C. Falters in Doping Bids as Summit Ends.” *New York Times*, February 5, 1999.

Neckermann, Josef. “Die Abkehr von Normen.” *Deutsche Schwimmsport*, no. 1 (1977): 6.

Neufeld-Spassov, Renate, Dimitrov Pentschon, and Johannes Hampel. *Politik und Sport*. Munich: Olzog, 1980.

Niese, Holger. “Stiftung National Anti-Doping Agentur.” In *Schiedsgerichtsbarkeit im Sport*, edited by Ulrich Haas, 61–74. Stuttgart: Boorberg, 2003.

Nolte, H. “Presserklärung des Sportausschusses Niedersachsen.” *Radsport*, no. 26 (1973): 10.

Nolte, Martin. “Dopingbekämpfung in Deutschland: Prototyp einer Verantwortungsteilung von Staat und Gesellschaft.” In *Die Freiheit des Menschen in Kommune, Staat und Europa: Festschrift für Edzard Schmidt-Jortzig*, edited by Utz Schliesky, 771–82. Heidelberg and Hamburg: Müller, 2011.

———, ed. *Persönlichkeitsrechte im Sport*. Stuttgart: Boorberg, 2006.

———. *Staatliche Verantwortung im Bereich Sport: Ein Beitrag zur normativen Abgrenzung von Staat und Gesellschaft*. Kiel: Lorenz-von-Stein-Institut für Verwaltungswissenschaften, 2004.

O’Leary, John, ed. *Drugs and Doping in Sport: Socio-Legal Perspectives*. London: Cavendish, 2001.

Oswald, D. "A Lesson to the Moralizers." *Olympic Review* 26 (1999): 21–23.

Pawlenka, Claudia. *Ethik, Natur und Doping*. Ethica 19. Paderborn: Mentis, 2010.

Pelshenke, Günter. *Stiftung Deutsche Sporthilfe. Die ersten 25 Jahre (Europäische Hochschulschriften Band 17)*. Frankfurt/M., Berlin, Bern, New York, Paris, Wien: Peter Lang, 1999.

Pitsch, Werner. "Dopingkontrollen zwischen Testtheorie und Moral: Nicht intendierte Folgen prinzipiell nicht perfekter Dopingtests." In *Sport und Doping: Zur Analyse einer antagonistischen Symbiose*, edited by Eike Emrich and Werner Pitsch, 95–110. Frankfurt am Main: Lang, 2009.

Pitsch, Werner, Eike Emrich, and Michael Klein. "Doping in Elite Sports in Germany: Results of a www-survey." *European Journal of Sports and Society* 4, no. 2 (2007): 89–102.

———. "Zur Häufigkeit des Dopings im Leistungssport: Ergebnisse eines www-surveys." *Leipziger Sportwissenschaftliche Beiträge* 46, no. 2 (2005): 63–77.

Pitsch, Werner, Peter Maats, and Eike Emrich. "Zur Häufigkeit des Dopings im deutschen Spitzensport: Eine Replikationsstudie." In *Sport und Doping: Zur Analyse einer antagonistischen Symbiose*, edited by Eike Emrich and Werner Pitsch, 19–36. Frankfurt am Main: Lang, 2009.

Porrit, Arthur. "Doping in Sport: Chairman's Opening Remarks." *British Journal of Sports Medicine* 4, no. 2 (1969): 105–8.

Pound, Richard W. *Inside Dope: How Drugs Are the Biggest Threat to Sports, Why You Should Care, and What Can Be Done about Them*. Mississauga, Ontario: J. Wiley & Sons Canada, 2006.

Prokop, Clemens. "Probleme einer nationalen Anti-Doping-Agentur." In *Doping-forum: Aktuelle rechtliche und medizinische Aspekte*, edited by Volker Röhricht and Klaus Vieweg, 77–85. Stuttgart and Munich: Richard Boorberg Verlag, 2000.

Prokop, Ludwig. "Das Dopingproblem im Sport." *Leibesübungen/Leibeserziehung* 9, no. 5/6 (1955): 6ff.

———. "Praktische Erfahrungen mit dem Doping in Österreich." *Sportarzt und Sportmedizin* 17, no. 2 (1966): 56–60.

———. "Sport und Sauna." In *Training, Leistung, Gesundheit: Vorträge und Referate anlässlich des Sportärztekongresses Berlin 1952*, edited by Deutscher Sportbund, 37–40. Frankfurt am Main: Limpert, 1953.

———. "Zur Geschichte des Dopings und seiner Bekämpfung." *Sportarzt und Sportmedizin* 21, no. 6 (1970): 125–32.

Prokop, L., and F. Radbauer. "Die Placebowirkung der Injektion beim Doping." In *XVI. Weltkongress für Sportmedizin 1966 in Hannover 12. bis 16. Juni 1966: Kongressbericht: Generalthema: Funktionsminderung und Funktionsertüchtigung im modernen Leben*, edited by Günter Hanekopf, 635–37. Cologne: Deutscher Ärzte Verlag, 1966.

Rabenstein, Rüdiger. "Some Facts about the History of Doping in Cycling History Competition." In *Proceedings 8th International Cycle History Conference, 1997*, 119–30.

Reindell, Herbert. "Begrüßung durch den Präsidenten des Deutschen Sportbundes." *Sportarzt und Sportmedizin* 17, no. 2 (1966): 45ff.

Reinold, Marcel. "Arguing against Doping: A Discourse Analytical Study on Olympic Anti-Doping between the 1960s and the Late 1980s: Final Research Report of the IOC Postgraduate Research Grant Program 2011." In *Final Research Report of the IOC Postgraduate Research Grant Program 2011*, edited by the International Olympic Committee, https://doc.rero.ch/search?ln=de&sc=1&p=Reinold+Arguing+against+doping&action_search=. http://doc.rero.ch/record/29383?In=fr2012. Accessed 24 August 2014.

Reinold, Marcel, and John Hoberman. "The Myth of the Nazi Steroid." *International Journal of the History of Sport* 31, no. 8 (2014): 871–83.

Reissinger, Fabian. *Staatliche Verantwortung zur Bekämpfung des Dopings*. Baden-Baden: Nomos-Verlags-Gesellschaft, 2010.

Resolution on the Doping of Athletes, Adopted by the Ministers' Deputies on 29th June 1967. Committee of Ministers of the Council of Europe. 1967.

Rigauer, Bero. *Sport and Work: European Perspectives*. New York: Columbia University Press, 1981.

Rittberger, Volker, and H. Boekle. "Das International Olympische Komitee: Eine Weltregierung des Sports?" In *Olympischer Sport: Rückblick und Perspektiven*, edited by Ommo Grupe, 127–57. Schorndorf: Hofmann, 1997.

Ritter von Halt, Karl. "Olympia." *Leibesübungen—Sportarzt—Erziehung* 4, no. 6 (1952): 34.

Röhricht, Volker, and Klaus Vieweg, eds. *Doping-forum: Aktuelle rechtliche und medizinische Aspekte*. Stuttgart and Munich: Richard Boorberg Verlag, 2000.

Rosen, Daniel M. *Dope: A History of Performance Enhancement in Sports from the Nineteenth Century to Today*. Westport, Conn., and London: Praeger, 2008.

Röthel, A. "Neues Doping-Gesetz für Frankreich." *SpuRT*, no. 1 (1999): 20–21.

Ruhemann, W. "Doping." *Sportmedizin*, no. 2 (1953): 26.

———. "Einführung." In *Sportmedizin und Gesundheitserziehung*, edited by Deutscher Sportbund, 7–12. Frankfurt am Main: Limpert, 1954.

Schaepdryver, A. F. de, ed. *Doping: Proceedings of an International Seminar Organized at the Universities of Ghent and Brussels, May 1964, by the Research Committee of the International Council of Sport and Physical Education (U.N.E.S.C.O.)*. Oxford: Pergamon Press, 1965.

Schenk, P. "Bericht über die Verpflegung der im Olympischen Dorf untergebrachten Teilnehmer an den XI. Olympischen Spielen 1936 zu Berlin." *Die Ernährung* 2, no. 1 (1937): 1–24.

Schiller, Kay, and Christopher Young. *The 1972 Munich Olympics and the Making of Modern Germany*. Berkeley: University of California Press, 2010. In German: *München 1972: Olympische Spiele im Zeichen des modernen Deutschland*. Göttingen: Wallstein, 2012.

Schliesky, Utz, ed. *Die Freiheit des Menschen in Kommune, Staat und Europa: Festschrift für Edzard Schmidt-Jortzig*. With the assistance of Edzard Schmidt-Jortzig. Heidelberg and Hamburg: Müller, 2011.

Schmidt, Judith A. *Internationale Dopingbekämpfung: Grundlagen und nationalstaatliche Umsetzung*. Stuttgart and Zurich: Boorberg; Schulthess, 2009.

Schnyder, P. "Erfundene Ursprünge und sprechende Bilder: Historische, etymologische und metaphorologische Bemerkungen zum Dopingkurs." In *Doping: Spitzensport als gesellschaftliches Problem*, edited by Michael Gamper, Jan Mühlethaler, and Felix Reidhaar, 69–88. Zurich: NZZ Verlag, 2000.

Schrange, C. "'Kompliment, Herr Hangstein . . . Das war präsidentisch!' Verhandlung gegen Dieter Leitner." *Radsport*, no. 34 (1971): 7–8.

Schulz, Stefan, Klaus Steigleder, Heiner Fangerau, and Norbert W. Paul, eds. *Geschichte, Theorie und Ethik der Medizin: Eine Einführung*. Frankfurt am Main: Suhrkamp, 2006.

Sievert, Hans-Heinrich. "Aufgaben und Grenzen staatlicher Hilfe für den Sport." *Die Leibeserziehung* 4 (1954): 73–74.

Singler, Andreas. *Doping und Enhancement: Interdisziplinäre Studien zur Pathologie gesellschaftlicher Leistungsorientierung*. Göttingen: Cuvillier, 2012.

Singler, Andreas, and Gerhard Treutlein. *Doping im Spitzensport*. Sportentwicklungen in Deutschland 12. Aachen: Meyer & Meyer, 2000.

———. *Doping im Spitzensport: Sportwissenschaftliche Analysen zur nationalen und internationalen Leistungsentwicklung*. Part 1. 6th ed. Aachen: Meyer & Meyer, 2012.

———. "Doping in der Bundesrepublik Deutschland: Historische und soziologische Aspekte abweichenden Verhaltens im Spitzensport." In *Hormone und Hochleistung: Doping in Ost und West*, edited by Klaus Latzel and Lutz Niethammer, 41–65. Cologne: Böhlau, 2008.

Sperryn, P., ed. "Proceedings of the International Symposium on Anabolic Steroids in Sport: Special Issue of the Symposium in London." Special issue, *British Journal of Sport Medicine* 9, no. 2 (1975).

Spitzer, Giselher, ed. *Doping and Doping Control in Europe: Performance Enhancing Drugs, Elite Sports and Leisure Time Sport in Denmark, Great Britain, East and West Germany, Poland, France, Italy*. Aachen: Meyer & Meyer, 2006.

———. *Doping in der DDR: Ein historischer Überblick zu einer konspirativen Praxis; Genese—Verantwortung—Gefahren*. Cologne: Sport und Buch Strauß, 1998.

———, ed. *Doping in Deutschland: Geschichte, Recht, Ethik, 1950–1972*. Cologne: Strauß, 2013.

———. "Gab es in der DDR Spionage des Bundesnachrichtendienstes?" *Sozial- und Zeitgeschichte des Sports* 13, no. 3 (1999): 28–40.

———. *Siegen um jeden Preis: Doping in Deutschland: Geschichte, Recht, Ethik, 1972–1990*. Göttingen: Verlag Die Werkstatt, 2013.

Spitzer, Giselher, and Harald Braun, eds. *Der geteilte deutsche Sport: Tagung der DVS-Sektion Sportgeschichte vom 24.–26. März 1995 in Potsdam*. Berichte und Materialien des Bundesinstituts für Sportwissenschaft 97/3. Cologne: Sport und Buch Strauss, 1997.

Steiner, Udo. "Schutz des Sports: Verbands- oder Staatsaufgabe?" In *Wettkampfmanipulation und Schutzmechanismen*, 45–52. Stuttgart: Boorberg, 2012.

Teetzel, Sarah. "The Road to WADA: Seventh International Symposium for Olympic Research (S. 213–224)." Unpublished manuscript. http://library.la84.org/SportsLibrary/ISOR/ISOR2004t.pdf.

Teichler, Hans J. "Die Ausspähung des westdeutschen Sports durch das Ministerium für Staatssicherheit der DDR." In *Der geteilte deutsche Sport: Tagung der DVS-Sektion Sportgeschichte vom 24.–26. März 1995 in Potsdam*, edited by Giselher Spitzer and Harald Braun, 65–98. Berichte und Materialien des Bundesinstituts für Sportwissenschaft 97/3. Cologne: Sport und Buch Strauss, 1997.

Thompson, Christopher. *The Tour de France: A Cultural History*. New ed. Berkeley: University of California Press, 2008.

Thyssen, S. *Manfred Donike und das Institut für Biochemie der Deutschen Sporthochschule Köln: Geschichte und Leistung im Kampf gegen Doping*. 2010.

Todd, Terry "Anabolic Steroids: The Gremlins of Sport." *Journal of Sport History*, no. 14 (1987): 87–107.

UNESCO. *Records of the General Conference. 33rd Session. Paris, October 3rd–21st*. Vol. 1: Resolutions. 2005.

———. *UNESCO Media Services: Meeting of States Parties to the International Convention against Doping Sport*. 2011.

Venerando, Antonio. "Patalogia del doping e mezzi di controllo." *Medicina dello sport* 3, no. 9 (1963): 30–40.

Venerando, A., and F. de Sio. "Organisation et résultats du control antidoping." In *Doping: Proceedings of an International Seminar Organized at the Universities of Ghent and Brussels, May 1964*, edited by A. F. de Schaepdryver and Marcel Hebbelinck, 133–45. Oxford: Pergamon Press, 1965.

Vettenie, E. "Runners, Rumors, and Dreams of Representations: An Inquiry into Drug Use by Athletes in the 1920s." *Journal of Sport History* 37, no. 3 (2010): 401–15.

Vögele, Jörg. "Zur Entwicklung der Gesundheitsverhältnisse im 19. und 20. Jahrhundert." In *Geschichte, Theorie und Ethik der Medizin: Eine Einführung*, edited by Stefan Schulz et al. Frankfurt am Main: Suhrkamp, 2006. 165–182.

Voy, Robert O., and Kirk D. Deeter. *Drugs, Sport, and Politics*. Champaign, Ill.: Leisure Press, 1991.

Waddington, Ivan. "Changing Patterns of Drug Use in British Sport from the 1960s." *Sport in History* 25, no. 3 (2005): 472–96.

———. "The Development of Doping and Doping Control in Britain". In Doping and Doping Control in Europe. Performance enhancing drugs, elite sports and leisure time sport in Denmark, Great Britain, East and West Germany, Poland, France, Italy, Oxford, edited by Giselher Spitzer, 115-144. Aachen: Meyer & Meyer, 2006.

———. *Sport, Health and Drugs: A Critical Sociological Perspective*. London and New York: E & FN Spon, 2000.

Waddington, Ivan, and Andy Smith. *An Introduction to Drugs in Sport: Addicted to Winning?* London: Routledge, 2009.

Weber, C. "Die Stiftung Nationale Anti-Doping Agentur." In *Persönlichkeitsrechte im Sport*, edited by Martin Nolte, 71–85. Stuttgart: Boorberg, 2006.

Weidemann, H. "Internationale Konferenz über Doping bei Sportlern vom 23.–25. September in Straßburg." *Sportarzt und Sportmedizin* 17, no. 2 (1966): 49–50.

Wettkampfmanipulation und Schutzmechanismen. Stuttgart: Boorberg, 2012.

Wilson, Wayne, and Edward Derse, eds. *Doping in Elite Sport. The Politics of Drugs in the Olympic Movement*. Champaign, Ill.: Human Kinetics, 2001.

Woodland, Les. *Dope: The Use of Drugs in Sport*. Newton Abbot: David & Charles, 1980.

World Anti-Doping Agency. Cape Town Declaration on Anti-Doping in Sport.

———. World Anti-Doping Code.

Wrynn, A. "The Human Factor: Science, Medicine and the International Olympic Committee, 1900–1970." *Sport in Society* 7, no. 2 (2004): 211–31.

Wülfing, Walter. Zum Jahreswechsel. Gedanken um 1953, ein Jahr der Bewährung. *Rudersport* 1 (1953): 3.

Yesalis, C. E., A. N. Kopstein, and M. S. Bahrke "Difficulties in Estimating the Prevalence of Drug Use among Athletes." In *Doping in Elite Sport: The Politics of Drugs in the Olympic Movement*, edited by Wayne Wilson and Edward Derse. Champaign: Human Kinetics, 2001. 43–62.

PUBLISHED BOOKS AND ARTICLES OF THE MUENSTER RESEARCH GROUP ON DOPING HISTORY

Krüger, Michael, Becker, Christian, Nielsen, Stefan, Reinold, Marcel. *Doping und Anti-Doping in der Bundesrepublik Deutschland 1950-2007. Genese – Strukturen – Politik*. Hildesheim: Arete, 2014.

Krüger, Michael & Reinold, Marcel. Doping, Sport und Staat – zur Genese eines komplexen gesellschaftlichen Systems. In *Nicht nur Sieg und Niederlage. Sport im deutschen Südwesten im 19. und 20. Jahrhundert*, edited by Arbeitsgemeinschaft für geschichtliche Landeskunde am Oberrhein e.V., 231-243. Ostfildern: Thorbecke, 2011.

Krüger, Michael, Becker, Christian & Nielsen, Stefan. The Munich Olympics of 1972: Its Impact on the Relationship between State, Sports and Anti-Doping Policy in West-Germany. *Sport in History*, no 32 (2012) 4: 526-550.

Krüger, Michael, Becker, Christian. Doping and Anti-Doping in the Process of German Reunification. *Sport in History*, no 34 (2014) 4: 620-643.

Krüger, Michael/ Nielsen, Stefan. Die Entstehung der Nationalen Anti-Doping Agentur in Deutschland (NADA) im Kontext der Gründung der Welt Anti-Doping Agentur (WADA). *Sport und Gesellschaft*, no 10 (2013) 1: 55-94.

Meier, Henk Eric & Reinold, Marcel. Performance enhancement and politicisation of high performance sport: The West German 'air clyster' affaire of 1976. *The International Journal for the History of Sport*, no 30 (2013) 12: 1351-1373.

Meier, Henk Eric, Reinold, Marcel, Rose, Anika (2012). Dopingskandale in der alten Bundesrepublik. Öffentlicher Diskurs und sportpolitische Reaktionen. *Deutschland Archiv. Zeitschrift für das vereinigte Deutschland*, no 45 (2012) 2: 209-239.

Meier, Henk Eric, Rose, Anika, Woborschil, Stefanie (2012). Der Dopingdiskurs der fünfziger und sechziger Jahre in den Leitmedien Der Spiegel und Die Zeit. *Sportwissenschaft*, no 42 (2012) 3: 163-177

Reinold, Marcel. Doping. In *Handbuch Sportgeschichte*, edited by Michael Krüger & H. Langenfeld, 362-377. Hofmann: Schorndorf, 2011.

Reinold, Marcel. *Arguing against doping: A discourse analytical study on Olympic anti-doping between the 1960s and the late 1980s* (Final Research Report of the IOC Postgraduate Research Grant Programm 2011), 2012. Access: http://doChristianrero.ch/record/29383?ln=fr

Reinold, Marcel / Becker, Christian/ Nielsen Stefan. Die 1960er Jahre als Formationsphase von Modernem Doping und Anti-Doping. *Sportwissenschaft*, no 42 (2012) 3: 153-162.

Reinold, Marcel / Meier, Henk Eric. Difficult Adaptions to Innovations in Performance Enhancement: 'Dr. Brustmanns Power Pills and Anti-Doping in German Post-war Sport. *Sport in History*, no 32 (2012) 1: 74-104.

Index

Adenauer, Konrad, 10, 17
amateurism, 17; and Olympic Games, 18, 79, 136, 191
Anquetil, Jacques, xxix
anti-doping: as counterpart to doping (definition), 23; government involvement, 24, 25, 26, 40–42, 45, 55, 58, 63–65, 66, 68, 69, 70, 71–72, 99, 105, 107, 112, 137, 138–140, 145, 146, 147, 148–150, 156, 163–164, 166–168, 170–175, 177, 180; involvement of organized sport, 24–26, 35–38, 39, 56, 62–63, 65–66, 73, 76, 108, 122–123, 124, 142, 146–147, 159, 163; laboratories and research, 38–39, 66–70, 71–72, 84, 107, 108, 113, 121, 136, 168, 173; moral issues, 32, 34, 75, 77, 78, 141, 154, 191, 192, 200; policies, testing and effectiveness, 26, 54, 62, 65, 66, 72, 73–74, 76, 78, 79, 80–81, 103, 107, 113–114, 115–116, 122–123, 124, 137, 159, 169. *See also* Olympic games, doping laboratories; Sport policy of FRG, and anti-Doping/ involvement in European and international initiatives
Anti-Doping Commission. *See* Anti-Doping-Kommission (ADK)
Anti-Doping-Kommission (ADK), 123, 166–167
Arbeiter-Turn- und Sportbund (ATSB), 7
Armstrong, Lance, 22, 170
Arzneimittelgesetz (AMG) (German drug law), 173
Astaphan, George (Jamie), 157
athletics, xiv, xxiv, xxix, 7, 8, 18, 21, 22, 25, 26, 28, 35–36, 56, 65, 73, 96, 101, 104, 107, 108, 111–112, 115, 137–138, 153, 157, 166, 174, 190, 196
Augustin, Roland, 169
Australia, 158
autonomy of sports: partnership, xvi, xvii, xx, 11, 71, 138, 140, 149, 156, 164, 177–179; subsidiarity, 11, 12, 13, 15, 142, 156, 166, 179

Bahrke, Michael, 62
Balbier, Uta Andrea, 15, 58
Banks, Tony, 163–164
Baumann, Dieter, 152–154, 153
Bechthold, Inge, 111
Becker, Howard, 23
Beckett, Arnold, 62, 69, 108
Belgium, 26, 38, 40, 63, 95, 120, 160, 166, 172
Benda, Ernst, 42
Berendonk, Brigitte, xxix, 20, 42, 47n41, 64, 76, 91, 93, 96, 104, 112, 143, 144, 182n7
Bergner, Christoph, 175
Berlioux, Monique, 62
Bette, Karl-Heinrich, xviii

Beyer, Harm, 149
Bode, Hans-Jürgen, 81–82
Brandt, Willy, 92
Braun, Jutta, 140
Brooks, Raymond V., 88
Brundage, Avery, xxv, 18, 25, 62, 63
Brustmann, Martin, 30, 31–32, 33, 192
Bund Deutscher Radfahrer (BDR), 65, 76, 95, 110
Bundesausschuss Leistungssport (BA-L), 58, 81, 82, 84, 98, 103
Bundesinstitut für Sportwissenschaft (BISp), xi, xxxn1, 60, 98, 109, 118, 119, 168
Bundesleistungszentrum (BLZ), 97, 170
Bundesminister/-ium des Innern (BMI): and anti-doping 36, 40, 40–42, 45, 63, 64, 66, 68, 69, 70, 121–122, 138, 145, 148, 148–149, 149, 151, 156, 163, 170, 172, 173, 175; implementation of the German NADA, 166, 167, 180–181, 181; relationship to sports (principle of subsidiarity of sports), 10, 14, 15, 19, 57–58, 60, 71, 107, 136, 138, 156, 175; "Sportförderung" as financial sponsor of sports, 10, 11, 19, 57–58, 82, 96, 106, 107
Bundesnachrichtendienst (BND), xxiii, 85, 87, 90
Bundesverband Deutscher Gewichtheber (BVDG), 73, 106–107
Bundesverwaltungsamt (BVA), 156

Canada, 158; government inquiry (Dubin commission), 62, 150, 157
Christian Democratic Union of Germany (political party). *See* Christlich Demokratische Union Deutschlands (CDU)
Christian Social Union of Bavaria (political party). *See* Christlich-Soziale Union (Bayern) (CSU)
Christlich Demokratische Union Deutschlands (CDU), 148, 149
Christlich-Soziale Union (Bayern) (CSU), 64
Clasing, Dirk, 69–70
Cold War: impacts on sport and effects on doping, 16, 18, 19–20, 43, 45, 53–54, 55, 123, 193, 196, 200; involvement of the FRG/rivalry with the GDR, xv, xxi, 2, 3, 14, 16, 19, 45, 53, 54–55, 59, 82, 83–84, 97, 100, 135, 141, 149, 193; sportive nationalism/politicization of sport, 18–19, 43, 54; superpower rivalry in sports, 37, 53, 123, 125n3, 160
commercialization of sports, xxvii, 21, 55, 57, 124
Connolly, Harold, 56
contemporary witness, xxiii
Coubertin, Pierre de, xxiv, 18, 201
cycling, xiv, xxiv, 3, 21–22, 25–26, 32, 35, 37, 38, 65, 73, 77, 78, 95, 110, 115, 118, 119, 161, 168

Danckert, Peter, 148, 175
Danz, Max, 88
Daume, Willi, 5, 9, 12, 14, 17, 27, 28, 97, 112, 135, 150
Dennis, Mike, 147
Deutsche Demokratische Republik (DDR): after reunification, xiii–xiv, 136–137, 143, 144, 145, 146–147, 149, 152, 155, 161, 177, 201; as antagonist and also model to the west German sports system, xx, 17, 19, 54, 58, 59, 71, 81, 85, 92, 97, 98, 122, 124, 130n109, 198, 199, 200; (political) sports system, 2, 4, 8–9, 15, 16, 19, 53, 101, 135, 140–141, 193, 195; "Sportwunder DDR," international success, 53, 53–54, 84, 135; "Staatsdoping," state-sponsored doping program, 19, 43, 44, 53, 56, 66, 73, 75, 76, 81, 84, 86, 92, 113–114, 136, 137, 143, 144, 145, 182n5, 182n7, 195, 197; Staatsplan 14.25 (GDR), xii, 144, 182n7; supervision of east German athletes and western sports systems by the Stasi, xxiii, 85–92; "Unterstützende Mittel" (UM) in the GDR (sustaining means), 75, 136
Deutsche Gesellschaft für Sportmedizin und Prävention (DGSP), 64. *See also* Deutscher Sportärztebund (DSÄB)
Deutscher Amateur-Boxverband (DABV), 35
Deutscher Leichtathletik-Verband (DLV), 8, 26, 35–37, 65–66, 73, 76, 78, 96, 97,

104, 108, 109, 111, 112, 153, 167
Deutscher Olympischer Sportbund (DOSB), xi, 8, 146, 175. *See also* Deutscher Sportbund (DSB)
Deutscher Ruderverband (DRV), 31
Deutscher Schwimm-Verband (DSV), 82, 120, 149
Deutscher Sportärztebund (DSÄB), 27, 31, 32, 32–34, 35, 40, 43, 70, 101, 194. *See also* Deutsche Gesellschaft für Sportmedizin und Prävention (DGSP)
Deutscher Sportbund (DSB), 5, 7–9, 11, 12, 13–15, 17, 28, 35, 39, 40, 42, 55, 58, 60, 63, 64, 70, 73, 78, 81, 87, 97, 100, 101, 103, 105, 106–107, 109, 112, 117, 120, 121, 138, 140, 142, 145, 147, 148, 149, 156, 166–167, 173, 181, 192, 195. *See also* Deutscher Olympischer Sportbund (DOSB)
Deutscher Turn- und Sportbund der DDR (DTSB), 91
Deviance in sport/deviant subculture, 22, 23, 34, 102, 146, 197
Dieckmann, Bärbel, 181
Diem, Carl, xxv, 7, 10, 14, 16, 36, 142
Digel, Helmut, 174
Dimeo, Paul, xxvii–xxviii, 56, 63, 72
Dixon, John, 7
Donike, Manfred, xxx, xl, 38, 66, 67, 68, 68–70, 72, 79, 82, 88–89, 103, 107, 108, 109, 113, 114, 116, 120, 121, 122, 127n49, 128n57, 142
doping: court cases and suspensions, 31–32, 96, 138, 153, 161, 173; definitions, 32–34, 38–39, 43, 44, 54, 80, 124, 192, 193, 194; drug-related deaths, 24, 42, 56, 63–64, 111, 112, 142, 143, 157, 159, 197–198; moral issues, 20, 23, 29, 30, 34–35, 44, 61, 77–79, 101, 176, 191, 192; networks, xx, xxi, xxvi, 22, 24, 30, 54, 97, 98, 112, 144, 146, 150, 152, 154, 155, 158, 176; structural reasons, 20–21, 22, 23–24, 84, 98, 101, 102, 104, 105, 107, 189; tests, xxix, 20, 22, 24–25, 26, 34, 35, 36–39, 62, 62–63, 65, 69, 70, 73, 74, 76, 78, 79, 80, 81, 82, 88, 92, 110, 112, 114–116, 118, 120, 159, 166, 169, 194, 197
Dorando, Pietri, xxiv
Drees, Oscar, 7
Dressel, Birgit, xli, 110–112, 111, 115, 125, 137, 142, 143, 150, 157, 198
Drug Law of the FRG. *See* Arzneimittelgesetz (AMG)
drug scandals, xxvii, xxix, 79, 81, 111, 112, 115, 125, 137, 138, 143, 144, 150, 155, 159, 161, 162, 170, 172, 197. *See also* Olympic games, doping cases
drugs in sports: alcohol, xxiv, 39, 69, 189; amphetamines, xxiv, xxvi, 3, 21–22, 25, 26, 32, 35, 39, 63, 77, 78, 197; anabolic steroids. *See* steroids; caffeine, xxiv, 116, 189; Captagon, 77; ephedrine, 26, 39, 77; protein powders and pills, 73, 93, 189, 196; relation to medicalization of life, 20, 21, 93–95, 177; stimulants, xxiv, xxv–xxvi, xxix, 22, 24, 32, 35, 39, 42, 43, 62, 63, 65, 69, 73, 74, 75, 76, 107, 189, 191
Dubin, Charles Leonard, 157
Dunning, Eric, 30

East Germany. *See* Deutsche Demokratische Republik (DDR)
education of athletes, xxi, 3, 9, 10, 13, 19, 26, 102, 116, 122, 152, 167, 169, 201
Eigenweltcharakter des Sports (sport as a world of its own), 9
Elias, Norbert, xiv, xviii, xix, 4, 30, 177
Eligibility Code, xxv, 63
Elze, Josef (Jupp), xxxix, 24, 42, 64, 142
Emrich, Eike, 20
Endkampfchance (finals opportunity), 61, 103–104
Engelhardt, E., 29
Eppelmann, Rainer, 182n5
equestrian sports, 25, 32, 190, 191
Erhard, Ludwig, 98
Erythropoietin (EPO), 108, 162, 198
European Council (EC), xxi, 35, 40, 45, 74, 115, 121–122, 150, 156, 158, 160, 163, 165, 172, 177, 199
Evers, Hans, 99
Ewald, Manfred, 90, 91, 182n3, 195

Fallak, Heinz, 100

Federal Association of German Weightlifters. *See* Bundesverband Deutscher Gewichtheber (BVDG)
Federal Committee for Achievement Sport. *See* Bundesausschuss Leistungssport (BA-L)
Federal Institute of Sports Science. *See* Bundesinstitut für Sportwissenschaft (BISp)
Federal Ministry of Interior. *See* Bundesministerium des Innern (BMI)
Federal Office of Administration. *See* Bundesverwaltungsamt (BVA)
Federal Training Center. *See* Bundesleistungszentrum (BLZ)
Fédération Équestre Nationale/Deutsche Reiterliche Vereinigung (FN), 35, 65, 100
Fédération Internationale de Médicine du Sport (FIMS), 25
Fédération Internationale de Natation (FINA), 37, 82
Federazione Medico Sportiva Italiana (FMSI), 25
Figuration (figurational sociology), xiv, xv, xviii, xix, 4, 21
Finland, 120
Foucault, Michael, 37
France, 1, 26, 40, 56, 63, 75, 95, 140, 160, 161, 166, 172, 176
Francis, Charles (Charlie), 157
Francis, Dick, 50n93
Franke, Werner, 42, 96, 144, 154, 182n7
Free German Trade Union of the GDR. *See* Freier Deutscher Gewerkschaftsbund der DDR (FDGB)
Free German Youth of the GDR. *See* Freie Deutsche Jugend der DDR (FDJ)
Freie Deutsche Jugend der DDR (FDJ), 8, 140
Freier Deutscher Gewerkschaftsbund der DDR (FDGB), 8, 140

Gaede, Eberhard, 96
Gauck, Joachim, 182n5
Gehrmann, Christian, 96
German Amateur Boxing Federation. *See* Deutscher Amateur-Boxverband (DABV)
German Association for Sports Medicine and Prevention. *See* Deutsche Gesellschaft für Sportmedizin und Prävention (DGSP)
German Athletics Federation. *See* Deutscher Leichtathletik-Verband (DLV)
German Cycling Federation. *See* Bund Deutscher Radfahrer (BDR)
German Democratic Republic. See Deutsche Demokratische Republik (DDR)
German Gymnastics and Sports Associtaion of the GDR. *See* Deutscher Turn- und Sportbund der DDR (DTSB)
German Olympic Sports Federation. *See* Deutscher Olympischer Sportbund (DOSB)
German Rowing Federation. *See* Deutscher Ruderverband (DRV)
German Sports Doctors Association. *See* Deutscher Sportärztebund (DSÄB)
German Sports Federation. *See* Deutscher Sportbund (DSB)
German Swimming Federation. *See* Deutscher Schwimm-Verband (DSV)
Gerschler, Woldemar, 28
Gieseler, Karl Heinz, 12
Gläser, Rolf, 84
Gleaves, John, xxv
Gorbachev, Mikhail, 136
Great Britain, 1, 2, 5, 157, 192
Grix, Jonathan, 147
Grupe, Ommo, xl, 60, 98, 100, 101, 103, 117
Guillaume, Günter, 92
Gummel, Margitta, 91
Günthör, Werner, 143
Guttmann, Allan, xiii, 18, 30
Gymnastics, xii, xiv, 3, 4, 6, 7, 9, 11, 13, 16, 17, 20, 60–61, 135, 140. *See also* Turnen (as specific German sport)

Haas, Ulrich, 167
Halt, Karl Ritter von, 16, 27, 28
Hansen, Hans, 138
Hanstadt, Dag Vidar, 162
Hartmann, Robert, 92

health of athletes, xvi, xvii, xix, xxiv, xxvii, 4, 13, 15, 16, 21, 25, 27, 29–30, 43, 44, 74, 75, 77, 79, 82, 92, 95, 142, 176, 177, 179, 189, 191, 192, 194, 196, 200
Heinilä, Kalevi, 30, 56
Heuss, Theodor, xii, xxxn3, 10, 14, 17
Hicks, Thomas, xxiv
Hoberman, John, xxv, 18, 29, 144, 160
Hollmann, Wildor, 36, 69, 81, 84, 85, 88–89, 116, 118
Home Office. *See* Bundesministerium des Innern (BMI)
Honecker, Erich, 91
Höppner, Manfred, 88–90, 144
horse doping, 25, 32, 190, 191
Houlihan, Barrie, xviii, 18, 150, 158, 159, 161, 164, 165, 175
Huber, Georg, 109, 110, 120
Hunt, Thomas, 56, 114

ice hockey, xxiv, 65
International Amateur Boxing Federation, 25
International Association of Athletics Federations (IAAF), 25, 56–57, 65, 73, 78, 88, 108, 138, 153
International Conference of Ministers and Senior Officials Responsible for Physical Education and Sport (MINEPS), xxi
International Fencing Federation (FIE), 25
International Olympic Committee (IOC), xix, xxi, xxv, 8, 16, 23, 24–25, 33, 39, 53, 56–57, 62–63, 65, 66, 67, 67–68, 69, 70, 73, 74, 79–80, 82, 88, 91, 108, 112, 113–114, 114, 115, 116, 120, 121, 128n51, 128n67, 137, 150, 154, 157, 159, 161–164, 175, 176, 183n13, 191, 192, 195, 199
International Organization of Sports Medicine. *See* Fédération Internationale de Médicine du Sport (FIMS)
International Swimming Federation. *See* Fédération Internationale de Natation (FINA)
International Union of Modern Pentathlon. *See* Union Internationale de Pentathlon Moderne (UIPM)
internationalization of sport, xxi
Iron Curtain, xii, xiv, 53, 89, 92, 136, 144, 148, 195
Italian Association of Cyclists. *See* Unione Velocipedistra Italiana (UVI)
Italian Federation of Sports Medicine. *See* Federazione Medico Sportiva Italiana (FMSI)
Italy, 22, 25, 40, 176

Jensen, Knud Enemark, xxxviii, 24, 142, 159
Johnson, Ben, xli, 22, 112, 115, 125, 150, 157, 159–160
Jokl, Ernst, 36
Jones, Marion, 37
Jung, Kurt, 71

Karppinen, Pertti, 80
Kehoane, Robert, 159
Keul, Joseph, 36, 40, 41, 68, 69, 82, 93, 115, 116–117, 118, 120–121, 127n49, 143
Kindermann, Wilfried, 118
Kirsch, August, 96, 108, 109, 120
Klamma, Erich, 77, 78
Klehr, Horst, 96
Klein, Michael, 20
Klöden, Andreas, 170
Klümper, Armin, 69, 92–93, 94, 95, 110–111, 112, 114
Koch, Alfred, 27
Kofink, Hansjörg, 20, 47n41, 65–66, 96, 104
Kohl, Helmut, 136, 138
Kohlhaas, Max, 40, 127n43
Kolbe, Peter Michael, 80, 81, 190–191, 192
Krabbe, Katrin, xlii, 137, 138, 139, 152, 174, 201
Krahl, Hartmut, 111
Kramp-Karrenbauer, Annegret, 181
Krasner, Stephen, 159

Landessportbund (LSB), 6, 7
Landsberg-Velen, Dieter Graf von, 100
Leitner, Dieter, 77
Lenk, Hans, 98
Liesen, Heinz, 109–110, 111, 118, 120

Lintner, Eduard, 147, 151
Llewellyn, Matthew, xxv

Maats, Peter, 20
Mader, Alois, xl, 81, 84, 85–87, 143
Maizière, Thomas de, 180
Mecklenburg, Herzog Adolf von, 16
Mengden, Guido von, 14, 15, 46n18
Merckx, Eddie, 37
Merk, Beate, 175
Merode, Alexandre de, 25, 62, 73, 128n51
Meyer, Helmut, 81, 82
Ministerium für Staatssicherheit der DDR (Stasi), xxii–xxiii, 85–89, 90, 92, 98, 131n117, 144–145, 154, 182n5, 183n20
Ministry of State Security of the GDR. *See* Ministerium für Staatssicherheit der DDR (Stasi)
Møller, Verner, xxviii
Munzert, Eberhard, 112

National Anti-Doping Agency. *See* Nationale Anti-Doping Agentur (NADA)
National Equestrian Federation of Germany. *See* Fédération Équestre Nationale; Deutsche Reiterliche Vereinigung (FN)
National Olympic Committee for Germany. *See* Nationales Olympisches Komitee für Deutschland (NOK/NOC)
National Olympic Training Center. *See* Olympiastützpunkt (OSP)
Nationale Anti-Doping Agentur (NADA), xiii, xiv, 20, 151, 166, 167–170, 171–172, 174, 175, 177, 179–180, 180, 181, 199
Nationales Olympisches Komitee für Deutschland (NOK/NOC), 7, 8, 17, 28, 58, 60, 64, 65, 66, 97, 107, 112, 121, 145, 147, 148, 167, 181
Neckermann, Josef, 98, 104
negative doping, 31–32, 190
Netherlands, 95, 121, 158
Neufeld, Renate, 143
Neumann, Alfred, 91
New Zealand, 158
nongovernmental organizations (NGOs), 158, 162, 164, 165, 175–177
Norway, 120, 158
Nurmi, Paavo, 31

Olympiastützpunkt (OSP), 170
Olympic Games: 1904 Saint Louis, xxiv; 1936 Berlin, 4, 5, 7, 16, 28, 55, 141; 1948 London, 7, 12; 1952 Helsinki, 5, 11, 12, 18, 28, 31, 53, 141; 1960 Rome, 24, 98, 142, 159; 1964 Tokyo, 104; 1968 Grenoble, 24–25, 62; 1968 Mexico City, 24–25, 62, 73, 91, 159; 1972 Munich, xv, 3, 14, 19, 38, 45, 55–56, 57, 59, 60, 61, 65, 66, 69, 70, 72, 73, 79, 84, 92, 97, 103, 106, 135, 141; 1972 Sapporo, 63, 69; 1976 Montreal, 60, 72, 73, 76, 79, 84, 92, 103, 104, 106, 112, 123, 135–136, 142; 1980 Lake Placid, 135; 1980 Moscow, 110; 1984 Los Angeles, 84, 114, 182n3; 1988 Seoul, 112, 115, 125, 150, 157; 1992 Albertville, 149; 1992 Barcelona, 149, 152, 153; 2000 Sydney, 153, 171; 2002 Salt Lake City, 162; and doping (cases), xvii, xx, xxiv, xxviii, 24, 62–63, 65, 74, 78, 79, 101, 107, 138, 142, 146, 147, 161, 167, 169, 170, 173; doping laboratories, 66–70, 113; meaning of and change of image, 53, 161–162, 163; national rivalry, 53, 71; political significance, 18, 29, 63, 68, 161
Ommer, Manfred, 96
Opel, Georg von, 32, 33
Ottey, Merlene, 137
out-of-competition tests, 62, 76, 88, 92, 103, 107, 112–113, 115, 117, 120–121, 122, 146, 148, 150, 198

performance-enhancement, 21, 30, 43, 57, 61, 80–82, 87, 103, 119, 194; blood doping, 88; genetic doping, 198; oxygen, xxiv, 108
Peltzer, Otto, 31
Pitsch, Werner, 20, 169
Porritt, Arthur, 62
Pound, Richard (Dick), 157, 170, 184n58
principle of subsidiarity, 11, 12, 13, 15, 16, 142, 166, 179
Prokop, Clemens, 167
Prokop, Ludwig, 18, 26, 29, 69, 74

Reagan, Ronald, xiv, 136
Regional Sports Association. *See* Landessportbund (LSB)
Reindell, Herbert, 36, 40, 66, 68, 69, 81, 101, 104
Reiter, Heinrich, 145, 148
Renger, Annemarie, 28
Reunification, German, xi, xiii, xiv, xv, xxi, xxii, 4, 104, 119, 122, 135, 138–140, 142, 152–155, 168, 177, 195, 200
Richthofen, Manfred von, 147, 181
Riedel, Hartmut, 120
Riedl, Erich, 64
Rogge, Jacques, 120
Ruhemann, Werner, 34
rules : in professional sports, xxiv, xxv, 3, 24–25, 42, 62, 141, 191, 201; of sports associations, xvii, 8, 11, 15, 40, 42, 43, 56, 57–58, 59, 63, 65, 70–71, 72, 73, 101, 103, 158, 166; related to banned substances, 25, 192, 197, 200

Samaranch, Juan Antonio, 162, 163–164
Sauer, Helmut, 149
Schäuble, Wolfgang, 136, 170, 175
Scheel, Walter, 109
Schiller, Kay, 55
Schily, Otto, 163–164, 166–167, 168, 173, 181
Schimank, Uwe, xviii
Schlickenrieder, Franz, 128n51
Schmidt, Wilhelm, 147, 149
Schmidt, Judith, 160
Schnyder, Peter, xxvii
Schöbel, Heinz, 91
Schüller, Heidi, 112
Schumann, Otto, 106
secret services, 85–92
Seiters, Rudolf, 138, 149
Sievert, Hans-Heinrich, 10, 11, 12
Silvester, Jay, 70
Simpson, Tom, xxxix, 24, 142, 159
Singler, Andreas, 140
Slupianek, Ilona, 89, 113
Smith, Andy, 162
soccer/football, 5, 7, 8, 17, 21, 22, 26, 35, 77, 109, 180
Social Democratic Party of Germany (FRG). *See* Sozialdemokratische Partei Deutschlands (SPD)
Socialist Unity Party of Germany (GDR). *See* Sozialistische Einheitspartei Deutschlands (SED)
Sommer, Ron, 168
Sorg, Heinrich, 7
Soviet Union. *See* Union of Soviet Socialist Countries/Soviet Union (USSR)
Sozialdemokratische Partei Deutschlands (SPD), 15, 149
Sozialistische Einheitspartei Deutschlands (SED), xii, 4, 8, 85, 91, 135, 140, 182n5, 195
Spain, 176
spirit of sport : appeals to, xix, 123, 197; Coubertinian view of, xxiv, 18, 201; fairness as moral issue ("fair play"), xxiv, 19, 43, 44, 83, 196, 197
Spitzer, Giselher, 76
sports medicine: development and professionalization of, 27–31, 54, 60, 93–95; engagement in anti-doping, 24, 25, 26, 27–28, 31, 32, 34–35, 43, 44, 54, 64, 66–70, 73, 80–81, 92, 100–101, 107, 109, 116–117, 122–123, 148, 150, 158, 160, 166, 174, 175, 176, 194, 196; medicalization of sports, 20, 21, 44, 93–95, 177; Regenerationsstudie (doping research), 117–120; role in doping/doctors as providers, 30, 31–32, 54, 55, 75, 84, 92–95, 100, 109–112, 136, 170, 194, 195–196, 198; sport officials, 3, 5, 12, 13, 15, 17, 27, 34, 35, 44, 45, 54, 56, 58, 59, 60, 61, 74, 81, 82, 84, 87, 89–90, 96, 98, 100, 101, 109, 110, 112, 120, 123, 124, 145, 148, 155, 157, 161, 167, 170, 172, 173–174, 179, 191, 193, 195, 196, 198, 199, 200
sports policy of FRG: change of policy of, 16, 18–19, 20–21, 54, 57, 58, 79, 97–98, 136, 138, 141–142, 156, 158, 166, 199; involvement in anti-doping, 24, 40–43, 58, 63–65, 66, 69, 70, 71, 99–100, 105, 107, 112, 121, 137, 138–140, 142, 143, 145–146, 147, 148–150, 155–156, 161, 163–164,

166–169, 170–175, 177–179, 180–181, 199; involvement in European and international initiatives, 24, 40, 45, 121–122, 150–151, 158–159, 160–161, 163–164, 166, 172, 177, 199–200; law against doping (debates), xx, xxxin10, 40, 42, 63–64, 64, 127n43, 146, 151, 156, 166, 172–175, 180–181
Springstein, Thomas, xlii, 138, 152
Stalin, Joseph, 1, 4, 125n1
Steiner, Udo, 156
steroids: detection of and attempts to avoid, 25, 62, 73, 74, 76, 88, 92, 107, 108, 114, 115, 118, 124; danger of use, 74, 75, 77, 92, 102; hormones, xxvi, xxix, 21, 31–32, 39, 45, 73, 74–75, 76, 95, 96, 108, 109, 115, 118, 124, 137, 138, 182n7, 192, 196, 198; human growth hormone, 108; impact on performance, 54, 66, 73, 75, 98, 118, 190; Oral Turinabol, xxxin11, 73; research into, 73, 75–76, 77, 86, 88, 89, 92, 108, 116, 118, 159, 196–197; spread in sports, xxvi, 18, 23, 25, 62, 70, 72, 73, 76, 84, 86, 92, 93, 97, 107, 124, 157, 196–197; Stromba, 110; testosterone, 73, 88, 108, 110, 115, 116, 117–120, 178; Testoviron, 31–32, 190, 191. *See also* drugs in sports
Stoph, Willi, 91
Strittmatter, Gerhard, 114
Sweden, 120, 158

Tennis, 180
Thiele, Wolfgang, 96
Tillmann, Ferdinand, 148
top-level sports, xi, xiii, xvi, xx, xxiii, xxvi, 3, 5, 10, 11, 12, 16, 17–21, 22, 24, 27, 29–30, 43, 44, 54, 73, 75, 79, 80, 81, 82, 83–84, 86, 87, 88, 90, 92, 93, 95, 97–98, 100, 101–102, 105, 107, 110, 117, 121, 124–125, 135–136, 138, 142, 144, 145, 147, 148, 149–150, 155–158, 164, 167, 168, 169, 172, 174, 177–180, 190, 193, 194, 195, 196, 197, 198, 199, 200
Torrence, Gwen, 137
Treutlein, Gerhard, 140
Tröger, Walther, 181
Turnen (as specific German sport), 3, 16, 61

Ueberhorst, Horst, 28
Ulrich, Jan, 170, 171
Union Cycliste Internationale (UCI), 26, 38
Union Internationale de Pentathlon Moderne (UIPM), 37
Union of Soviet Socialist Countries/Soviet Union (USSR), xiv, 1, 2, 4, 16, 18, 53, 66, 84, 121, 125n1, 125n2, 135–136, 182n3, 195, 200
Unione Velocipedistra Italiana (UVI), 25
United Nations Educational, Scientific, and Cultural Organizations (UNESCO), xxi, 158, 160, 165–166, 174, 177, 199
United States of America:, 1, 2, 5, 19, 36, 57, 114, 135, 178, 193, 195
US Olympic Committee (USOC), 57, 162

voluntary commitment, xvii
Voy, Robert, 57

Waddington, Ivan, 162
weightlifting, 21, 22, 73, 107, 115, 118
Weyer, Willi, 97, 109, 195
Wildung, Fritz, 7
World Anti-Doping Agency (WADA), xiv, xviii, xxii, 34, 114, 151, 154, 157, 160, 161, 163, 164–165, 166, 167, 169–170, 173, 175–176, 177, 179, 180, 184n58, 195, 199, 201
World Anti-Doping Code (WADC), 34, 154, 165, 166, 169, 175–176, 190
Wülbeck, Willi, 112

Yesalis, Charles E., 62
Young, Christopher, 55

Zabel, Eric, 170

About the Authors

Dr. Michael Krüger is professor of physical education and sports history at the University of Münster in Germany. He is council member of the International Society for the History of Physical Education and Sport (ISHPES).

Christian Becker is a sports historian and publisher in Hildesheim, Germany.

Dr. Stefan Nielsen is a historian and editor in Münster, Germany.

www.ingramcontent.com/pod-product-compliance
Lightning Source LLC
LaVergne TN
LVHW101446200926
848483LV00001B/59
9781442249202